Second Edition

Rosemary Rogers,
Jane Salvage and
Roger Cowell

Nurses at Risk

A Guide to Health and Safety at Work

Nurses at Risk

A Guide to Health and Safety at Work

Second Edition

Rosemary Rogers
Jane Salvage
and
Roger Cowell

Foreword by Harriet Harman, MP

Cartoons by Kipper Williams

MACMILLAN

First edition published 1988 by Butterworth-Heinemann Ltd
Halley Court, Jordan Hill, Oxford OX2 8EJ

This edition published 1999 by
MACMILLAN PRESS LTD
Houndmills, Basingstoke, Hampshire RG21 6XS
and London
Companies and representatives
throughout the world

ISBN 0–333–73185–9

A catalogue record for this book is available from the British Library.

This book is printed on paper suitable for recycling and made from
fully managed and sustained forest sources.

10   9   8   7   6   5   4   3   2   1
08 07 06 05 04 03 02 01 00 99

Copy-edited and typeset by Povey–Edmondson
Tavistock and Rochdale, England

Printed in Great Britain by Creative Print and Design Wales

Contents

The authors and publishers are grateful to the Editor-in-Chief of *Nursing Times*, Emap Healthcare Ltd, for permission to reproduce copyright material from that journal.

Foreword

A decade ago, in the foreword to the first edition of this book, I said that nurses were one of the most valuable resources of the National Health Service. They are hard-working and dedicated people who deserve the best possible conditions in which to carry out their vital work. Ten years on these words still apply. The health and well-being of staff are integral to the well-being of the NHS. If they are off sick or injured, they cannot treat patients at all.

This book raises nurses' own concerns about the hazards they face and suggests ways of tackling them.

The most frequently reported type of injury is caused by lifting and handling. Research in one trust has shown that as the result of a safer handling policy, time off for injuries sustained by handling patients was reduced by 84 per cent. This saved £400,000 a year in replacement nursing costs alone.

Research also shows that stress at work is a widespread problem in the NHS and this rightly falls within the remit of health and safety. Current research will lead to the issuing of guidance to the service on ways of coping with organisational stress.

Fourteen per cent of recorded accidents to staff involve physical assault, making it the third most common type of accident to staff. Violence can cause pain, suffering and disability, and verbal abuse and threats can damage health through anxiety or stress. The issue of violence to staff must be managed as a health and safety risk.

These problems are difficult ones, but the fact that so much work-related illness – mental and physical – can be prevented should give us hope. This book offers valuable guidance to nurses and to their employers and managers on how to improve matters. The authors' research into the problems is backed by sound practical advice on how to tackle them.

The NHS is taking action on a number of issues relating to staff. The framework for human resources currently being developed will raise the profile of staff health and welfare as core management issues. The Health at Work in the NHS project has been disseminating guidance and good practice information; 80 per cent of NHS employers are participating, and NHS Estates have been working on benchmarking and risk management tools.

The NHS is determined to tackle these areas to ensure that nurses are able to work properly, safely and happily, thus helping them to give better care while enjoying greater job satisfaction and better morale.

RIGHT HONOURABLE HARRIET HARMAN MP

ix

Introduction

It is a decade or so since the first edition of *Nurses at Risk* – a decade which has seen many changes in health care and nursing. Yet much of what we wrote in that first edition is, sadly, still relevant today. In revising this book, we found that all the issues researched then remain topical now - indeed there appear to be more rather than fewer hazards, while the failure of the Conservative government to tackle the key issues concerning the well-being of the NHS workforce has taken an even greater toll, especially on nurses – its front-line workers.

Rarely a week passes without new evidence of old and new hazards. *Improving the Health of the NHS Workforce*, published by the Nuffield Trust and the biggest ever report on the health of NHS staff, was issued just after our manuscript was completed in March 1998. It provides compelling research-based evidence of how little has changed in the last decade and points out the appalling human and financial consequences of this systematic and shameful neglect.

There have of course been some positive developments. New Labour has yet to prove its Bevanite credentials as the saviour of the health service, but it has more card-carrying credibility in this area than its Tory predecessors and a lot more to lose in public credibility should it let the NHS down. Initiatives such as the Health at Work in the NHS project, described in Chapter 12, may eventually prove to have no teeth but at least on the surface promise a greater commitment to the health and welfare of the NHS workforce. Meanwhile a raft of much tougher European legislation affecting health and safety at work, covering the whole spectrum of workplaces where health care is delivered, has come into effect in the UK since 1988.

Despite these hopeful signs, however, we found the persistence of many familiar hazards to health and well-being – such as back injuries caused by staff shortages, poor training and lack of equipment – as well as the emergence or escalation of new ones: glutaraldehyde, latex allergy and methicillin-resistant *Staphylococcus aureus* (MRSA), to name just a few.

Some of these problems are attributable to new evidence or to changes in clinical practice. Use of the sterilising solution glutaraldehyde, for example, has risen in the past decade because of the increasing use of endoscopes for diagnostic and therapeutic surgical procedures; at the same time, evidence-based awareness of the risks it poses has risen dramatically. Latex allergy is a massively more significant health and safety problem than it was ten years ago, thanks to the introduction of universal precautions and the consequent increase in glove use. The effects of widespread and often indiscriminate

antibiotic use are being seen in outbreaks of antibiotic-resistant organisms –
MRSA, vancomycin-resistant enterococci and newly virulent strains of TB.

Nurses meanwhile are taking on increasingly advanced technological roles
and procedures, and thus exposing themselves to more hazards. They are
practising in a growing range of settings, for different employers and across
hospital and community boundaries. They are working in higher education,
in GP surgeries, in corporate business, in the burgeoning nursing home
sector and on their own as independent practitioners. The risks to which
they are exposed, and the framework in which their health and safety is
protected, is shifting all the time.

Other emerging problems have been directly caused by the policies of the
previous government. The introduction of the internal market, the growing
use of management consultants, the endless search for efficiency savings and
the rampant managerialism which characterised the NHS of the early 1990s
impacted on the NHS workforce in countless ways: some of the worst effects
were gagging clauses, bullying, less favourable job contracts and redundan-
cies, all inevitably affecting staff's mental health and well-being.

Meanwhile, despite the shortages of suitably qualified staff faced by the
NHS throughout the UK, many work-injured and disabled nurses are
unable to find suitable employment when they are ready to return to work,
thus wasting valuable skill and experience and forcing a dependency on
benefit that would shame New Labour's welfare to work platform. Nursing
continues to be a mainly female profession (the largest female workforce in
the UK) yet the NHS has so far made little progress in helping its women
workers cope with the so-called double shift of home and work. Violence
against nurses at work – an issue highlighted in the first edition of this book –
has increased.

By its very nature, the health care sector is a risky and stressful place to
work. Yet employers too often ignore the many simple steps they could take
to reduce the risks inherent in the job, to improve the working environment
and job satisfaction of their employees and to help recompense and
rehabilitate those injured at work.

So in researching this second edition, there was no shortage of issues to
revisit or to explore. There remains little published on health and safety
aimed specifically at nurses. The subject is in general under-researched and
nowhere more than in health care, apart from one or two notable exceptions,
such as back injury, which has been the focus of active campaigning. When
revising the book all relevant reports, case studies and references were
reviewed thoroughly and new material and contemporary references have
been incorporated in the original text. Some sections will therefore be readily
recognisable; others, where the nature of the hazard or the focus of
protection has changed, have been completely rewritten.

Uncovering individual examples of good practice which safeguard the
health and safety of workers or improve their working environment was one
of the more heartening aspects of this project. As in the previous edition, we

have highlighted as many as possible. All too often they are isolated examples rather than consistent good practice, but they illustrate how, with commitment, it is possible to tackle the threats posed to the health and safety of nurses at work, ensuring that they are able to work properly, safely and happily – thus giving better care to their patients while enjoying their jobs more.

The views in this book are our own and should not be attributed to the organisations for which we work or the many people who have helped us. It is satisfying, however, to acknowledge the generous and unstinting support, information and practical assistance provided by so many organisations and individuals, in particular Carol Bannister, Sheelagh Brewer, Wendy Lopatin and Shirley Slipman. Our biggest thanks, however, go to our co-author Roger Cowell for the enthusiasm and commitment which prompted us to tackle this revised edition, and for the painstaking research and thought he put into compiling the revisions and updating. As we go to press it is a pleasure to report that the Royal College of Nursing has acknowledged Roger's sterling contribution to nurses' welfare by bestowing on him a Merit Award.

ROSEMARY ROGERS
JANE SALVAGE

About the authors

Roger Cowell, RGN, BA, held various clinical nursing posts including Primary Nurse at Burford Community Hospital, Oxfordshire. He is now a freelance writer, and edits the quarterly newsletter of the RCN Work Injured Nurses Group. He is an active member of the Royal College of Nursing.

Rosemary Rogers, RGN, BA, is editor of the monthly journal *Professional Nurse*. She has worked in nursing publishing for some years, holding posts on *Senior Nurse, Nursing Standard and Paediatric Nurse*. She has published extensively, including open learning texts, and was chief advisory editor of the *Dictionary of Nursing*.

Jane Salvage, RGN, BA, MSc, HonLLD, is editor-in-chief of *Nursing Times*. She has worked as a nurse journalist and project leader, including posts at the King's Fund and the World Health Organization. Her many publications include the best-selling book *The Politics of Nursing*.

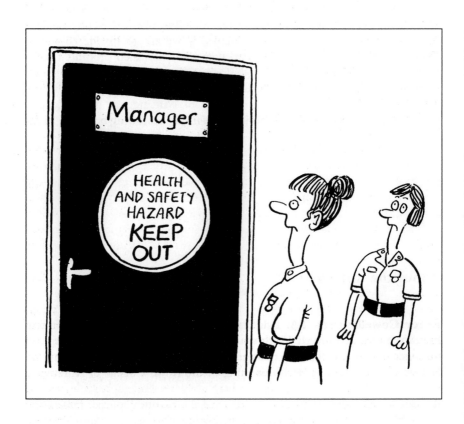

1 Health services: bad for your health?

Are you inspired by health and safety at work? If not, it's likely you are not alone. It conjures up visions of tedious regulations and being told to do your work in ways which seem utterly impractical in the daily hurly-burly of health care. Yet what could be more important to each nurse than her or his own welfare? Evidence suggests that the mental and physical health of the nurse is frequently put at risk by work, and that many nurses suffer serious problems, sometimes resulting in the loss of a job or permanent disability. Why, then, is a subject which should be near the top of the nursing agenda so often neglected or ignored?

This neglect of occupational health and safety is not peculiar to nurses, the NHS or the UK. The lack of government-funded research and statistics on all kinds of work-related ill-health is a reflection not only of official indifference but also of society's frequent failure to acknowledge that work can be bad for you. We seem to have travelled such a long way from the dismal factories and coalmines of the Industrial Revolution that it is hard to perceive many of the more insidious modern hazards to health and safety. Indeed many of them cannot be seen, for the visible horrors of dangerous machinery or heavy loads have largely given way to invisible risks such as microbes, viruses, radiation and stress.

A further difficulty in dealing with health hazards is the fact that they often affect workers slowly and quietly over many years. Risks may not be apparent immediately , especially when – as is often the case – no rigorous monitoring, research or follow-up is carried out by the employer. Without legislation and procedures which require health and safety audits and the assessment and management of risks, the worker remains ignorant of the dangers, and the link between damage to health and particular occupational hazards remains unexposed. Cancers triggered by working with carcinogenic substances and damage to the unborn child from chemicals are two examples. Furthermore the symptoms of work-related disease resemble those of other illnesses, making the cause difficult to trace. Accidents at work, of course, are immediately obvious, but here attempts are often made to blame the individual worker for carelessness, rather than looking critically at working conditions and safer systems.

Working conditions have been repeatedly identified as an important factor in inequalities of health, notably in the Black report (Townsend and Davidson, 1982) and *The Health Divide* (Whitehead, 1988), and are central to the independent inquiry launched in 1997 by the new Labour government to update the Black findings and underpin the White Paper on public health,

Our Healthier Nation, promised for 1998. The Black working party's suggestion of 'a tendency to accept poor working conditions as an inevitable accompaniment of particular jobs' still has the ring of truth, although it was unpalatable to the government of the day, which downplayed the importance of the report.

This blindness to occupational ill-health has persisted in the years since the Black working party, despite growing awareness. It does not occur by chance, but suits certain vested interests very well. There are also historical reasons for the neglect of the health and safety of nurses. Apart from a few exceptional employers, most of the positive action on health and safety has come from trade unions and pressure groups, and, not surprisingly in view of the traditional pattern of union membership, this has concentrated on male factory workers. Moreover women's work has been commonly assumed to be less dangerous than men's. Although far more recognition is now given to the risks faced by women at work, and by those doing less obviously dangerous work, much remains to be done in health services, and for nurses. Doyal (1995) states that women do not enter the labour force on equal terms with men, and this is reflected in a male bias in occupational health research and research methods, which underplay or ignore hazards which jeopardise women's health. As she notes, 'it is widely believed that "female" jobs are neither physically hazardous nor particularly stressful'.

Writers on health and safety often use statistics to try to convey the magnitude of the problem. For example back injury to nurses loses the NHS officially over one and a half million working days every year, at a cost of between £265 million and £383 million a year (RCN, 1996; Centre For Health Economics, 1995). Such figures are supplemented by a mass of unreported work-related illness, particularly that of a psychological nature, which is usually regarded as an unacceptable excuse for taking time off. Although stress-related illness is still stigmatised as a form of skiving or scrounging, it is argued (for example by Doyal, 1979, 1995) that diseases such as tuberculosis, which formerly accounted for much sickness absence, have been replaced by more subjective, psychosomatic illnesses – so much so that sickness rates have actually been rising in Britain since the early 1960s. Problems such as headaches and stress should be taken far more seriously as indicators of the largely preventable psychological dangers of certain kinds of work; nursing is a prime example.

On the positive side, occupational health and safety has become an even more prominent cause for social concern in the 1990s. There are many reminders that work should not be assumed to be safe until proved dangerous – scandals such as the death of workers in the asbestos, cotton and other industries, many years after the hazards were first noted; the debate about nuclear power and public health; and Gulf War Syndrome – the symptoms, possibly organophosphate-derived, experienced by some troops and support workers during and after the 1990 conflict. In the NHS, the less dramatic but nevertheless serious problems of back injury,

HIV, MRSA and cytotoxic drugs have been highlighted through pressure from workers and their organisations, with awareness probably greater than it has ever been. We hope to raise it further by alerting nurses to the many hazards they face, and suggesting ways of tackling them.

Contexts

Europe

With the expansion of the European Union and the opening up of Eastern Europe in the post-communist period, much discussion, research and legislation is undertaken in a broader spirit of cooperation. It is no longer considered satisfactory for governments to operate alone, and Europe-wide study of hazards, together with common minimum standards, is envisaged as the way forward.

In 1989 the then European Community laid down the basis of Europe-wide safety laws in the EC Framework Directive, consolidated through the 1992 directives, which were implemented in six sets of regulations in the UK. This does not mean these common standards have been achieved – perceptions of risk, and of the importance of occupational health, still vary widely, even within single nations – but there is increasing awareness that common standards are needed across Europe. Throughout this book we indicate where EU regulations are having an impact on health and safety.

The United Kingdom

The NHS and health care in general have undergone tremendous change in the 1990s, with far-reaching implications for staff health and safety. The establishment of NHS trusts, both acute and community, the internal market, and health service commissioning and provision (the purchaser–provider split) have fragmented health care and created inequalities, some foreseen, others not. The enforced separation of hospitals into competing trusts within single towns and regions, and the two-tier health provision of fund-holding and non-fund-holding GP practices, damaged the once co-operative and amicable relationship between health providers, put research in jeopardy, and set budgetary considerations – the competitive advantage – above clear clinical sense. It has become increasingly difficult for health care workers to maintain open links with colleagues in neighbouring patches, and trade unions are less able to cooperate regionally in promoting rigorous standards of health and safety.

According to Jean Bailey, RCN adviser in nursing management, 'trusts are getting away with ignoring DoH good practice guidelines. . . . If a unit or ward or department develops something that's useful in nursing practice . . . there's a growing unwillingness on the part of the chief executive to allow that to be talked about without a price being put on it.'

For some managers, health and safety is a low priority, even a luxury to be trimmed to help balance the books. 'Short-termism is almost inevitable because of the internal market. Trusts are only looking six to 12 months ahead and that's being imposed on them because of the contracting process', said John Humphreys, RCN labour relations officer. Some trust executives have said openly that they have been selective in following Department of Health guidance 'if we felt it was inappropriate or did not fit in with our philosophy' (Downey, 1994).

The 1997 White Paper *The New NHS* promised to dismantle the internal market and attempt to reverse some of these trends. It will take some time for the new policies to take effect, however, and even longer for the negative effects on staff welfare of the years of 'reforms' to be put right.

A more welcome recent trend is the emphasis on bringing services closer to where the patient lives and works – a World Health Organization goal, which is reflected in the wide range of settings where care is delivered. The perception of the NHS as a collection of acute hospitals is gradually changing as the range of providers and settings expands. Throughout this book we show that health and safety is significant in all settings – the community, GP practices, acute medical and surgical units, mental health care and so on. They embrace not only the NHS but social services, private and non-profit services.

Although the NHS still dominates health provision in the UK, there is a growing private hospital industry and, with the NHS drifting away from the provision of long-term elderly care, a burgeoning multinational, multi-million-pound nursing and residential home sector. Additionally, nurses work in many new areas, from industry and commerce to higher education and NHS community care, in inner-city streets and housing estates, in the non-profit and voluntary sectors.

Health and safety, and occupational health, should be examined by employers and employees in all settings. There are minimum legal requirements, and desirable standards beyond the minimum, and it could become increasingly complex and difficult to assess the standards and requirements for improvement in all places where nurses work.

Nursing procedures and systems of work

The Health and Safety at Work Act 1974, as well as telling employers to provide and maintain safe premises, also says they must establish 'systems of work', which should, 'so far as is reasonably practicable', be safe and without risk to health. Employers' duties in relation to these regulations are clarified in The Management of Health and Safety at Work Regulations 1992 (HSE, 1993). The RCN defines 'systems of work' in the nursing context to mean all practices and procedures, a definition which should provide maximum protection for the employee as well as the patient. One topical example, highlighted by the incidence of HIV/AIDS, hepatitis B and MRSA, is infection control policies; nurses' worries about contracting these viruses have brought to light the failure of many employers to draw up practicable policies and make sure that workers are familiar with them.

The Act requires arrangements for employers to consult employees over health and safety issues (this, with other legislation and safety guidance, is covered in more depth in Chapter 2, 'Health and Safety: the legal framework') and for ensuring safety and the absence of health risks in connection with the use, handling, storage and transport of all articles and substances. This covers everything used at work and all work activities and settings. The RCN and the Institute for Employment Studies say that 85 per cent of a surveyed sample reported the need to lift or move people or things at work which they found heavy, but 57 per cent have never had access to manual handling equipment (Smith and Seccombe, 1996). If staff – in whatever context, hospital, health centre or community – are asked to handle patients, or handle and store such items as continence pads or weighing scales, then managers must in law provide and maintain necessary items such as hoists.

Policies and procedures on such issues as infection control, moving and handling, staff vaccination and equipment are discussed in more detail in the chapters on hazards. The principles are the same in all settings, and legislation applies equally to the self-employed and to peripatetic staff such as community nurses. Guidance should be drawn up with specific reference to the particular conditions of work outside hospital, and to local factors.

The role of the nurse

Some of the roles included under the umbrella of 'nurse', such as nurse practitioner and clinical nurse specialist, are relatively new, while others, such as community mental health nurse and primary nurse are becoming more widespread and understood. Yet others, for example district nurses, have long traditions but are changing in response to current needs. Recent official reports such as *A Vision for the Future* (NHSE, 1993) and *The challenges for nursing and midwifery in the 21st century* (DoH, 1993a) discuss the effects of NHS reforms and their implications for nursing, and, with UKCC documents on guidelines for and the scope of professional practice, suggest stepping beyond established boundaries to provide a better service.

The UKCC widened the discussion of extended or extending roles in *The Scope of Professional Practice* (UKCC, 1992), suggesting that the terms were 'no longer suitable since they limit, rather than extend, the parameters of practice . . . it is the Council's principles for practice rather than certificates for tasks which should form the basis for adjustments to the scope of practice'. However, 'new work' should still be properly delegated, and training must be given and recognised as satisfactory if the nurse acting alone is not to find herself unsupported – she should follow established policies and procedures, and if there are none, she should insist they are drawn up. Equally, if the nurse is asked to do an unaccustomed task, she should make sure she is appropriately trained and feels comfortable and confident in what she is doing; her accountability requires it.

Nurses in clinical practice are obliged to take account of health and safety issues, as are their managers and employers. As nursing education moves into the environment of higher education, nursing students still need to be taught about health and safety as an integral part of their curriculum, both in the classroom and in clinical placements. Indeed it might be argued that the education authorities are obliged by law to inform them of hazards and risks and how to deal with them, just as they are obliged to do with the lecturers and tutors, their employees. It might anyway prove beneficial in the long run to produce graduate nurses who have been comprehensively informed of their rights and responsibilities by the end of their undergraduate courses.

Continuing education is a major preoccupation among nurses in the UK, the more so since the UKCC's Post-Registration Education for Practice (PREP) scheme introduced mandatory requirements for updating, and defined categories for study within a statutory requirement to demonstrate competence to practise. Health and safety issues are an important aspect of continuing education and professional development.

The Health and Safety at Work Act states that the employer should provide such information, instruction and training and supervision as is necessary to ensure the employee's health and safety; the RCN interprets this to mean that managers should ensure nurses are kept up to date on new products, drugs and equipment. Refresher courses, distance learning packages and conferences/study days should be provided on all aspects of health and safety.

The politics of occupational health

Employers have often interpreted health and safety legislation in an individualistic way, enabling them to shift responsibility away from themselves and to blame the employee for being lazy, feckless or otherwise failing to protect herself properly. Clearly the employer's self-interest is involved, and helps to perpetuate a linked set of ideas which are echoed in society's general attitudes towards health, built around the notion that if you are ill or injured, it's your own fault. The order to 'look after yourself' and the prevailing medical emphasis of our health services paint a misleading picture of health as a personal responsibility – in spite of a growing body of evidence that the bulk of ill-health is caused by social, economic and environmental factors.

It is perhaps a sign of the times that publicity and money may be the main incentives for health service managers to take collective responsibility for occupational health and safety. The adverse publicity surrounding security incidents (such as violence and baby-snatching), food poisoning, breach of health and safety regulations or perioperative mortality rates, is often followed by rapid review of existing systems of work and public declarations of the steps being taken to remedy problems. The steps are often inadequate and the raised standards short-lived.

In 1996 the Health and Safety Executive (HSE), which works actively to encourage good management through risk assessment, began a scheduled audit of risk management in all NHS trusts, and later announced a six-month-long series of visits (termed a 'blitz' by HSE staff) to 40 trusts. HSE sources spoke of including clinical areas in their visits, and of a readiness to issue prohibition and improvement notices – legal actions which would force trusts to take immediate action or face fines.

One trust, prosecuted in 1997, attributed its breaches of health and safety regulations to a repair backlog that predated its attaining trust status in 1994. Such explanations illustrate a common thread already mentioned in respect of litigation, bad publicity and security problems – that the NHS reforms (the internal market and trust status in particular) fragmented a once unified service. Collective responsibility and liability has been devolved to local trusts, magnifying the pressure to control budgets, apply regulations selectively and blame individuals for accidents.

The increased incidence of litigation by staff and patients has forced almost all NHS hospital trusts into a clinical negligence scheme (established in 1995) to which each can expect to pay about £65 000 a year in premiums. This could rise to £1 million as the number of claims rises (Burbedge, 1997). Negligence litigation costs are currently estimated at £200–500 million a year, and are expected to rise by 25 per cent a year between 1997 and 2002 (Chad-Smith, 1997).

Blaming the victim

The tendency to blame the victim rather than the author of the problem persists in stereotypical attitudes towards health and safety which are reiterated by management, traditional health educators and sometimes workers themselves. Yet ignoring the hazards, justifying them or shifting the responsibility for them does nothing to tackle the roots of the problem, and permits the continuation of an unacceptable state of affairs.

Like other forms of ill-health, occupational diseases and injuries are largely preventable, but the dominant ideology tells us something different. Doyal (1995) expresses it powerfully: 'Workers are presumed safe unless their exposure to a dangerous substance exceeds what has been set as the "safe level".' But as she points out, medical and legal 'knowledge' – and power – tend to be kept in the hands of 'experts'. This creates particular problems for health service staff, who work with or as 'experts' every day; it seems incongruous to think that services established to look after a nation's health could themselves cause harm. If harm does occur, it seems reasonable to assume that the worker would receive instant skilled attention.

The truth is that the NHS has a poor record in looking after its staff, and the lack of 'care for the carers' remains proverbial. For nurses the lack of money, awareness and management action on health and safety (many fine policy statements; less action) are compounded by the persistent idea that they should put 'service before self' and sacrifice their own needs for the good of the patients. Despite the risk assessment requirement of the Manual Handling Operations Directive 1992, which should stop any nurse lifting manually in most situations, the nurse who lifts a patient on her own when no help is available, risking permanent injury, is acting with the silent approval of a value-system which has exploited the dedication and neglected the welfare of generations of nurses. Successive governments have reinforced such sentiments by saying that health workers' pay rises must be funded from service budgets, in the hope that pay claims will be kept to a minimum when bartered against patients' interests. Short-term and trust contracts, the attempted imposition of local pay, terms and conditions, and a defensive or oppressive work climate are further disincentives to staff action.

Thus health workers are placed in a double bind when trying to improve their own working conditions. It is one thing to demand improvements from an employer who is making large profits, but another to put pressure on an underfunded and vulnerable service to which they are morally committed. Statements from trusts and managers show that they are uncomfortable about being obliged to make choices between different but equally pressing needs, yet the result of their compromises is often pressure on the workforce to drop its demands. Health and safety therefore also raises the issue of democracy in the workplace; what part do and should health service staff play in reaching these decisions?

The problem of resources

The politics of occupational health touch on central issues about power and control at work, and relations between workers. These are particularly complex in a service such as the NHS where most people, even the minister, are employees of the state; but the health service shares with other public sector services a poor record on staff welfare. The fact that the NHS is seen as being owned by the people has proved no guarantee of better treatment of employees or of more democracy. In fact, since the mid 1980s the establishment of NHS trusts, the internal market and service purchasing and commissioning has resulted in even more arbitrary treatment of staff, more secrecy and less democracy.

Many of the arguments about power focus on resources; while everyone blames the lack of money, some groups of staff, notably doctors, managers, information technology consultants and accountants, have fared better than others and some sectors have gained disproportionate shares of the resources. The chronic underfunding of parts if not all of the NHS, which reflects and is compounded by most employees' powerlessness, has had serious effects on staff health and safety, and on morale.

Every day the media carry news of how underfunding is damaging the provision of health care. Hospital closures, long waiting lists, rising prescription charges and all the other adverse effects on users are readily documented, but the plight of staff receives less attention. Cuts and zero growth do not simply reduce services. There is not enough money for:

- Repair and maintenance of buildings and equipment.
- Replacement of damaged and outdated equipment.
- New equipment or apparatus that would improve systems of work.
- Upgrading old buildings.
- New building.
- Education and training of all staff and their representatives in health, safety and other relevant topics.
- Staffing levels that will ensure work is done at a reasonable pace.
- Staff to take proper breaks, and complete the workload without overtime.
- Provision of a first-class occupational health service.
- Pay rises that would free health care staff from the stress of low incomes.
- Good staff accommodation, rest and leisure facilities and restaurants.

How little changes: as in the 1980s, the screw continued to be tightened in the 1990s by Conservative government policies which, by imposing strict cash limits on already underfunded health authorities, forced them to cut corners and defer improvements. Privatisation – bringing in outside contractors to do NHS work – was blamed by the trade unions for reduced standards of cleanliness and safety which impinge directly on the welfare of staff and patients. Ten years on, according to Mohan (1995), most domestic services contracts are awarded in-house, and two thirds of those held privately are held by two major firms, with cost-cutting enabled by staff reductions, lost holiday entitlements and so on. 'Creeping privatisation', 'privatisation by the back door' and similar phrases continued to be used by trade unionists and Labour politicians in opposition, up to the 1997 general election, pointing to a decline in cleanliness and staff terms and conditions. At the time of writing, it seems probable that the Labour government will continue the Private Finance Initiatives to enable new hospital building, though the private contracting of clinical services remains sensitive. Throughout the NHS, short-term financial expediency is the order of the day, to the detriment of longer-term investment. Labour ministers have promised action but will not be rushed into quick-fix solutions, so the future remains uncertain.

The agencies responsible for advice and enforcement of the law are being cut back, to the consternation of the trades union movement. 'There are only about 1572 HSE inspectors in the field to cover over 650,000 workplaces. Since 1979 the [Conservative] government has cut staff numbers in the HSE to pre-1974 levels, meaning that some workplaces will now never receive a visit again unless there is an accident or a complaint' (TUC, 1997). The number of HSE preventive workplace inspections dropped from over 156,000 in 1993–4 to fewer than 100,000 in 1997, a reduction of almost two thirds in five years. The proportion of investigations into major injuries fell from 15 per cent of the total in 1994–5 to 4 per cent in 1996–7 , and the 1997 HSE figures showed a rise in fatal accidents at work, from 258 to 302. John Monks, TUC general secretary, commented, 'These tragic figures show we cannot be complacent about health and safety at work. . . . Cuts in the HSE are a dangerous and false economy', while according to Bill Morris, general secretary of the Transport and General Workers' Union, 'The HSE is simply failing to get to grips with the rising tide of reckless disregard by employers for workers' safety.'

In 1997 the HSE reported a total of 4077 staff, with 79 per cent 'on operational work' (HSE, 1997, p. 6), and 108,174 planned inspections – about a fifth of the total number of workplaces in the UK. HSE director-general Jenny Bacon called the investigation policy 'more targeted', and acknowledged the damage done to the HSE by falling resource and staff levels under the Conservative government, which could cause 'significant problems' without further resources.

No extra money was made available to health authorities to enforce the minimum standards required of employers in the Health and Safety at Work Act, and until crown immunity was removed in early 1987 they were let off the hook by immunity from prosecution. Since then, there has been greater pressure on them to take action, but it is expensive and once again no special funds are forthcoming. Successive governments have said that money can be found within the existing budgets, but this cannot happen without cutting back other services, since there is little fat to trim for the 'efficiency savings' which are supposed to be the answer to every financial director's prayer. When in opposition, the Labour health spokesman Frank Dobson estimated that enforcing the food hygiene regulations alone could cost the NHS around £100 million. In government, he talked in 1997 of possibly restoring crown immunity in order to save NHS insurance costs.

Health authorities cannot fail to be aware that if private sector experience is anything to go by, fines for offences are likely to be negligible compared with improvement costs. Hard-up NHS employers may follow the example of those who prefer to risk prosecution than to spend more on the staff or premises.

Occupational health in the NHS

The neglect of occupational health in the health services, and the failure to tackle preventable problems, is demonstrated by the high levels of illness, stress and accidents suffered by thousands of nurses. This is documented throughout this book in our discussions of specific hazards. We have already looked at some of the reasons why the NHS is so reluctant to look after the welfare of its most precious resource, its own staff. There is a further linked factor which contributes to the problem: the continuing lack of a proper occupational health service for all NHS workers.

There is a key difference between an occupational health (OH) service and a staff clinic. The latter primarily gives on-the-spot treatment and care to health workers, often as an alternative or adjunct to local casualty and general practitioner services. It may offer surgeries and immediate treatment for minor injuries or accidents incurred at work, and may also carry out immunisation and other screening. Such services may be useful, but they are more limited in scope than a full occupational health service.

Recent government guidelines (see Box 1.1) are in tune with the policies of the RCN and the British Medical Association. The RCN (1991) defined the key functions of an OH service as surveillance of workers' health, health promotion at work, the management of illness and injury at work, and environmental monitoring and assessment under the Control of Substances Hazardous to Health (COSHH) regulations. The BMA, in a 1994 report on the risks of health care, stated that 'the low priority given to occupational health services in the NHS is unacceptable'. It underlined the need to establish a comprehensive, consultant-led OH service, which would be a prerequisite of trust status and required in all private hospitals, and urged that OH services should have a coherent approach across each region, based on central guidance from the NHS Executive.

Box 1.1 *An occupational health service for the NHS*

Department of Health guidelines (1993b) set out the following functions of the NHS Occupational Health Service:

- Provision of expert medical, nursing and health and safety advice on occupational health matters.
- Health assessment on recruitment, including advice to management on immunisation policy.
- Health surveillance of in-service employees, other contractors employed, student nurses and other students on practice placements.
- Health promotion and education in the workplace.
- Education of staff in the necessity of compliance with health and safety legislation in association with health and safety advisers and line managers.

(See Chapter 12 for a more extended discussion.)

Nurses' sick rooms, part-time physicians and other ad hoc arrangements found in the NHS today clearly fall short of a comprehensive preventive service. We return to the question of the ideal OH service in our final chapter, with our recommendations for 'the healthy nurse'. But what of the current situation?

There is no lack of official guidelines, but the actual provision of OH services remains patchy and woefully inadequate. In the first place, there is no unified or agreed concept of the role of the OH service within the NHS, and 'present provision . . . could perhaps be most kindly described as haphazard', as Lunn and Waldron (1991) and successive studies and reports have pointed out. Its organisation, aims and functions and even levels of acceptance continue to vary from one trust or one hospital to another. The mistaken idea that health workers are somehow immune from ill-health, and the widespread practice of 'corridor consultation', have undoubtably contributed to this lack of coherence.

Comprehensive studies show that OH services in both the private and the public sector remain poorly funded, and that managers lack awareness of and motivation towards staff health issues. Health professionals provide only 8 per cent of care in the private sector, with a further 15 per cent having 'first aiders' only and the rest having no provision. In the public sector, 72 per cent of employees have access to a doctor and 86 per cent to a nurse, though often only part-time. Fingret and Smith (1995) found that only 53 per cent of OH staff in the public sector have OH qualifications, and only 19 per cent in the private sector are appropriately qualified; OH staff are generally less well qualified than others and the emphasis is on treatment and medical examination, not prevention or environmental surveillance.

Yet another problem with the existing staff health services is that too often they operate, or are seen to operate, as an arm of management (Davies, 1995). There are many stories of staff clinics failing to observe scrupulous confidentiality, an issue that is especially important to ill or injured nurses who already feel isolated and poorly supported. A welcome if unintended consequence of nursing education's move into higher education is a more mature and truly confidential approach to the nursing student's private life.

Unsurprisingly, breaches of confidentiality and ethics go largely unremarked and unpunished. On the whole, the individual nurse who is already feeling vulnerable will not feel like taking on the role of whistle-blower, understandably and sometimes justifiably fearing that the staff clinic acts more as a surveillance service for management than a support for the staff. Collecting information on sickness and accident rates is an important way of assessing and preventing accidents, but such data appear just as likely to be used to berate an individual nurse for her poor record, while gimmicks such as 'air miles' for 100 per cent attendance records are not encouraging.

The Allitt inquiry and the subsequent Clothier report demanded more rigorous pre-employment screening of nursing candidates (HMSO, 1994). Carol Bannister, the RCN's occupational health adviser, suggests that such policies could produce illegal discrimination, and urges that independence from management and strict confidentiality must come first in a good OH service.

Mental health issues

In 1989 I was seen as an emergency case at psychiatric outpatients, and was immediately admitted to hospital under section with severe depression. I had been at work until two days before. Had my normally high standards at work dropped, I have no doubt it would have been noted. There were a few comments about me not being my usual 'cheery' self, but my colleagues seemed oblivious to my suffering. . . . Depression is isolating and creates a profound sense of guilt. The last thing likely to be helpful is to be reported to the UKCC. . . . It is possible that a nurse could present a danger to patients, but it remains very unlikely. And mentally ill people have as much right as anyone else to be considered as individuals (Veronica Burton, letter to *Nursing Standard*, 11 June 1997, vol. 11, no. 38, p. 10).

This story is typical of the experience of nurses with mental health problems, and as Hammond (1995) has said, 'the state of the NHS is . . . accurately mirrored by the mental health of those working in it'. Sadly, we must conclude that health services are failing their staff spectacularly: nurses do not get the sensitive and appropriate support they need to do their job without excessive stress, fatigue and illness. Even when they recover from mental health problems, they are not helped to resume their career.

Burton and many others give similar accounts of the difficulties they have faced when returning to work. Irene Challoner, a paediatric ward sister, had to leave her work because of depression. She was able to resume nursing a few months later, but as a staff nurse in a gynaecology ward. 'They just don't want to take the risk and they see you as a liability . . . I was told: "This is all we're going to let you do because you have had time off sick. We cannot possibly give you a job with the same level of stress."'

Nurses who have had mental health problems, whether work-related or not, talk of a loss of confidence, and of employers who fail to take account of the damaging stress levels in nurses' work. Yet the remedies are obvious – a recognition at all levels that health care work is inherently stressful, and that staff need adequate education, management support and confidential counselling services. Further, managers should acknowledge that mental health problems are not infections for which people should be isolated and treated with universal precautions, but part of the normal fabric of human life and deserving of sensitivity, respect and trust. Nurses who have time off with mental health problems should be given the confidence to return to work and develop their careers.

Unfortunately, exceptional cases such as that of Beverley Allitt have stirred up panic. Instead of asking for help when they need it, nurses are afraid to acknowledge mental health problems for fear of reprisal or victimisation. People are classed into 'good' and 'bad' , 'safe' and dangerous' – instead of it being acknowledged that working in health services may be bad for your health.

Pre-employment screening (PES) is seen by some as a way of ensuring that only 'good nurses' are selected for nursing posts. This was brought into focus by the Clothier report , which recommended that PES be adopted by health service occupational health departments: 'We recommend that no candidate for nursing in whom there is evidence of major personality disorder should be employed in the profession'. Unfortunately 'there is no reliable marker of that sort of dangerousness' (*Nursing Times*, 1997) (see also RCN, 1994; Naish, 1997).

The idea of screening out 'mad' or dangerous nurses is flawed, and 'absolves health services of their responsibility to maintain an environment in which dangerous practice is minimised' (*Nursing Times*, 1997). Minimising dangerous practice is a surer approach to a problem which cannot be solved by blaming individuals. Well-intentioned but overzealous pre-employment screening may cause more problems than those it aims to solve. Focusing on individuals and not the whole environment may produce more casualties, stigmatising anyone who has experienced stress, stress-related concerns, or other mental health problems. As RCN occupational health adviser Carol Bannister warns, 'You can't take a group such as people who have had mental health problems and say "We don't employ them". Any trust which did that would automatically be found guilty of discrimination under the [Disability Discrimination] Act.' She suggests that most current pre-employment and periodic health assessments also fall foul of the Act.

Others acknowledge the legitimacy of trying to identify and support nurses of borderline competence or who are vulnerable to work stress, but similarly dismiss links between mental illness and dangerousness (House, 1997). They also draw attention to the risk of victimisation if breach of the confidentiality rules reveals a nurse's mental health history to employers and colleagues. House concludes that 'occupational health services could state that they do not intend to implement the Allitt inquiry recommendations on screening for psychiatric disorder'.

A history of inaction

The provision of an occupational health service is an integral aspect of maintaining health and safety at work, yet the record of the NHS is even worse than that of industry. This is not for want of official recommendations or acknowledgement of the need, but these paper proposals have never been backed with hard cash. The authors of the 1994 BMA report and experienced OH researchers such as Bamford (1995), Fingret and Smith (1995) and Burbedge (1997) all cite lack of resources and managerial will as the main reasons for inaction, and point out how shortsighted this failure is. Apart from the individual benefits to staff, a good OH service would be cost-effective in reducing sickness absence, legal claims and compensation, and in raising morale, reducing staff turnover and improving productivity.

The stream of official guidance started even before the NHS was established, with a 1945 Ministry of Health booklet, *Staffing the Hospitals*. Over 20 years later the RCN set out the aims, functions and practical requirements of an OH service for NHS staff. This helped maintain the pressure that culminated in the report of the Tunbridge committee, established to examine the standards and scope of the existing services. Its 1968 recommendation that hospital authorities should set up an OH service for all employees was accepted in principle, but action was piecemeal and sporadic among both management and senior nurses.

Official reports continued to underline the need, with the Briggs commit-tee on nursing supporting the Tunbridge proposals and devoting attention to occupational health problems, including stress. Yet in 1979 the RCN complained to the Royal Commission on the NHS that in spite of some experiment and advance, 'for the most part not only are the cobbler's children badly shod, in many cases they have no shoes'.

The Royal Commission itself deplored the delay and uneven progress in setting up services and called for guidelines. These appeared in 1982; the Department of Health and Social Security reiterated its support for the Tunbridge proposals, admitted that 'some general guidance' would appar-ently be useful, but said that no additional resources would be available. 'Many authorities have introduced OH services for some or all of their staff, but there is considerable variation in the functions undertaken and the way in which the services are organised', it said. This circular had already watered down draft proposals and it hardly seemed calculated to galvanise already hard-pressed authorities into action. However the subsequent appearance of guidelines from the Health and Safety Commission's health services advisory committee may have built up more momentum.

In the late 1980s some NHS managers tried to combat criticism of inaction on staff health by calling on the private sector, and private health companies began to offer OH services on contract. However, under the pressures of the internal market, NHS trusts became more likely to offer OH services elsewhere to generate income. The continuing negative picture is exacerbated by the lack of employer support for educational programmes to develop specialist practitioners (illustrated by the decline in nurses gaining OH nursing qualifications since degree programmes began – from 300 in 1995 to 148 in 1997), continued variations in OH provision, the HSE's isolated work on it and the lack of attention to OH in the government review of health inequalities.

Amid this generally bleak landscape there have been some bright initia-tives, such as in Sheffield, the NHS Healthy Workplace Initiative in the

South and West Region, and the Christchurch Occupational Health Project (see Bannister and Coakley, 1995, and our discussion in Chapter 12, 'The Healthy Nurse'). The International Labour Organisation Convention 161, 1985, required member nations to develop OH services for all workers, and led to significant change in the UK's voluntary approach to such provision. Following consultation, the Health and Safety Commission advised the government to ratify the convention, and launched a programme to improve OH services in general. The Health Services Advisory Committee (HSAC) has been producing guidance on OH in the health services, with the participation of OH nurses, and in 1996 the TUC launched a National OH Forum. Yet it is ironic that larger numbers of nurses and more dynamic OH practice might be found in companies such as Sainsburys or local authorities such as Sheffield City Council, while in the NHS it remains under-resourced and underdeveloped – there is still a very long way to go before the shoemaker's children get their due.

Trade union pressure

This poor record on OH services has been partly compensated for, and to some extent improved by, the activity generated by the Health and Safety at Work Act of 1974. This helped stimulate more workplace and worker-initiated action on health and safety, largely through the efforts of staff organisations. The Act is based on the principle of joint employer–employee responsibility, following the Robens report (HMSO, 1972), which drew attention to the UK's high rates of work-related death, disease and injury. It places statutory duties on all employers – for the first time the NHS was legally required to provide for the health and safety of its staff. In particular, the establishment of union-appointed safety representatives and committees offered a framework for improvement via worker participation, which opened new doors in the NHS.

The Act was rightly hailed as a major advance, not least in extending protection to a further eight million workers. But its emphasis on persuasion, education and the responsibility of the individual employee, rather than on enforcing standards, ignored the politics of the issue and left too many loopholes, including the major drawback of crown properties originally being immune from prosecution for breaking health and safety laws. This immunity was only withdrawn from the NHS in 1987 after a hard campaign. The TUC's comment on the development of health and safety legislation is apposite: 'Much of the pressure for change came from the trade union movement – but laws were passed in a haphazard way . . . [they] had many weaknesses' (TUC, 1997). Most employers – and the state is no exception – will only make improvements, and often only the minimum, when forced to do so.

OH services may be seen everywhere as a foundation stone for improving health and safety issues, and the absence of an adequately funded, autonomous and proactive occupational health service in the NHS has contributed to the lack of official focus on health and safety issues. Watterson (1986) noted, ironically, that the Act affected OH education not through enforcement of provisions or the government machinery set up to administer it, but through the way in which the trade union movement responded; this was equally true in the NHS. The stewards, officials and safety representatives of all the health unions have done a sterling service in persuading managers to improve conditions.

The growth in unionism in the 1970s was linked to a more modest but nevertheless influential flowering of interest in the politics of health. Fresh enthusiasm for the neglected area of OH, and an awareness of the action workers could take to improve their health and safety, led to a mushrooming of local groups, campaigns, newsletters, conferences and skill sharing. Many of the resources we recommend in this book were produced by such groups to tackle the deficiencies in official information, usually done in people's spare time with minimal funds. In health services the high point was perhaps reached in 1988, when nurses initiated widespread industrial action, faced with severe staff shortages, increased workloads and greater responsibilities. This radicalism faded in the early 1990s as the NHS reforms brought a 'market culture' to the workplace and unions concentrated on 'conservative' membership policies.

The radical health movement of the 1970s and early 1980s encouraged some unions to employ full-time health and safety officers and researchers, who provide vital knowledge and support for the workplace activity. Most of the safety officers employed by NHS trusts have been unable to match their commitment, expertise or collective approach – they are under great pressure not to rock the boat and to keep politics under wraps (for 'public relations' reasons and 'commercial confidentiality'). The unions, on the other hand, are autonomous in theory and have relatively independent resources, as Watterson points out, which enables them to evolve a more wide-ranging and radical analysis of ill-health and risk.

The trade union emphasis on the 'safe workplace' rather than the 'safe worker in a dangerous workplace' puts the chief responsibility back where it belongs – with the employer. According to the Watterson, this is reflected in the key elements of occupational health education provided by the unions. These are:

- An emphasis on workplace solidarity and organisations involving members.
- A policy of collective action to solve problems.
- A teaching approach that is built on group work and the experiences of members, and is student-centered rather than tutor-centred.

- Materials and analysis based on the real problems of the workplace but located in a wider economic, political and educational framework.
- The development of skills to organise, communicate and negotiate within the workplace.

The emphasis is clearly on the workers becoming well informed and taking collective action, rather than waiting for 'expert' professional opinions from employers. As our discussion of particular hazards shows, the conflict of interests – even within NHS trusts – means that staff cannot safely assume that their welfare will be a prime consideration. The unions' approach springs from a clear understanding of the politics of occupational health, refusing to adopt the victim-blaming approach that still dominates traditional health education.

The development of a positive health and safety culture should be a shared process between employee and employer, according to the Institute of Occupational Safety and Health (1997), which defines this culture as including:

- The demonstrated commitment and leadership of directors and senior managers.
- The acceptance among managers at all levels that health and safety is a line management responsibility.
- Participation in health and safety decisions by personnel at all levels.
- Training to promote competencies in health and safety.
- Shared perceptions of the nature of hazards, magnitude of risks and the practicality and effectiveness of preventive plans.

Experience shows that legislation may be used as a lever but does not of itself solve the problems, especially if there are powerful countervailing forces at work, such as vested interests and lack of money or political will. Many such forces are apparent in health services today, and the quest for better health and safety for nurses will achieve little if it fails to grapple with the underlying politics of occupational health.

Media influences on health and safety

Health services have always attracted media attention, but media influences have become more prominent since the 1970s. The impact of print and broadcast media on health policy and practice, and in turn on health and safety issues, is obvious and has occurred principally in two ways: through media scrutiny of health care and health services, and through media images of nursing, medicine and health.

Since its inception over 50 years ago, the NHS has been regarded with particular public esteem and affection, more, perhaps, than any other national institution. Any news story about the NHS excites similar public interest, and influences political decision making. Numerous TV and radio documentaries and current affairs programmes have resulted in public demands for government action. Reports of critically low staff levels in paediatric intensive care and special care baby units in 1989 reputedly prompted Margaret Thatcher's call for NHS 'reforms'. There have been influential documentaries on legionnaires' disease, salmonella, hepatitis B, HIV and AIDS, methicillin-resistant *Staphylococcus aureus*, 'contracted-out' hospital cleaning services, fire hazards in hospitals and the decay of hospital buildings. Some of these programmes have been made with the cooperation of health managers, some covertly and without the clinical staff's knowledge.

The nursing press has initiated campaigns on the health and safety of nursing staff (back injury, manual handling, hepatitis), nurses' accommodation, sexual harassment, racism and bullying. These have been launched by experienced nurse journalists in consultation with clinical and union experts, and were therefore timely, accurate and effective.

Nurses should not be misled into thinking that the motives behind media scrutiny are always altruistic: television companies and advertisers want audiences, newspapers and magazines want to sell more copies. Nurses should be equipped to take advantage of media interest without expecting automatic coverage and support in their efforts to influence health and safety policy. Support from the nursing press is more consistent; newspaper journalists will run with an issue as long as it is current, but with few exceptions drop it as quickly as they picked it up. Many trust managers, realising this, and anxious to avoid adverse publicity, have appointed media relations officers and insisted on 'gagging clauses' in staff contracts to inhibit or prevent whistleblowing and media access to clinical staff. This increases the pressure on staff.

To ensure your actions are effective, it is advisable to follow some ground rules. First, it is vital to have accurate information and to discuss your concerns in advance with your managers before you consider telling them to the media. Second, nurses should ask their union representatives and bodies such as the Health and Safety Executive for advice and support on their proposed actions, because it is far better to act with others than alone, risking isolation and personal attack. Third, plan a strategy of what you hope to achieve, and be prepared to compromise to reach agreement with your managers: losing your job as a martyr benefits nobody, least of all the individual. Finally, nurses, especially union stewards and safety representatives, should receive training in media awareness, so that they can be informed and effective campaigners for their colleagues. Nurses cannot control media scrutiny, but with information and experience they can strengthen their influence over it.

Public perception of health services is also affected by media images. Television drama has developed significantly since the days of 'Dr Kildare', 'Emergency Ward 10' and 'Angels', with the slick, fast pace and detail of 'Casualty', 'ER', 'Chicago Hope' or even 'Cardiac Arrest'. Yet the images of the nurse as ministering angel or sex symbol are difficult, perhaps impossible to erase from the press or public mind, and are both a hindrance to the development of nursing as a profession, and detrimental to the health and safety of nurses.

These images, however objectionable, might indicate a level of public sympathy that is greater than that shown for politicians, lawyers, estate agents or even doctors. This sympathy may be turned to the nurse's advantage, perhaps, in campaigning for the elimination of hazards, the promotion of health and the prevention of ill-health. In addition, the dramatic realism of health environments in fictional series such as 'Casualty', and factual ones such as 'Children's Hospital', has done much to raise awareness of professional issues and the complexities and changing nature of nursing and health provision. Health care environments shown in gory detail and colour are scarcely glamorous or romanticised, and leave a lasting impression of nursing as a 'dangerous occupation'.

Whether in fictional or factual settings, nurses are shown to be using knowledge, expertise and judgment in providing care for people needing acute or chronic interventions, and nurses are shown to be risking their health and safety in providing that care. It is only a short jump from these images to an understanding that it is not only the situations nurses face that are hazardous, but the environments too.

Nurses have a role, perhaps underestimated and underused, in interpreting the media images of health and health care from an individual one of discussing the realities of health services with members of the public – their family and friends – to a collective one as members of a union and an occupation, informing and correcting errors and misinformation in the political and media arenas. In exercising this role, nurses may also influence the enforcement of health and safety legislation and the progressive development of a more effective legal framework.

References, contact organisations and further reading on health service management

Bamford, M. (ed.) (1995) *Work and Health: an introduction to occupational health care.* London: Chapman & Hall.

Bannister, C. and Coakley, L. (1995) 'The best laid schemes', *Occupational Health*, vol. 47, no. 9 (September), pp. 428–9.

BMA (1994) *Environmental and Occupational Risks of Health Care.* London: British Medical Association.

Bunt, K. (1993) *Occupational Health Provision at Work.* HSE Contract Research Report no 57. London: HSE.

Burbedge, J. (1997) 'Life or death decisions put NHS in the front line', *Occupational Health*, vol. 49, no. 7 (July), pp. 265–6.

Centre for Health Economics (1995) 'Back Pain: its Management and Cost to Society', press release, 1 March 1995, University of York.

Chad-Smith, J. (1997) 'Pro-active claims management, *Health Care Risk Resource*, vol. 1, no. 3, pp. 4–5, in *Health Service Journal*, vol. 107, no. 5582 (4 December).

Chard, C. (1993) *Health and Safety for Nurses.* London: Chapman & Hall.

Clay, T. (1987) *Nurses: Power and Politics.* London: Heinemann Nursing.

Davies, C. (1995) *Gender and the Professional Predicament in Nursing.* Buckinghamshire: Open University Press.

DHSS (1982) *Health Services Management. Occupational Health Services for NHS Staff,* HN(82)33. London: DHSS.

DoH (1993a) *The challenges for nursing and midwifery in the 21st century. The Heathrow debate.* London: Department of Health.

DoH (1993b) *The management of occupational health services for health care staff.* NHS MEL 97. London: HMSO.

Downey, R. (1994) 'Autonomy or accountability?', *Nursing Times,* vol. 90, no. 27 (6 July), pp. 31–2.

Doyal, L. (1979) *The Political Economy of Health.* London: Pluto.

Doyal, L. (1995) *What makes women sick: gender and the political economy of health.* London: Macmillan.

Fingret, A. and Smith, A. (1995) *Occupational Health: a practical guide for managers.* London: Routledge.

Hammond, P. (1995) 'Unhealthy attitudes', *Nursing Times,* vol. 91, no. 20 (17 May), p. 55.

House, A. (1997) 'Damned if you do . . .', *Nursing Times,* vol. 93, no. 46 (12 November), pp. 38–9.

Hazards (1997) 'Some watchdog', *Hazards,* vol. 60 (October), p. 5

HMSO (1972) *Safety and Health at Work,* Report of the [Robens] Committee 1970–72 (Cmnd 5034). London: HMSO.

HMSO (1994) *The Allitt Inquiry: Independent inquiry relating to deaths and injuries on the children's ward at Grantham and Kesteven Hospital during the period February to April 1991.* (The Clothier Report). London: HMSO.

HSE (1993) *Management of Health and Safety at Work Regulations 1992,* Health Services sheet no.1. Sudbury: Health and Safety Executive.

HSE (1995) *Health and Safety at Work etc Act: Advice to employers* (HSC5); *Advice to employees* (HSC3). Sudbury: Health and Safety Executive.

HSE (1997) *Annual Report 1996/97 Summary, Health and Safety Commission,* Misc. 094 (November). Sudbury: HSE Books.

IOSH (1997) *Policy Statement on Health and Safety Culture.* Wigston: Institute of Occupational Safety and Health.

Lunn, J. A. and Waldron, H. A. (1991) *Concerning the Carers. Occupational health for health care workers.* London: Butterworth Heinemann.

Mackay, L. (1989) *Nursing a Problem.* Milton Keynes: Open University.

Mohan, J. (1995) *A National Health Service?* London: St Martin's Press (Macmillan Press).

Naish, J. (1997) 'Dangerous assumptions', *Nursing Times,* vol. 93, no. 46 (12 November) p. 37–8.

NHSE (1993) *A Vision for the Future. The Nursing, Midwifery and Health Visiting Contribution to Health and Health Care.* London: NHSE.

Nursing Times (1997) 'Comment', *Nursing Times,* vol. 93, no. 46 (12 November), p. 4.

RCN (1991) *A Guide to an Occupational Health Nursing Service,* 2nd ed. London: RCN Society of Occupational Health Nursing.

RCN (1994) *The Care of Sick Children: a review of the guidelines in the wake of the Allitt Inquiry.* Re-order no. 000 369. London: Royal College of Nursing,

RCN (1996) *Hazards of Nursing,* Personal Injuries at Work, re-order no. 000 692. London: Royal College of Nursing.

RCN (1997) *Your Rights and Responsibilities,* Health and Safety at Work 5, re-order no. 000627. London: Royal College of Nursing.

Salvage, J. (1985) *The Politics of Nursing.* London: Heinemann Nursing.

Smith, G. and Seccombe, I. (1996) *Manual Handling: Issues for nurses.* London: Institute for Employment Studies with the RCN.

Townsend, P. and Davidson, N. (1982) *Inequalities in Health – The Black Report.* London: Penguin.

TUC (1997) *Hazards at Work: TUC guide to health and safety.* London: Trades Union Congress.

UKCC (1992) *The Scope of Professional Practice.* London: United Kingdom Central Council for Nursing, Midwifery and Health Visiting (UKCC).

Watterson, A. (1986). 'Occupational health and illness: the politics of hazard education', in (Rodmell, S. and Watt, A., eds), *The Politics of Health Education.* London: Routledge & Kegan Paul.

Whitehead, M. (1988) *The Health Divide: inequalities in health in the 1980s.* London: Penguin.

Contact organisations

MIND, 15–19 Broadway, London E15 4BQ. Tel.: 0181 519 2122.

Depression Alliance, 309 The Chandlery, 50 Westminister Bridge Road, London SE1 7QY. Tel.: 0171 721 7411

2 *Health and safety: the legal framework*

The most important piece of legislation affecting occupational health and safety in the United Kingdom is the Health and Safety at Work Act, passed in 1974. The 1974 legislation underpinned all other health and safety legislation and provided, for the first time, a broad and integrated legislative framework to promote, encourage and enforce high standards of health and safety in the workplace. The Health and Safety Commission (HSC) was established as a result of the Act, and government inspectorates were unified into the Health and Safety Executive (HSE). And for the first time, NHS employers were required by statute to provide for the health and safety of their employees.

However, in the case of the NHS at least, implementation of the Act was patchy, with some authorities taking their legal responsibilities far less seriously than others, especially before the removal of crown immunity, which the NHS enjoyed until 1987. This meant that health authorities could not be prosecuted for neglecting the legislation and maintaining unsafe places of work. Therefore, although health authorities were obliged by the Health and Safety at Work Act to provide a safe system of work – and were subject to inspection by the Health and Safety Executive – before 1987 they could not be prosecuted for failing to do so.

It is remarkable that it was not until 1997, ten years after the removal of crown immunity, that the HSE brought the first general prosecution (that is, not for specific incidents or breaches, but for many), without prior warning, against the Swindon and Marlborough NHS Trust for failing to lay down guidelines to ensure the safety of staff and patients.

Before the removal of crown immunity the HSE was forced to rely on the system of crown notices, which were issued to call for specific improvements but were not legally enforceable. For example environmental health officers could visit hospital kitchens but only recommend improvements. They could not even make surprise visits to 'crown premises', but had to apply for permission. In the case of kitchens, this resulted in an absurd situation: health authorities could continually flout food hygiene regulations without fear of prosecution, unlike hotels and other public facilities.

It took the tragedy of the 1984 outbreak of food poisoning at Stanley Royd Hospital, Wakefield, in which 19 elderly patients died, to bring about change. The government finally bowed to mounting pressure and lifted NHS crown immunity, initially from the food hygiene laws only. A subsequent Lords amendment forced its extension to the Health and Safety

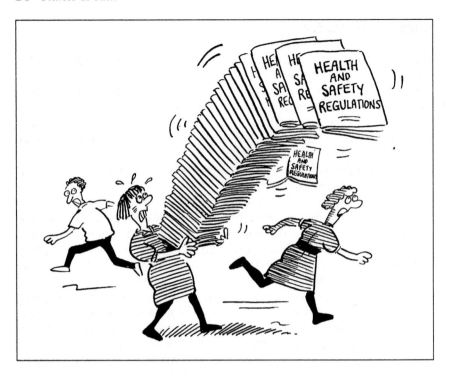

at Work Act. The resulting legislation, the NHS (Amendment) Act, came into operation in February 1987.

Trade unions regarded it as the most important piece of legislation on this subject since 1974 and hoped it would have far-reaching effects. By April the same year, one hospital, the Hammersmith in West London, had already had a compulsory closure order served on its kitchens and was facing legal action.

However no extra cash was provided by the government upon the removal of crown immunity, and, faced with huge bills – estimated at the time by the GMB to total £100 million – health authorities were forced to choose between postponing badly needed upgrading of premises and facing prosecution, or siphoning money away from patient care.

Clearly some took a gamble: between 1988 and 1997 the HSE ordered 61 prosecutions in the health services and issued 55 improvement notices (HSE, 1997c). These ranged from failing to comply with improvement notices or failing to provide safe systems of work, to poor maintenance of gas boilers, resulting in fatal accidents.

The removal of crown immunity and a raft of detailed further legislation, regulation and guidance – generated largely by virtue of the UK's membership of the European Union and considered in detail later in this chapter – has given real teeth to the UK's health and safety legislation, with primary responsibility for the protection of employees' health, safety and welfare resting firmly with the employer.

Employers' duties

The health and safety legislation says that employers must safeguard, as far as is reasonably practicable, the health, safety and welfare of the people who work for them, and a whole raft of detailed and specific legislation, regulations and codes of practice (all described below) now exists to try to ensure that this is so. In the case of nurses, the employer is usually an NHS trust, but may include GPs, local authorities, universities, schools, commercial companies or government departments.

Examples of how the health and safety legislation applies to health services include the following:

- Systems of work: for example procedures for the control of infection, the wearing of protective clothing, being taught and using safe lifting techniques, training in safety procedures and in the use of potentially dangerous equipment, and the principles and practice of food hygiene regulations.
- A safe working environment: for example good standards of hygiene, monitoring to ensure there is no toxic or radioactive contamination, the safe disposal of sharps and other clinical waste, the elimination of – or proper protection when working with – hazardous substances, proper heating and lighting, safe means of entry and exit from clinical areas, equipment which conforms to safety standards and is properly maintained.
- Training: for example in infection control procedures, the safe handling of drugs and chemicals, the use of protective clothing, the use of equipment and appliances, protection from radiation, and how to move and handle patients safely. Employers are responsible for assessing training needs and regularly updating training; failure to do so leaves employers justifiably open to litigation by employees with work-related injuries or illness.

Risk assessment

Risk assessment – the identification of risks and hazards in the work environment to the health and safety of staff, patients and others on health services premises – is a key responsibility of employers under the health and safety at work legislation. It is the central purpose of the Management of Health and Safety at Work Regulations (1992) (see below).

Risk assessment is required by the regulations to be 'suitable and sufficient' – a management obligation which the HSE defines as 'a careful examination of what, in your work, could cause harm to people, so that you can weigh up whether you have taken enough precautions or should do more to prevent harm' (HSE, 1996).

The GMB advises its safety reps that 'suitable and sufficient' [means that] whoever carries out the assessment must be thorough, and sometimes may require specialist advice' (GMB, 1995). The HSE believes that risk assessment should be straightforward and manageable, and suggests a five-step approach. This advice is aimed at employers, but if you are aware of what is required, you can assess if adequate risk assessments exist in your workplace.

1. Look for the hazards. Take a walk around the workplace to consider what are significant hazards which could cause serious harm, taking manufacturers' data sheets and accident and ill-health records into account.
2. Decide who might be harmed and how, including cleaners, visitors, contractors, maintenance personnel and others with whom the workplace is shared.
3. Evaluate the risks arising from hazards. Decide whether existing precautions are adequate or if more should be done. For each significant hazard, employers must decide the level of risk (see Box 2.1), consider whether generally accepted standards exist (for example radiation exposure limits, noise levels) and what precautions are reasonably practicable. They must ask if they can get rid of the hazard altogether, or if not, control the risk so that harm is unlikely. If the work varies, or employees move from site to site (a good example might be health visitor clinics), these possible hazards must be considered. In a shared workplace the other occupants must be informed of work hazards which might affect them.
4. Record the findings. If there are five or more employees, employers *must* record the main findings of a risk assessment and inform their employees.

Box 2.1   *What is risk?*

The TUC defines a hazard as 'something with the inherent potential to cause harm or injury', and risk as 'the likelihood of harm or injury arising from a hazard' (TUC, 1997).

A rough guide to the different levels of risk is as follows:

- Low: remote or unlikely to occur.
- Medium: will occur in time if no preventive action is taken.
- High: likely to occur immediately or in the near future.

The likely consequence of these different levels of risk is:

- Low: may cause minor injury/illness/damage – no lost time.
- Medium: may cause lost time, injury/illness.
- High: may cause serious or fatal illness/injury.

5. Review and revision of assessments. Assessments must be reviewed if they are no longer valid. Unison suggests that the reasons might include complaints from employees or union reps, accident or illness records, warnings from enforcement agencies or – if there has been a major change in work methods – staffing, shift patterns, equipment and management structures (Unison, 1994).

Safety policy statements

Employers of more than five people must draw up a safety policy, detailing what they intend to do to protect the health and safety of their employees and identifying the key managers responsible at various levels. It should be prepared in consultation with union, safety and staff representatives, and should be regularly reviewed as a result of organisational changes, experience or new hazards. There should be effective arrangements for informing staff about it and it should be translated if English is not the first language of a significant proportion of the workforce.

Health service employers do not have a good record in this area and there is little evidence of any energetic efforts by NHS trusts to draw safety policies to the attention of staff. Common faults in existing safety policies include a lack of detail on specific hazards and procedures and an overemphasis on employees' responsibility for their own safety.

Drawing up a safety policy involves:

- Risk assessment (see above): identifying the hazards (for example toxic chemicals, radiation, microbiological hazards, the risk of violence) to staff and others (such as visitors), who may be at risk or exposed to potential risk.
- Detailing the measures necessary to control or eliminate those hazards, for example infection control policies and arrangements for the safe purchasing, storage and use of toxic substances.
- Identifying the officers accountable for monitoring the safety arrangements for each work process, as well as the responsibilities of committees such as the trust safety committee and the infection control committee.

The Safety Policy should include:

- Procedures for maintaining equipment and the work environment, and reporting hazards to management.
- Procedures for reporting accidents and keeping records of accidents and incidents.
- Procedures for keeping staff informed of known dangers, necessary precautions and any changes in policy and procedure, and for monitoring and revising policies.
- Systems for identifying training needs and ensuring that training is carried out.

The Health Services Advisory Committee document *Management of Health and Safety in the Health Services* (HSAC, 1994), provides special guidance for health services. The HSE leaflet *Writing a safety policy statement: Advice to employers* (HSE, 1996), while general to all employers, is very useful.

Reporting accidents and dangerous occurrences

More than 10000 accidents were reported to the HSE in 1991–2, but according to the RCN (1995) only one third of accidents are likely to be reported, so a more realistic figure might be 30000.

Reporting accidents is a legal requirement of UK health authorities and trusts under the Reporting of Injuries, Diseases and Dangerous Occurrences Regulations 1995 (RIDDOR) (see below), which cover all work activities but not all incidents (HSE, 1996). These replaced the 1985 regulations, which in turn replaced previous ones. Each successive set has been more comprehensive. Under the 1995 regulations, the list of specified injuries and dangerous occurrences which must be reported is longer and all injuries resulting from accidents at work that cause incapacity for more than three days must be reported direct to the HSE. People in training are covered in precisely the same way as employees and there are requirements for reporting cases of certain diseases associated with specified work activities. Guidance leaflets on employers' and employees' responsibilities are available from the HSE, as is detailed information for doctors, on reportable diseases, infections and substance-derived conditions. Full details are given at the end of this chapter.

It should be emphasised that failure to report an accident under RIDDOR is a criminal offence. The employer is also required to keep an accident book under the Social Security Regulations (1979).

Following an injury or accident at work, the UK employee must fill in an accident form. This serves three purposes. First, it provides a legal record should the employee subsequently claim injury benefit or compensation, or if a prosecution is brought against the employer. But remember, not having filled in a form should not affect your claim and you may fill in a form retrospectively, even though employees have been discouraged from seeking compensation or injury benefit through not having filled in an accident form immediately after the incident.

Second, the information is used in the national monitoring of work-related accidents and injuries. Third, if used properly accident forms can provide local management and staff organisations with a very useful tool for identifying why accidents are occurring and for carrying out preventive measures. Management have traditionally been very bad at using the wealth of information these forms provide, often because of their poor design and wording. A good accident form should be agreed with union and safety reps. It should separate opinion from fact, help in any further investigation of the accident and feed back useful information for prevention. Guidance on accident forms is available from the HSE; an example of one which is approved by the Health Services Advisory Committee, and is being used increasingly, is outlined in Figure 2.1.

An employee injured at work should also register the incident with the Department of Social Security (DSS) as an industrial accident, using form B195. If the DSS accepts it as such, it will confirm it in writing as an industrial injury, entitling a claim for Industrial Injuries Benefit, a non-means-tested benefit which may continue to be paid even after the employee returns to work. It is also important to contact your local union representative as soon after an accident as possible. (Further details of this procedure are provided in Chapter 11.)

First aid at work

This is another of the employer's statutory responsibilities, under the 1981 First Aid Regulations Approved Code of Practice (HSE, 1997c). It requires employers to ensure there is adequate first-aid provision for employees if they are injured or become ill at work. In the case of the NHS, this requirement is usually fulfilled by a trust's occupational health service, ideally with qualified and specialist nurses and doctors, or by the accident and emergency department. Nurses working in clinics, health centres, industrial and commercial or other non-NHS premises should make sure that the first aid facilities are adequate.

Employees' duties

Employees have a duty to 'take reasonable care' to avoid injury to themselves or others by their work activities. For example if your health is affected through not wearing protective clothing when you are aware that safety policies require it, when the clothing is available and you have been taught the correct way of wearing it, you will probably not be successful in claiming any compensation. This clause in the legislation has been a great let-out for many employers, most strikingly when nurses have claimed compensation for back injuries. The EU *Manual Handling Guidelines* require staff to use lifting equipment if available.

If by your action you cause harm to other employees, you may individually be liable for prosecution. Employees must also cooperate with employers in meeting statutory requirements. This includes reporting hazards and accidents.

A nurse has other professional responsibilities imposed upon her by the body responsible for registration and for setting and maintaining professional standards – in the United Kingdom, the UK Central Council for Nursing, Midwifery and Health Visiting (UKCC). Clause 13 of the UKCC *Code of Professional Conduct* states that a nurse must 'report to an appropriate person

Figure 2.1   *Example of a Model Incident/Accident Form*

A. Which of the following best describes the incident?

1. Personal accident; 2. Violence, abuse or harassment; 3. Ill-health; 4. Security incident; 5. Vehicle incident; 6. Other.

B. Was any individual affected by the incident?

If *Yes*, complete details (name/title/sex/date of birth; status of person: e.g. staff, in-patient, out/day patient, visitor). If *No* go to Section E.

C. Did the person receive any attention (e.g. treatment, advice, counselling, etc.)?

Select from: None/First Aid/Seen by resident doctor/Occupational health/ Accident and Emergency Dept/Advised to see own GP/Other.

D. Did the person suffer physical injury, ill-health or other adverse effect?

If *Yes*: Which part of the body was affected? What nature of injury was sustained (e.g. abrasion, bruising, laceration, sprain/strain, needlestick, fracture)? If *No*, go to Section E.

E. Where and when did the incident occur?

Primary location (e.g. hospital, clinic); Secondary location (e.g. department, ward); Exact location; Management unit; Clinical speciality; Date and Time.

F. Outline apparent circumstances of incident. Outline what happened, together with any relevant circumstances. Where applicable, what was the person doing? Were there any contributory factors?

If any property/equipment involved, give details. For accidents involving patients, give details on patient condition; for clinical incidents, indicate the staff and speciality.

G. Outline any remedial or other action taken following the incident.

H. Where applicable, identify any witnesses.

RIDDOR reportable? *Yes/No*; Complaint potential? *Yes/No*; Claim potential? *Yes/No*

Risk evaluation:
Severity: Minor/Serious/Major/Fatality.
No. people: None/1–2/3–15/16–50/>50
Recurrence: None/Remote/Possible/Likely/Highly likely/Certain.

Further investigation might require some more detailed study of circumstances, equipment, cost of staff time, remedial action etc.

Source: *NHS Incident Record*, Mid Essex Hospitals (Forms IR1 and IR2).

or authority where it appears that the health and safety of colleagues is at risk, as such circumstances may compromise standards of practice and care'. A nurse charged with professional misconduct may be called before the UKCC Professional Conduct Committee, which has the power to remove her from the register. Since it was set up, however, the committee has shown a consistently humane attitude towards the cases called before it, often preferring to blame managers for imposing conditions of work on staff that were very likely to lead to mistakes or misdemeanours. Many cases are referred instead to the UKCC Health Committee, for example if misconduct has been brought about by illness – mental or physical – or by drugs or alcohol. So although it is viewed by many nurses as a disciplinary body, the UKCC can act as a resource and support.

Duties of manufacturers and suppliers

Under Section 6 of the Health and Safety at Work Act, designers, manufacturers, importers, suppliers and installers of articles or substances used at work must ensure as far as possible that they are safe when used. They must test articles for safety in use, or arrange for this to be done, carry out research on the design and manufacture of articles, and supply any available information about the use of the article, any known hazards in its use and any safety precautions that should be taken.

Safety representatives

From the employee's point of view, possibly the most significant aspect of the health and safety legislation is the right it gives to trade unions to appoint safety representatives with wide-ranging legal rights. It was the most contentious clause in the passing of the Health and Safety at Work Act and the House of Lords tried to remove it, believing it would erode the rights of employers to run their own businesses.

Even after the legislation was passed, the reps' rights were resisted, with employers trying to limit their effectiveness by refusing paid time off for health and safety duties or to attend health and safety courses, and refusing to allow inspections and to provide information. Safety reps have nevertheless proved an enormously useful resource in highlighting problems and achieving change: TUC studies of injury statistics show that half as many injuries occur in workplaces that have safety reps as in those that do not. It is not always easy for a member of staff to complain directly to his or her line manager. The safety rep can be more approachable, should know how to get hold of relevant information, and will have more clout in getting things done than the average member of staff. So find out who your safety reps are and use them.

The roles of safety reps are laid down by law in the Safety Representatives and Safety Committees Regulations (1977). Safety reps have the right to:

1. Obtain full information from the employer about potentially harmful practices, substances or items of equipment, including details of manufacturers' trials, known or suspected hazards and necessary safety precautions. If the employer refuses to make particular information available, the safety rep can make a formal complaint to the HSE inspectorate.
2. Obtain information from HSE inspectors about the results of their checks.
3. Investigate accidents, injuries or dangerous occurrences with full access to any relevant information, ensuring action is taken to prevent recurrences.
4. Examine the causes of accidents in the workplace.
5. Investigate employees' complaints about unsafe conditions and practices, with full access to any relevant information.
6. Negotiate with the employer over employees' complaints and work practices; for example, for the substitution of a particular chemical or the supply of more lifting aids.
7. Carry out safety inspections – at least once every three months, more often by negotiation or if there is a change in working conditions, such as the introduction of new equipment, a notifiable accident, injury or dangerous occurrence, or new official information on a hazard.
8. Liaise with occupational health nurses, infection control nurses and HSE inspectors.
9. Attend safety committee meetings.
10. Have paid time off to carry out these functions.
11. Have paid time off to attend health and safety training courses. If either of these are refused, the safety rep is entitled to take the issue to an industrial tribunal.
12. Be provided with facilities to operate effectively, including a room for meetings, office equipment such as a filing cabinet and desk, notice board space and access to a telephone.

Workers in any workplace with more than two employees are entitled to elect safety reps or to appoint them through a recognised trade union. There is no recommended ratio of safety reps to number of employees. The TUC estimates that there are more than 200,000 union safety reps throughout the UK. Among non-TUC unions the RCN currently has about 1500 safety reps, and the RCM 313. All have produced guidelines for safety reps, either in separate manuals or incorporated into stewards' or regional officers' handbooks, and they run training courses for safety reps. The TUC has developed a training programme, which is organised by its Education Service and held at local education institutions which run courses for trade unionists.

The legislation

The health and safety of all employees is protected by a mixture of legislation, regulations, approved codes of practice and guidance. Regulations are legal requirements, often concise, that must be complied with. They may be qualified by words such as 'adequate' or 'suitable'. Examples are the Ionising Radiation Regulations 1985, the Noise at Work Regulations 1989, the snappily titled Reporting of Injuries, Diseases and Dangerous Occurrences Regulations 1995 (RIDDOR 95) and the 'Six Pack' Regulations – there are many more.

Approved codes of practice (ACoPs) represent practical advice, provided by the Health and Safety Commission (HSC), on how to comply with the law, and fill the unanswered gaps in the regulations. Although employers need not follow the ACoPs, they must demonstrate that their systems are as good or better. Both the HSC and the HSE may issue guidance on legislation; outlining the expectations of health and safety inspectors – the information, amount of detail and standards necessary to conform to the laws. The ACoPs are not legally enforceable, but ignoring them would probably risk breaching the law (Unison, 1994).

The Health and Safety at Work Act (1974)

Although this legislation has been considerably strengthened since 1974 – by the removal of crown immunity, as described above, by the introduction of new regulations and approved codes of practice, and by the role of the European Union (EU) – it remains the most important and unifying piece of legislation affecting occupational health and safety.

Before the Health and Safety at Work Act, health and safety was tackled in a piecemeal way through numerous single-purpose Acts such as the Factories Act 1961, the Clean Air Act and the Offices, Shops and Railway Premises Act. Eventually, most pre-1974 legislation will be replaced by new European regulations and codes of practice.

The general purpose of the Act, as outlined in its first section, is to maintain or improve the standards of health, safety and welfare of people at work; to protect people against risks to health and safety arising from work activities; and to control the storage and use of dangerous substances.

Section 2 imposes the general duty on employers to ensure the safety, health and welfare of employees, to consult employees about joint action on health and safety, to establish safety committees at the request of appointed or elected trade union safety representatives and to prepare and publicise a written safety policy statement. Other sections deal with the duty not to endanger coworkers or the public and not to misuse items provided for health and safety purposes, as well as requiring HSE inspectors to provide information on health and safety to workers and workers' representatives.

Since the removal of crown immunity, a number of new Acts and regulations have been introduced, generally elaborating on specific issues in relation to the Health and Safety at Work Act and to European Union legislation. These are described in chronological order below.

Control of Substances Hazardous to Health (COSHH) Regulations (1988) (amended 1994)

The COSHH regulations form a legal framework to protect people against health risks from hazardous substances used at work. These include those which are classed as very toxic, harmful, corrosive or irritant and all other hazardous substances encountered at work. Amendments in 1994 brought 'biological agents' – micro-organisms, including those from hospital inpatients – under this umbrella.

The substances covered by the COSHH regulations include pastes, powders, liquids, oils, gases, aerosols, sprays, fumes, dust, micro-organisms and pathogens. At present, asbestos, lead and radiation are covered by separate regulations, although this may change.

According to the GMB, more guidelines have been published on the COSHH regulations than on virtually any other health and safety regulations. Despite this, the union estimates that only 56 per cent of UK companies have complied with the regulations since their inception (GMB, 1995).

The key provision of the COSHH regulations, from which other elements follow, is for the employer to carry out a 'suitable and sufficient' assessment of likely risks (TUC, 1997). The first step after assessment is to eliminate the risk, or if this is not possible, to control it. The GMB calls this a 'safe place' approach to risk management (GMB, 1995) and emphasises that personal protective equipment must not be used as a substitute for the elimination or control of risks.

The COSHH regulations also call for regular workplace monitoring of hazardous substances, using HSC recommended procedures and current maximum exposure limits (MELs) and occupational exposure limits (OELs) for specific substances listed in a COSHH schedule. The environmental hazard guidance note (EH40) states that 'exposure limits should not be used as an index of relative hazard or toxicity'. They are not sharp dividing lines between 'safe' and 'dangerous' concentrations (TUC, 1997). Records of tests, showing the dates, procedures used and results, should be kept and be available to employees.

The regulations also require employers to ensure that appropriate and free health surveillance of people exposed to hazardous substances is carried out when necessary. Schedule 6 lists substances to which exposure requires a statutory medical examination. The GMB states that risk assessments should identify when surveillance is necessary under statute, and when it is necessary because of an identifiable, work-associated disease or health condition, or a reasonable possibility of it (GMB, 1995). Examples are people exposed to waste anaesthetic gases in operating departments, or to glutaraldehyde in, for example, endoscopy units.

Employees are entitled to sufficient information, instruction and training in hazardous substances to enable them to be aware of the risks and the precautions which should be taken. When a new hazardous substance is introduced into a workplace, the employer should ensure that those affected are given new information and instructions. This might be graded according to the level of risk to which groups of people are exposed, therefore the fullest amount of information would be given to the staff handling or most directly exposed to a substance, with less being given to other groups, always ensuring that safety is not compromised.

The HSE provides detailed guidelines on good practice in relation to the COSHH regulations, in writing, on video, via the Internet and in response to telephone, fax and local office inquiries.

The Health and Safety Information for Employees Regulations (1989)

These require a summary of the main legal requirements to be made available in workplaces in the form of a poster or a leaflet circluated to all employees. The poster must give the address of the local Health and Safety Executive (HSE) office and the Employment Medical Advisory Service (EMAS), which is responsible within the HSE for providing advice about professional, nursing and medical issues.

The Noise at Work Regulations (1989)

These regulate noise measurement and control, the issuing of hearing protectors and indication of noisy areas. Employers must assess employees' exposure to noise, and when necessary provide information and protective equipment such as earmuffs. Employees are required to use any equipment which is provided.

The 'Six Pack' Regulations (1992)

The so-called 'Six Pack' Regulations of 1992 – six regulations based on EU directives – probably represent the most robust reinforcement of the Health and Safety at Work Act that has occurred over the past decade.

1. Management of Health and Safety at Work Regulations (1992). These apply to all health service activities and detail how employers should manage health and safety in the workplace by carrying out risk assessments, monitoring and reviewing working practices, dealing with serious or imminent danger and providing information and training. Their central purpose is risk assessment, but under the regulations employers also have a duty to appoint competent people to help ensure health and safety and set up emergency procedures. Employees must use equipment and dangerous substances according to training, and report dangerous situations and shortcomings in the health and safety arrangements (Unison, 1994).

The regulations were amended in 1994 and 1997 to include additional 'preventive and protective measures' for 'new and expectant mothers' (defined as employees who are pregnant, have given birth within the previous six months or are breastfeeding), and 'young people' (under 18 years). Employers are obliged to assess the potential health and safety risks to these groups. In the case of new or expectant mothers, they must adjust their working hours and conditions, or offer suitable alternative employment or paid leave for as long as is necessary to protect them and/or their children (see also Chapter 9: 'Reproductive hazards').

2. The Manual Handling Operations Regulations (1992).   These deal with the prevention of injuries caused by pulling, lifting, pushing, carrying or moving loads or people. They apply to any manual handling operations that may cause injury at work and require employers to:

- Avoid the need for hazardous manual handling operations.
- Assess the risk involved in unavoidable manual handling.
- Reduce the risk of injury, 'so far as reasonably practicable'.
- Provide general and specific employee training in manual handling.

A more detailed discussion of these regulations can be found in Chapter 10, 'Manual handling: Time to stop?'

3. The Personal Protective Equipment at Work Regulations (1992).   These cover the provision and use of all personal protective equipment and clothing worn or held at work for health and safety reasons. Under the regulations, employers are required to:

- Provide, maintain, store and replace suitable protective clothing and equipment, free of charge.
- Provide information and training in the use of protective clothing and equipment.

Employees are required to comply with protective clothing and equipment policies.

4. Workplace (Health, Safety and Welfare) Regulations (1992).   These cover almost all aspects of the working environment, excluding only transport, domestic premises and construction sites. The regulations established for the first time consistent workplace standards in all health care settings, setting standards for space, staff facilities, toilets, washing facilities, maintenance, ventilation and temperature. These regulations are discussed further in Chapter 3: The working environment.

5. Health and Safety (Display Screen Equipment) Regulations (1992).   These regulate the safe design and use of visual display units (VDUs) and workstations when they are a significant feature of the work. They aim to prevent health problems through the ergonomic design of equipment, furniture, workplaces and work. They emphasise the employer's role in risk assessment, minimum requirements, training and informing employees, as well as the statutory provision of free eye tests and protective equipment, which employees must use.

6. Provision and Use of Work Equipment Regulations (1992).   These deal with the safety of machines, tools and equipment in most occupations. Employers are obliged to maintain work equipment properly and to offer correct information and training in its use. Employees are obliged to use equipment correctly.

The Trade Union Reform and Employment Rights Act (1993)

This legislation protects safety reps and employees from unfair treatment if, for example, they object to the standards of health and safety in their workplace, or plan to act against a serious or imminent hazard.

Reporting of Injuries, Diseases and Dangerous Occurrences Regulations (RIDDOR) (1995)

These regulations cover the recording and reporting of accidents and so on in all workplaces for all workers, including trainees and those who are self-employed. Since 1996 they have also covered violence and an extended list of reportable diseases.

Health and Safety (Consultation with Employees) Regulations (1996)

These regulations enable employers who don't recognise trade unions to choose whether to consult their employees directly on health and safety issues or to arrange for independent worker reps to be elected. Like union safety reps, they should be allowed time off for training and protection from harassment, but they don't have the right to set up a safety committee or conduct inspections.

The Fire Precautions (Workplace) Regulations 1997

These cover the fire safety aspects of 1989 EU Workplace Directives and place the primary responsibility for fire risk assessment with the employer, who must integrate it within the risk assessments required by the Management of Health and Safety at Work Regulations (1992).

Enforcement of the health and safety regulations

As well as introducing new safety regulations, the 1974 Health and Safety at Work Act brought the responsibility for enforcing the new laws and inspecting safety standards under one body, the Health and Safety Commission (HSC). Made up of representatives from industry, trade unions and local authorities, the HSC is responsible for developing effective health and safety policies and for improving health and safety performance throughout employment.

Its operating arm is the Health and Safety Executive (HSE), which brought together and coordinated the activities of all the major health and safety inspectorates which had formerly worked independently within several different government departments. The factory inspectorate is the body responsible for inspecting health care premises in the UK. The HSE is responsible for enforcing health and safety legislation as well as providing an advisory service.

The three principal means of enforcement available to HSE inspectors are:

1. Improvement notices – the employer must make a specific change to working practice or conditions within a specified time span, or a prohibition notice will be issued.
2. Prohibition notices – these may be issued after failure to comply with an improvement notice, or sooner if the danger to employees or the public is immediate. An appeal for delay may be made through an industrial tribunal, but delay is unlikely if the inspector believes there is an imminent risk of serious injuries. If the inspector thinks there is no immediate risk, he/she may issue a deferred prohibition notice, which allows more time to comply.
3. Prosecution – this follows non-compliance with improvement or prohibition notices. Most cases are referred to magistrates rather than Crown courts, therefore the maximum fine can only be £5000.

The HSC has also set up a number of advisory committees to consider and report on health and safety issues relevant to a particular industry. The Health Services Advisory Committee was set up in 1980, and is made up of representatives of health authorities and trusts, employees, trade unions and professional organisations. It has produced some good work, notably reports on manual handling, violence to NHS staff, the management of clinical waste and occupational health services for health care staff.

The role of the European Union

The EU is of fundamental importance in modern health and safety policy and practice, both in the UK and in the broad European context. The most significant body in the EU is the Council of Ministers, a decision-making body made up of representatives of all member states. EU policy is carried out and overseen by the European Commission, which may act against any member state that does not comply with EU legislation.

The HSC is the UK body responsible for suggesting how the UK should comply with EU laws, which fall into three main categories: (1) European regulations, which are immediately binding at community and national level and do not need separate national legislation; (2) directives, which lay out general principles which national governments are obliged to implement, but as they see fit; and (3) decisions, which may be addressed to a single country, an organisation or an individual, and affect only those addressed.

The role of assisting the European Commission to prepare and implement health and safety falls to the Community Advisory Committee on Safety, Hygiene and Health Protection. This committee develops action programmes, and it drew up the measures that laid the foundations for Europe-wide standards of safety law, extended in legislation such as the 'Six Pack' regulations of 1992.

Of particular, though controversial, significance is the Social Chapter of the Maastricht Treaty, from which the UK has been exempt, although the present Labour administration is committed to signing it. Part of the Social Chapter, the EU Working Time Directive, is seen by its UK opponents as a threat to employer autonomy in setting working hours, and by its supporters as a valuable measure to protect workers from the adverse impact on health of overwork. If implemented in the UK, it could have positive benefits for the shift patterns and working hours of doctors and nurses, although there is provision for health care workers to be exempt from the directive's requirements.

Financial awards and injury benefits

In the past it was difficult for staff to sue health authorities and trusts for financial compensation if they were injured or made ill through their work. The existing legislation allowed for varied interpretation, in particular of clauses requiring employees to take 'reasonable care'. Thus claims for financial settlements following back injuries failed because employers claimed that the nurses were using an unsafe technique, putting the onus firmly on the staff members to look after their own safety. In those cases that did succeed, compensation tended to be small.

The EU guidelines, however, have changed the situation significantly. Health authorities and trusts are now required by law to provide adequate systems of risk assessment, adequate training in manual handling and equipment-assisted handling, and appropriate and readily available equipment. Failure in any of these areas by employers provides grounds for litigation in the event of injury and has resulted in higher awards.

Recently an increasing number of judgments have been going against health authorities and trusts, and many more cases have been settled out of court. Awards of £250,000 or more have been made in several back injury claims, with the RCN Legal Department achieving payments totalling £8.5 million in 1996 (RCN, 1997).

Industrial injury benefit is currently payable if an employee is injured or contracts a prescribed industrial disease through work. Payable from 15 weeks after an accident or onset of disease, it is assessed by a DSS medical examiner, there is a percentage disability scale and benefit is given only if a disability is assessed at 14 per cent or above.

If you are injured at work:

- Report the accident to your immediate superior.
- Record it in writing (on a standard accident form if this is adequate, expanded if necessary) and in the official accident book. Keep a copy of the accident form.
- A medical examination should be carried out straight after the accident and the results recorded, preferably by your general practitioner.
- Inform your union steward and safety rep.
- Keep the union informed of your progress.
- Notify the Benefits Agency by filling out Form B195.
- Keep a record of all extra expenses, correspondence, appointments, treatment, medication and investigations. These may be vital during discussions with your employer if redeployment or ill-health retirement become a possibility, or in relation to possible legal claims.

The situation has tended to be bleak for nurses who become disabled or chronically ill but wish to continue working. The Disability Discrimination Act 1996 has some potential to change this situation by placing a legal requirement on employers to consider making 'reasonable adjustments' to retain a disabled person, before pressing for dismissal or early retirement. There are, however, many exemptions. Until recently, few authorities tried seriously to find suitable alternative employment – a disabled nurse is usually an embarrassment (and considered a financial burden) to both her employers and her peers. 'Management is at best indifferent, at worst antagonistic' – this comment by one RCN officer remains true in most cases. The number of NHS staff who had to retire on ill-health grounds rose from 7387 in 1991–2 to 8613 in 1993–4, of whom an estimated 3600–6000 were nurses (Smith and Seccombe, 1996). It remains difficult to obtain accurate statistics. Until forced by law, many health authorities or trusts had no policy on the employment of disabled people.

Union officials, stewards and safety reps should be trained to negotiate on behalf of disabled nurses and be aware of jobs where a nurse could fulfill her personal and professional potential despite her disability. It is time that employers stopped discarding and disregarding the experience, knowledge and abilities of so many people in health care. Antidiscrimination legislation may force the issue to some extent, but surely, as far as is possible, is it not preferable to prevent work accidents and work-related ill-health through effective application of the legal framework?

References, further reading and resources on the legal framework

The Health and Safety at Work Act and related legislation

Croner (1996) *Croner's Health Service Risks* (August), F1-2 (Fire Safety).

GMB (1995) *Safety Reps Handbook*. London: GMB. The GMB also produces an information kit for safety representatives.

HSE (1992) *New Health and Safety at Work Regulations* (1993 EU regulations, alias 'The Six Pack'). Sudbury: Health and Safety Executive.

HSE (1993) *Management of Health and Safety at Work Regulations 1992*, Health Services Sheet no. 1. Sudbury: Health and Safety Executive.

HSE (1995) *Health and Safety at Work etc Act: Advice to employees* (HSC3), 'Advice to Employers' (HSC5). Sudbury: Health and Safety Executive.

HSE (1996) *A Guide to Information, Instruction and Training: Common provisions in health and safety law*, IND(G)2351. Sudbury: Health and Safety Executive

TUC (1997) *Hazards at Work: TUC guide to health and safety*. London: Trade Union Congress.

Unison (1997) 'New Fire Regulations', Health and Safety HS/41/97.

HSE (1997c) 'Health and Safety enforcement prosecutions in the health sector 1988 to date', HSAC typesheet (NIG)8/97. Luton: Health and Safety Executive.

Safety policies

HSE (1996) 'Writing a safety policy statement: Advice to employers', HSC6. Sudbury: Health and Safety Executive.

RCN (1994) *Safety Representative's Manual* (compiled by Sheelagh Brewer), Chapter 6, 'Safety Policies'. London: Royal College of Nursing.

TUC (1997) *Hazards at Work: TUC Guide to Health and Safety*. London: Trades Union Congress.

Reporting accidents

GMB (1995b) Safety Reps Kit: Accidents Checklist.

HSE (1996) 'Everyone's guide to RIDDOR 95. Reporting of Injuries, Diseases and Dangerous Occurrences Regulations'. HSE31. Available free from HSE Offices 'RIDDOR 95: Information for doctors', HSE 32.

RCN (1994) *An RCN Guide for Work Injured Nurses*, London. re-order no. 000 405. London: Royal College of Nursing. The RCN's Work Injured Nurses' Group has also produced a pocket sized, quick guide on what to do after an accident or incident at work.

RCN (1995) *Reporting Accidents*, Health and Safety at Work Series no. 2, re-order No. 000 344). London: Royal College of Nursing.

First aid

HSE (1981) 'Health and Safety (First Aid) Regulations' IND (G)3(L). Sudbury: Health and Safety Executive.

HSE (1997a) 'The Health and Safety First Aid at Work Regulations 1981, Approved Code of Practice and Guidance, L74. Sudbury: Health and Safety Executive.

HSE (1997b) 'General Guidance for Inclusion In First-Aid Boxes', IND(G)4(P). Sudbury: Health and Safety Executive.

TUC (1997) *Hazards at Work – TUC Guide to Health and Safety*, Chapter 4, 'First Aid and Welfare Facilities'. London: Trade Union Congress.

Crown immunity

Barker, R. (1992) 'Coping without Crown Immunity in the NHS', *Health and Safety at Work*, July, pp. 37-38.

Professional responsibilities: nurses

UKCC (1992) *'Code of Professional Conduct'*. London: United Kingdom Central Council for Nursing, Midwifery and Health Visiting (UKCC).

UKCC (1992) *'The Scope of Professional Practice'*, London: UKCC.

UKCC (1993) *Complaints about Professional Conduct.* London: UKCC.

UKCC (1996) *Guidelines for professional practice.* London: UKCC.

UKCC (1996) *Reporting misconduct – information for employers and managers; Reporting unfitness to practice. . .; Issues arising from professional conduct complaints.* London: UKCC. All available free from the UKCC. See also *Register*, the quarterly newsletter to all people on the UKCC Register.

The 'Six Pack' Regulations

GMB (1995) *Safety Reps Handbook.* London: GMB.

HSE (1993) 'Management of Health and Safety at Work Regulations 1992' Health Services sheet no. 1. Manual Handling Operations Regulations 1992, Health Services sheet no. 2. 'Personal Protective Equipment at Work Regulations 1992, Health Services sheet no. 3. Workplace (Health, Safety and Welfare) Regulations 1992, Health Services sheet no. 4. Health and Safety (Display Screen Equipment) Regulations 1992, Health Services sheet no. 5. Provision and Use of Work Equipment Regulations 1992, Health Services sheet no. 6. Sudbury: Health and Safety Executive.

TUC (1997) *Hazards at Work: TUC Guide to Health and Safety* (London: Trade Union Congress see especially Chapters 1, 5, 15, 25.

Unison (1994) *Unison Guides to Health and Safety Regulations* (one for each of the six sets of regulations). London: Unison.

Unison (1997) *Work – it's a risky business*, Stock no. 1351. London: Unison.

Control of Substances Hazardous to Health (COSHH)

Collier, S. (1987) 'COSHH policy-makers decide on cancer controls', *Health and Safety at Work,* January, pp. 37–9.

Glass, D.C., Hall, A. J. and Harrington, J. M. (1989) *The Control of Substances Hazardous to Health: Guidance for the initial assessment in hospitals.* London: HMSO.

GMB (1995) *Safety Reps Handbook.* London: GMB.

HSE (1996) 'COSHH: the new brief guide for employers. Guidance on the main requirements of the Control of Substances Hazardous to Health (COSHH) Regulations 1994', IND(G)136L. Sudbury: Health and Safety Executive. The HSE has published numerous other booklets and leaflets on COSHH.

The European Union

Ludvigsen, C. and Roberts, K. (1996) *Health Care Policies and Europe*. London: Butterworth Heinemann.
TUC (1997) *Hazards at Work – TUC Guide to Health and Safety*, see Chapter 1 in particular. London: Trade Union Congress.

Safety representatives

GMB (1995) *Safety Reps Handbook*. London: GMB.
HSE (1996) 'Consulting Employees on Health and Safety: A Guide to the Law', IND(G)232L. Sudbury: Health and Safety Executive.
HSE (1996) *Safety Representatives and Safety Committees*, L87. Sudbury: HSE Books.
RCN (1994a) *'Safety Representatives'* (Health and Safety at Work series no 1, re-order no. 000 215. London: Royal College of Nursing.
RCN (1994b) *Safety Representative's Manual: A Guide for Safety Representatives*. London: Royal College of Nursing.

The following are also worth looking at:

Hazards, bi-monthly magazine that provides information for safety reps. Available by subscription from PO Box 199, Sheffield S1 4YL. Has a wealth of news, articles and statistics. Also publishes an international newsletter on similar issues: *Workers' Health International Newsletter*
'Health and Safety Record', the T & G's health, safety and environmental bulletin, first published winter 1996.

Financial awards and injury benefits

RCN (1994) *An RCN guide for work injured nurses, RCN WING*. London: Royal College of Nursing. (RCN WING is a self-help group for RCN members and associate members, financed by RCN Membership Services: offers advice, support, information, financial grants, study days and a quarterly newsletter. Membership is open to full and associate members of the RCN.)
RCN (1994) *RCN Core Policies and Advice Notes for Stewards and Staff*. London: Royal College of Nursing.
RCN (1995) *Accidents at Work: Your Financial Rights*, Health and Safety at Work series, no. 3, re-order no. 000 344. London: Royal College of Nursing.
RCN (1997) *RCN Legal Services Report* [for] *1996*. London: Royal College of Nursing.
Seccombe, I. and Ball, J. (1992) *Back Injured Nurses: A Profile*. London: Royal College of Nursing.
Smith, G. and Seccombe, I. (1996) *Manual Handling: Issues for Nurses*. London: Institute for Employment Studies/Royal College of Nursing.

3 The working environment

The word 'nurse' still conjures up the image of someone working in a hospital, although one of the most remarkable recent changes in UK health services is the focus on delivering health care in any and every setting – wherever the patient lives or works and wherever she or he prefers to be treated. There is greater recognition that nurses can, should and do work in all settings. The idea of a 'hospital without walls' is now more familiar, with the shift of emphasis in mental health nursing to community teams; generalist nurses working in schools, health centres, universities, airports, in the air, at sea, in refugee camps, industry and commerce; working with homeless people and travellers, on housing estates, with women and men in the sex industry and with people with learning difficulties; and still as district nurses, health visitors, family planning advisers, Macmillan nurses and so on. Most nurse educators are now employed in higher education, and most nurses undergo their initial professional training outside hospital as full-time bursaried students.

This wide spectrum of settings has major implications for the protection and development of nurses' safety and health, which must be tackled in the context of all these settings and work roles, and not simply within the traditional physical structure of the hospital. While some of the issues in this chapter relate to specific settings, most can be considered in relation to anywhere that nurses work.

Reviewing your work environment may seem daunting, and it could be helpful to start with workplace guidelines and health and safety policies. All employing authorities are legally required to produce a document outlining health and safety for their staff – not just a generalised statement, but specific guidelines – and they must consult staff and their representative organisations on it. Drawing up, assessing and revising such a policy document could be a sensible starting point for a rigorous review of what is happening in your work place, and for stimulating local discussion and action. Inspection, hygiene and the other aspects of health and safety discussed in this book should all be included in a trust-wide policy, and implemented with equal care.

Buildings

Is the NHS falling down? During the years of Conservative government it was regularly claimed that the NHS was being dismantled. While the health service proved more resilient than predicted, there is much evidence that it is falling down in a more literal sense, owing to the age, poor construction or bad state of repair of many of its buildings. This has great relevance to the health and safety of its workers and users, for it is difficult to maintain high standards and promote good health in an environment which is itself positively harmful – not just in clinical areas, but also in staff accommodation and facilities.

When the NHS was established in 1948 it inherited around 3000 hospitals and clinics of enormously varied standards. Now there are around 1700 hospitals and clinics of differing ages, states of repair and suitability for use (Audit Commission, 1991). The age of the buildings need not itself be a problem, but regular maintenance and repairs – simply good housekeeping – has become something of a luxury in today's cash-starved health services. During the 1990s much staff accommodation was closed or sold. Some old hospital buildings were replaced by new, purpose-built units, but faulty design and shoddy construction have not been eliminated. A report on the state of hospital buildings (SAVE, 1997) estimated that by 1995–6 the NHS repairs backlog stood at a minimum value of £2.4 billion, with an upper estimate of £10 billion. Many trusts were reported not to have surveyed their building stock, contrary to the Audit Commission's recommendations to NHS Estates to conduct a five-facet survey (physical condition; energy performance; compliance with fire, statutory and non-statutory regulations; functional suitability; and space use).

It may have been assumed that directives to health authorities to produce and maintain a proper record of the condition of all their premises would lead to better management of the building stock, but the SAVE report contradicts that assumption. Successive official circulars emphasised the possibility of selling property rather than improving it, and encouraged authorities to have an eye to market value. No NHS hospital or clinic could be considered safe if it happened to be in a prime location.

Older buildings might need repair, but this is often postponed. For example the Cardiff Royal Infirmary, built in 1883, needs major repairs but is due to close in 1999. The report notes that it isn't only older buildings which are decrepit: some hospitals built in the 1960s, 1970s and 1980s have major structural problems. The University Hospital of Wales in Cardiff was built as recently as the 1970s but has continually leaking roofs, as well as cladding and heating system problems (Millar, 1997). New structures may also prove unsafe or unhealthy due to poor lighting, artificial ventilation and humidification – the sick building syndrome (Garvey, 1994).

NHS premises

NHS premises, whether health centres, clinics or hospitals, are all subject to the same legislation and should adhere to the same standards. The Workplace (Health, Safety and Welfare) Regulations 1992 established for the first time a consistent set of standards for all health care environments, covering topics such as temperature, ventilation, lighting, cleaning, maintenance, room dimensions and space, largely superseding the benchmarks of the Offices, Shops and Railway Premises Act. First aid provision is covered under the Health and Safety (First Aid) Regulations 1981, with an Approved Code of Practice (ACOP) updated in 1997.

Whether privately owned or not, a community nurse's car is legally defined as 'premises' and is therefore subject to the regulations which require the employer to maintain certain standards. When the employer provides a car it must keep the vehicle roadworthy, and crown cars should be regularly maintained and renewed. But all too many staff are being required to drive unroadworthy vehicles because of shortage of cash, plain misman-agement or both. There should be a policy outlining what to do when cars break down, and alternative arrangements when a car is off the road.

Non-NHS premises

Many nurses work in premises that are not owned by their employing authority, for example schools and village halls. They should not be expected to work in places that fall short of the minimum standards, and the employer must recognise its obligation to bring these up to scratch or find alternatives. The regulations outlined above also apply here, and to temporary or contract workers, and the employer – not the individual nurse – should check that cleanliness, lighting, heating, storage of equipment, rest and refreshment facilities and fire precautions are all adequate. The Workplace (Health, Safety and Welfare) Regulations 1992 do not cover domestic premises, but under the Health and Safety at Work Act employers must look after their employees' health and safety at work, and ensure that people not in their employ – including children and other visitors to their work premises – are protected from health and safety risks.

Staff accommodation

During the 1980s the shocking state of many NHS buildings was brought home to nurses by the condition of their own live-in accommodation, some of it appalling and highlighted in a series of campaigns. Since then many buildings have been sold or converted to other uses, such as education, research or administration. The remaining stock ranges from purpose-built nurses' homes of a high standard to homes where no improvements have been made. A recent case in Edinburgh highlighted the plight of 300 nursing students with flea-ridden beds in decrepit buildings. Only three of eleven toilets were operating, and fridges and cookers were broken. In 1996–7 nursing students at Thames Valley University, with the support of the RCN and Unison, campaigned publicly about their accommodation charges and poor conditions. One student had cockroaches and silverfish in his room; others mentioned a rusty bath aggravating eczema; paying £10 a month for cleaning which was done badly, if at all; and bags of rubbish, shopping trolleys and old furniture left in corridors. Similar anecdotes were told in an earlier survey (RCN, 1994).

The Conservative government introduced a policy of selling off NHS property which it considered 'surplus to requirements' – even homes where staff were living. Severe restrictions were imposed on the number and type of staff entitled to live in, and by the end of 1987 each health authority had assessed its need for accommodation and sold off the 'surplus'. It was accepted that some students would continue to need accommodation, and the authorities were urged to make plans to bring accommodation up to scratch – but each authority was free to decide how many places to provide. There was a storm of protest from nurses. Many pointed out that the already acute difficulty in recruiting nurses in London was being exacerbated by the policy, since few could afford the capital's private rents, let alone obtain mortgages on such low salaries. Other cities reported similar concerns.

The then Department of Health and Social Security admitted that 'some of the existing stock is in a poor state of repair and decoration . . . staff who need to be resident should be housed in accommodation of good quality'. But few nurses were able to remain living in and thus reap the benefits, while local policies failed to address the reasons why nurses would choose to live in despite the often bad conditions. These included travel problems created by

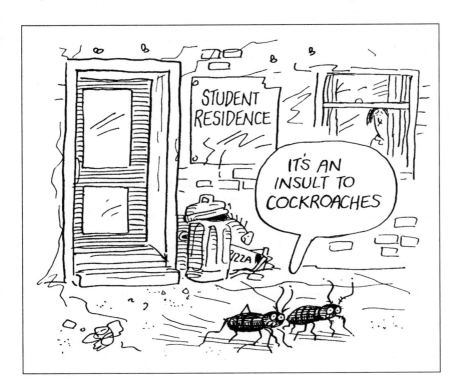

shift work and the danger and difficulty of travelling at odd times; the lack of alternative accommodation; the isolation of many hospitals; and, by no means least, small pay packets which made it impossible for most nurses to afford mortgages or high rents.

Nurses' accommodation problems have not diminished today. Their income has risen, but so have market rents, and not just in London. Cities such as Oxford now have such high living costs that the recruitment and retention of staff is a major and continuing problem, though one which many trusts seem reluctant to tackle head-on. Nursing students in higher education also face serious problems, as they enter courses on fixed bursaries and are forced to compete with other students for limited on-campus resources, or equally finite numbers of rental properties in inner city areas. Both environments have the hazards associated with poor security and poor maintenance, while the particular needs of students undertaking clinical placements are often not taken into account, bringing added disruption to sleep and study, and additional stress.

Obstacles have arisen even where trusts are prepared to build new staff accommodation, such as the Royal Free Hospital NHS Trust in London, where local residents opposed the planned new homes.

The reduced availability of live-in accommodation has coincided with a decline in the standards of public transport, compounding the problem of getting to and from work. Deficiencies in bus and train services have led to increased car usage and greater staff travelling time in many areas, often accompanied by the unwelcome introduction of parking charges for staff vehicles, with the added anxiety of having to arrive early for work in order to find a space. Preference is often given to visitors and top medical and management staff, with clinical staff parking – when it exists – relegated to distant locations, which puts staff increasingly at risk of violence, especially after evening or night shifts.

Current and future prospects

The government's policy of selling off NHS premises which have been allowed to run down into decrepitude has not been applied solely to staff accommodation. The government-dictated estates management priority has been to get the best price rather than to preserve NHS buildings. SAVE reports that many NHS buildings have been sold off to developers, who neglect or vandalise the properties as soon as the staff and patients move out. According to the head of policy for NHS Estates, 'It is not the mission of the NHS to find new uses for our surplus property – we just have to make sure it sells at a reasonable price.' In other words, once we've got the money, we don't care what happens to the buildings.

In London especially, it has been argued for some years – for example in the 1992 Tomlinson report – that there are too many acute hospital beds and too many hospitals, and that rationalisations and resource reallocations are essential to redress the balance in favour of community services, regional centres outside London, and new areas of need. However the failure to care for NHS stock has led to a vicious circle in which properties are not adequately maintained and fall into a state of decay, whereupon they are deemed too costly to renovate. Poor condition is often used as part of the justification to close hospitals or clinics for which there is no alternative service, as no one wants either to give or to receive care in substandard or inappropriate surroundings. The underlying lack of government investment in health services is a key reason behind such closures.

Selling off NHS resources raises serious questions about the ability of health services to cope with future demand, which is growing. The massive, continued backlog of repairs demonstrates that more money is needed for health services, and is a good example of how 'efficiency savings' can ultimately prove to be costly and jeopardise the welfare of employees and clients.

This, then, is the bleak background against which the quality of the nurse's environment must be considered. Those who live in the remaining staff accommodation face additional problems on top of the poor conditions endured by everyone who works in substandard, old, badly maintained or insufficiently repaired premises – and unfortunately they remain a significantly large group. Poor premises and insecure surroundings do not encourage people to work well or to enjoy their jobs. But although this picture is grim, it is possible for you to do something about it – not just by pressing for more spending on health services, but also by taking action in your own workplace against some of the hazards outlined in this book. This chapter will therefore continue by looking at a variety of problems associated with the places in which you work – the fabric of buildings, temperature, noise lighting and ventilation, as well as many other factors that affect the quality of the working environment.

References and further reading on buildings

Audit Commission (1991) *NHS Estate Management and Property Maintenance.* London: HMSO.
Garvey, J. (1994) 'Sick building syndrome: developing an integrated approach to SBS' *Occupational Health*, vol. 46, no. 2 (February), pp. 50–3.
Meara, R. (1992) *London's Legacy: aspects of the NHS estate in London.* London: King's Fund.
Millar, B. (1997) 'Assets or liabilities', *Health Service Journal*, vol. 107, no. 5572, *Special Report: Facilities Management*, p. 8.
NHS Estates (1996) *An exemplar estate strategy* (pamphlet). London: HMSO.
RCN (1993a) *London Needs All its Nurses: The Health Care Challenge for the 21st Century*, re-order no 000 212. London: Royal College of Nursing.

RCN (1993b) *Royal College of Nursing Response to the Report of the Inquiry into London's Health Service, Medical Education and Research.* London: Royal College of Nursing.

RCN (1994) *Must it be so hard? Hardship among nursing students.* London: Royal College of Nursing.

SAVE (1997) *Hospitals: a medical emergency*, London: SAVE Britain's Heritage.

Asbestos

Asbestos is a good example of a hazard made even more deadly by the poor condition and cut-price maintenance of so many health service buildings. Concern about its effects is not new: Lucy Deane, a 'lady inspector', wrote in 1898 that 'the evil effects of asbestos dust have also attracted my attention' (Yeendle, 1993). And although much asbestos has been removed since the 1980s, it remains true, as asbestos expert Alan Dalton once put it, that 'hospitals are alive with asbestos' (Dalton, 1979). The Health and Safety Executive estimates that asbestos-related diseases kill around 3000 people annually in the UK, and the number is expected to rise well into the twenty-first century.

Hospital maintenance, renovations, refurbishment and repairs mean there is a continued risk of exposure to asbestos particles. Particles may be found in wards, corridors, kitchens and laundries, and are spread via damaged and flaking insulation, ventilator shafts, clothing and food. Hospital fitters and plumbers have died of mesothelioma, a cancer that is nearly always caused by exposure to asbestos. The deadly fibres have been used in cement, pipes, sheeting, flooring, ceilings, roofing, insulation, fireproofing and even sprays to coat steel structures.

People who work with asbestos in industry and construction are clearly at risk of asbestosis, the lung scarring caused by inhaling the dust. It's unclear what levels of exposure cause disease, but just one day's exposure to the dust may be enough to cause cancer. But how likely is it that a nurse will be affected? Both the government and the HSE agree that there is no 'safe' level of exposure, and failure to deal with asbestos on health service premises could therefore harm nurses and patients, as well as workers actually handling the substance – an example of shared interests in health and safety.

Public concern has led to stricter regulations, with tighter controls introduced by the Health and Safety Commission: no more spraying or using asbestos in insulation, lower exposure limits, and new rules for its removal. Useful information may be found in *Managing Asbestos in Workplace Buildings* (HSE, 1996) and other references listed at the end of this section. The Asbestos (Licensing) Regulations 1983 and the Control of Asbestos at Work Regulations 1987 were followed by the Construction (Design and Management) Regulations 1994 and the Special Waste Regulations 1996. These govern working practice in areas with risk of exposure to asbestos, and the disposal of asbestos, which must normally be done by contractors licensed by the HSE.

Just tightening the rules, however, isn't enough. As Dalton has pointed out, asbestos is an avoidable hazard: there are less risky alternatives for nearly all its uses. Most trusts have embarked on programmes to remove old asbestos. They are legally obliged to label asbestos materials and maintain records of existing asbestos sites to give to planning supervisors – do you know your employer's policy and practice?

Furthermore the process of removing the deadly fibres can give rise to more problems. As recently as 1991, Mid Glamorgan Health Authority was prosecuted after two fitters were exposed to asbestos dust while removing steam pipes from a boiler room. Health trade unions, especially Unison, and building unions continue to campaign for tougher action, calling for continued local surveys and the monitoring of dust levels.

Asbestos is a difficult hazard to fight because of its low visibility. Yet it is so dangerous, and appears to be harmful after such a brief exposure, that nobody can afford to be complacent about it – nurses should be alert to any potential risk.

References and further reading on asbestos

Dalton, A. (1979) *Asbestos: Killer Dust*. London: BSSRS Publication.
HSE (1993) *The Control of Asbestos At Work: Control of Asbestos at Work Regulations 1987*, ACoP L27. Sudbury: Health and Safety Executive.
HSE (1996) *Managing Asbestos in Workplace Buildings*, IND(G)223(L). Sudbury: Health and Safety Executive.
TUC (1997) *Hazards at Work: TUC Guide to Health and Safety*. London: Trades Union Congress. Chapter 8, 'Asbestos', gives a comprehensive account of issues concerning asbestos; detailed information on maximum exposure limits, how to claim compensation for asbestos-related diseases etc; and an extensive list of HSE and other publications.
Unison has published the *Asbestos Hazards Handbook* (London Hazard Centre Guide) and *Registering Asbestos in Public Buildings* (Unison/TUC).
Yeendle, S. (1993) *Women of Courage: 100 Years of Women Factory Inspectors*. London: HMSO. This is a wonderful book on the almost forgotten story of women factory inspectors from 1893 to the 1950s, published for the HSE.

Fire

In sessions on fire safety, nursing students have often been shown films such as the graphic and memorable '*Hospitals don't burn*', followed by a lecture by the fire officer, and concluding with practical demonstrations and the handling of extinguishers and fire blankets – usually in a classroom, occasionally in a courtyard, where a small, controlled fire could sometimes be lit and extinguished with ease. These sessions are usually one-off events of doubtful value, laughed at by all participants. Yet the prospect of fire in health service environments is appalling.

Every year at least 2000 hospital fires are reported. They can have tragic results. Patients in mental health and elderly care units have been killed or severely burned, and nurses have suffered, too, as in the Kirkcaldy nurses' home fire in 1981, which caused the death of two students. The need to ensure that fires are prevented and that staff know what to do in a crisis applies to the nurse not just as a worker with vulnerable people in her care, but also as a potential victim.

The majority of hospital fires happen at night. One Scottish survey found that fires begin in kitchens (both hospital kitchens and those in staff residences), wards (chiefly elderly care and mental health), patient and staff lounges, cloakrooms and bathrooms, in that order. The careless disposal of cigarette ends and matches is an important cause, but human negligence often becomes fatal because avoidable hazards such as flammable materials, bedding and faulty electrical appliances continue to be used – a responsibility which lies firmly at the door of the employer.

Resources are crucial, and employers who are forced to count every penny are liable to cut spending to the detriment of safety standards: replacing flammable furniture or panelling, checking and replacing equipment, regular inspection of premises and staff training all cost money. The most expensive resource of all is people, and staff shortages, and reliance on part-time or agency staff, have implications for preventing and fighting hospital fires because of the availability of nurses familiar with the work environment and with fire procedures to help rescue patients if a fire breaks out. Staffing levels, moreover, need to be high enough to enable workers to attend courses, fulfil their responsibilities as employees and develop their commitment to high standards of safety.

The relevant regulations are banded together as the 'Firecode' regulations and cover all aspects of fire safety in health care premises. The health and safety and fire safety laws, and the principles and policies of the Firecode, are given below, and a list of selected Firecode documents is included in the References.

Fire legislation and regulations

Fire Services Act 1947

This gives local fire authorities a statutory duty to give advice on fire precautions if requested. Trusts are expected to make use of their expertise when drawing up fire safety plans (DHSS, 1987a).

Health and Safety at Work Act 1974

The general principles of the Health and Safety at Work Act 1974 form part of the legislation relating to fire, together with specific fire legislation.

Fire Precautions Act 1971

This applies to all patient areas in the health services, together with local authority fire and building regulations. Fire authorities can only recommend measures such as the installation of sprinklers and other fire suppression systems, but insurers have more comprehensive requirements.

Residential Care Homes Regulations 1984, and the Nursing Homes and Mental Nursing Homes Regulations 1984

The fire safety of nursing and residential care homes is prescribed by these acts, which have identical requirements.

The Fire Precautions (Workplace) Regulations 1997

These regulations implement the 1989 EC Workplace Directives, and bring UK fire legislation up to the minimum requirements of the directives, placing primary responsibility for fire safety on the employer. Employees are obliged to follow fire arrangements and avoid placing themselves or others at risk.

Employers' obligations are to:

- Assess fire risks (either specifically or within general health and safety risk assessments) under the Management of Health and Safety At Work Regulations 1992.
- Ensure the workplace has appropriate fire extinguishers, hoses, detectors and alarms, and that they are easily accessible, simple to use, checked and maintained in working order, and marked by clear signs.
- Nominate and train employees to carry out firefighting actions and contact external fire services in the event of fire; consult trade union safety reps before appointing a fire safety coordinator.
- Keep emergency exits clear, and ensure people can leave buildings safely in an emergency.
- Make sure people know what to do if a fire occurs.

The local fire authority or appointed fire inspectors enforce these regulations, which are a consolidation of existing UK fire laws. If an employer has a Fire Certificate and is assessed by the fire authority to comply with the current fire safety standards, this is considered adequate to comply with the new regulations. The fire authority may resolve minor breaches by informal discussions with an employer, or bring a civil action. More serious offences – failure to remedy known defects within a specified time, or 'reckless failure' to comply with the regulations – could lead to enforcement notices or criminal prosecution if informal discussions or notice of an application to serve a Crown Court order do not prompt the employer to make the required improvements (Croner, 1997; Health and Safety, 1996; Health and Safety, 1997; Unison, 1997).

Most of the general fire legislation applies to Scotland as well as England and Wales, but there are some differences. In Scotland there are no local Acts relating to fire safety; the Crown Premises Inspection Unit is in the HM Fire Inspectorate of Fire Services for Scotland. There is no statutory requirement for building regulations authorities to consult the fire authority about escape methods, because Scottish building regulations already include these aspects, and also provide for building completion certificates which confirm that a new building incorporates adequate fire precaution features.

In 1997 the government began consultations on developing fire legislation in the UK following the Fire Precautions (Workplace) Regulations 1997. The aim of the consultation was to rationalise existing legislation in 'a new modern approach . . . based on risk assessment, which will ensure that fire safety precautions are in proportion to the risk faced' (Home Office, 1997). The proposals included:

- Placing the general duty of care on employers, occupiers and owners (except of private dwellings), with fire authority validation of safety in high-risk premises.
- Consideration of existing fragmented legislation: the so-called 'Holroyd distinction' – made by the Holroyd Committee in 1970 – between fire safety measures incorporated during construction (building regulations) and those required in occupied buildings by the Fire Precautions Act 1971 (enforced by fire authorities) and local Acts in England and Wales.
- The Health and Safety at Work Act 1974 should continue to cover fire precautions, but with separate legislation for general fire safety.

The Home Office noted the importance of the Fire Precautions Act 1997 being goal-based, so that the means of achieving fire safety could be adapted to circumstances, unlike the prescriptive approach of the 1971 Act. This may help to ensure that fire safety is seen as a continuous process, rather than one-off. The Home Office feels that statutory guidance is unsuitable for a goal-based approach, though it accepts that the Health and Safety Commission's use of Approved Codes of Practice might be a good model.

Fire certificates

Health authorities must obtain a fire certificate, which lays down the legal requirements for fire precautions, means of escape, fire-fighting equipment, warning equipment and training. Safety reps are entitled to have a copy of this document, which can be used as the basis for an inspection checklist and as a lever for action. Fire certificates are issued either by the Home Office (for 'crown premises') or local authorities, or by the Health and Safety

Executive (for 'special premises' – those with large amounts of flammable liquid, nuclear materials or explosives, or small building sites not requiring a fire certificate).

Preventive measures

There is an extensive literature on fire safety; much of it outlines the range of preventive measures which should be taken. Primary responsibility rests with the employing authorities, but nurses, stewards and safety reps concerned about the standards in their own place of work or residence can do a great deal to raise awareness and pressurise management into action.

The inquiry which followed the Kirkcaldy disaster could not pin down the cause of the fire, but did highlight various serious failures to comply with the fire regulations, which could have contributed to the nurses' deaths (Urquhart, 1982). Although the home was fairly new it did not meet the standards required by the Fire Prevention Act (Scotland) 1971, or the local building bylaws, or the Scottish Home and Health Department. As the building was crown property, though, those responsible for this neglect were immune from prosecution – a scandal which could have been repeated as the lifting of immunity then applied only to the Health and Safety at Work Act.

The horrifying point about Kirkcaldy is that the low standards there were by no means unusual – they just happened to be disclosed in the wake of a tragedy. The specific breaches in the regulations can be found today in health service premises everywhere: fire doors wedged open, fire escapes locked, faulty wiring on fire alarms, parts missing from the emergency release panel containing the fire alarm, and obstacles hindering rescue and the use of fire-fighting appliances.

Inspection and updating

Management should carry out regular inspections not just of fire precautions such as escape routes, but also of other aspects of prevention. Have all materials known to be hazardous, for example hardboard partitions, been removed? Information is available from the Department of Health and from the local fire service, and many authorities now employ fire prevention officers who are expert in the field. In addition, full reports should be made after any incident, however small, and remedial action taken when the causes are known; the reports should be studied systematically to assess trends and dangers.

Electrical appliances

Old wiring, outdated equipment and overloaded circuits can all lead to fires. Procedures for the regular checking of equipment and circuitry should be in place, with designated works staff and budget allocations for replacing hazardous items. Refer to the Electricity at Work Regulations 1989, current HSE Guidelines, and the Firecode.

Smoking

Smokers' materials are the major cause of hospital fires. Limiting smoking by patients and staff is therefore not only a matter of individual health, but also an important measure for the protection of the whole community. Many employers now have no-smoking policies, and most health premises designated smoke-free or have limited smoking areas; hazard notices, plus sandboxes and other safe disposal receptacles, may help to remind smokers of the need to be careful. The health risks associated with smoking and the passive inhalation of smoke mean that non-smoking employees may insist on the introduction of a no-smoking policy if it doesn't exist. There is a risk, however, that a new hazard may be created by confining smokers in small areas.

Removing hazardous materials

Fire prevention officers can give advice on dangerous materials which should be replaced and practices which should be amended or avoided; the DoH Safety Information Bulletins cover a range of fire hazards such as hospital beds, bedding and antihypothermia blankets, and these bulletins should be studied by all managers.

One potential hazard which has attracted publicity is flammable nurses' uniforms. Following claims that the national uniform was a fire danger, the then DHSS produced a report which concluded that 100 per cent flame-retardant polyester was the material best in terms of flammability, but no single material among those commonly used came out top in all the criteria tested. Health care employers should be aware of this when they order uniforms – and choose safer and more comfortable alternatives, such as cotton.

The growing use of continental quilts in hospitals in the 1980s also aroused fears about safety, especially following a fire in a Northampton hospital in which several patients died and duvets were thought to be a contributory factor. Supplies departments have information on current DoH specifications, and should be able to answer nurses' questions. There is also reference to fire safety standards for textiles, furnishing, bedding and mattresses in the Firecode documents.

Training

As already mentioned, another important facet of the employer's responsibilities is providing good staff training in fire prevention and dealing with fires. Regular instruction and practice are crucial not only in encouraging efficiency, but also in making the staff alert and aware. Perhaps the most effective initiatives are those with the emphasis on practical exercises – staff experiencing at first hand a complete lack of visibility and feeling of disorientation as they attempt to rescue patients from a smoke-filled ward. A good example is provided by nurses in the Brighton Nursing Development Unit, who simulated a fire to prove to management that the unit was unsafe for wheelchair users. They invited the general manager, who subsequently agreed to renovations.

Action points

What can nurses do if they are worried about safety standards or a lack of training and fire drills? They should seek out their safety rep and/or steward and together they can approach management. If no action is forthcoming, they can contact their health or local authority fire prevention officer and request an inspection – preferably with union backing. Fire authorities can take up complaints, locally or with the DoH, and if they think all or part of a building is dangerous they can apply to close it, or, as discussed earlier, take legal action against the employer.

What to look for

- Are there reasonable means of escape to the open air, and are they clearly indicated? Fire-resistant and smoke-retardant doors should be self-closing (not self-locking) and should never be propped open.
- Corridors and fire escapes are 'protected' areas in law, which means there should be no fire risks present, or obstructions (DHSS, 1987b).
- Is there a good fire alarm system, preferably linked to smoke detectors and with fire phones?
- Is there an emergency lighting system for public areas?
- Are fire drills held regularly, and are they assessed and the results fed back to staff?
- Are there management systems to ensure that new and temporary staff are given adequate fire instructions?
- Does every room on the premises have visible and up-to-date guidance notices on what to do in case of fire?
- Is there a plentiful supply of regularly maintained extinguishers, hoses, and patient moving gear such as straps and lines, and do people know how to use them?
- Are all fire exits and fire-related equipment marked clearly?

References and further reading on fire

Note: HTM = Health Technical Memoranda

Croner (1997) *Croner's Health Service Risks*. August, Fire Safety.
DHSS (1987a) 'Policy and Principles', ISBN 0 11 321109 0. London: HMSO.
DHSS (1987b) 'Fire Precautions in New Hospitals'. HTM81. London: HMSO.
DHSS (1988) 'Alarm and Detection Systems'. HTM82. London: HMSO.
DHSS (1988) 'General Fire Precautions'. HTM83. London: HMSO.
DHSS (1988) 'Fire Precautions in Existing Hospitals'. HTM85. London: HMSO.
DHSS (1987) 'Fire Risk assessment in hospitals' HTM86. London: HMSO.

DHSS (1988) 'Textiles and Furniture'. HTM87. London: HMSO.

DoH (1997) *Firecode: guide for fire precautions in hospitals*. London: Department of Health.

GMB (1996) 'Fire Legislation: Home Office rekindles controversial fire safety laws - more than three years late'. *Health and Safety Bulletin* no. 247 (July), p. 4.

GMB (1997) 'Fire Legislation: New workplace fire Regulations in place'. *Health and Safety Bulletin*, no. 262 (October), p. 2.

Home Office (1997) *Fire Safety Legislation for the Future. A Consultation Document*. Home Office ISBN 1 84082 006 3

HSE (1976) *Fire Certificates (Special Premises)Regulations, Health and Safety Executive*.

HSE (1991) *Assessment of fire hazards from solid materials and the precautions*. Sudbury: Health and Safety Executive.

HSE (1997) *Fire Precautions (Workplace) Regulations 1997* (replaces 55 pieces of legislation, and said to be the minimum necessary to conform to EU requirements). Sudbury: Health and Safety Executive.

RCN (1994) *Safety Representatives' Manual*. London: Royal College of Nursing.

Rosenthal, T. and Rosenthal, S. (1988) 'Foresight – secret of survival'. *Nursing Management*, vol. 19, no. 5 (May), p. 80.

Unison (1997) *New Fire Regulations*, Health and Safety Notice, December, HS/41/97. London: Unison.

Urquhart, S. (1982) 'Kirkcaldy nurses' home fire: countdown to tragedy'. *Nursing Mirror*, vol. 154, no. 24 (16 June), pp. 14–15.

Security

Security is an essential aspect of a healthy and safe working environment, whether staff live on or off health care premises. Staff are at risk not only from theft, which is rife, but also from violent assault. Nurses are a consistent target for sexual attacks, and a number of attempted or actual rapes have occurred in nurses' homes, or in hospital and health centre environs such as car parks. Violence is so widespread that in this book we have devoted a whole chapter to it, together with bullying.

Security matters in NHS trusts are regulated by the DoH and the NHS Confederation, whose previous incarnation, the National Association of Health Authorities and Trusts, produced an advisory resource, the *NHS Security Manual*. Security also falls under the Management of Health and Safety at Work Regulations 1992. As with so many issues, the problems of security are exacerbated by inadequate resources, staff shortages and lack of proper staff training.

Every health provider should have security staff who ensure that premises are safe and security measures are followed. Public areas such as accident and emergency units and clinics are especially vulnerable and usually require police supervision too, though high-profile 'baby snatching' incidents from maternity wards, shootings and stabbings of inpatients and visitors demonstrate the need for effective, well resourced security policies. The use of closed circuit TV in entrances and corridors has become more widespread, though as with all security measures a balance needs to be maintained between freedom of movement and protection of staff and the public. Hospitals are public places, and staff residences are home to their occupants, so the solution should not be sought in locking doors after dark and restricting or banning visitors from public areas or bedrooms, but rather in having trained security staff who are readily available when needed, with alarm buttons in all areas. Nurses whose roles are geographically mobile or community based may be justified in demanding that pagers and mobile phones are provided by their employers, and certainly safe systems of work and monitoring policies should be in place.

Training in security is available to help managers identify security problems and their solutions. If you have particular worries at your workplace, raise questions at health and safety meetings and ask for the security officer to be present – often this helpful source of expertise is overlooked. Other specialist groups such as the Suzy Lamplugh Trust (see below) can provide useful information and advice.

References, further reading, contact organisations and resources on security

Bibby, P. (1995) *Personal Safety for Health Care Workers*. Aldershot: Arena (commissioned by the Suzy Lamplugh Trust).

Elson, L. (1997) 'Hospital Watch', *Nursing Standard*, vol. 11, no. 26 (19 March), pp. 26–7

HSE (1987) *Violence to Staff in the Health Service*. Sudbury: Health and Safety Executive.

NAHAT (1993) *NHS Security Manual*; with audio and video tapes. Birmingham: National Association of Health Authorities and Trusts.

TUC (1997) *Hazards at Work: TUC Guide to Health and Safety*. London: Trades Union Congress.

The National Association of Healthcare Security is an advisory group set up by the NHS Executive, comprising security managers from hospitals and trusts. Its aim is the improvement of security through exchange of information and experience. NAHS, c/o NHS Executive, Quarry House, Quarry Hill, Leeds LS2 7HE. TEl.: 0113 254 5000.

The Suzy Lamplugh Trust was set up by Diana Lamplugh, mother of the estate agent whose disappearance was never explained, to campaign for better security for vulnerable staff at work. 14 East Sheen Avenue, London SW14 8AS. Tel.: 0181 392 1839.

Staff facilities

The quality of the facilities provided for staff is an important factor in determining whether they feel like valued members of the organisation or simply pairs of hands. This is particularly true of a job such as nursing, which makes heavy emotional and physical demands; so it is all the more important that nurses should have the use of comfortable and pleasant changing rooms, restaurants, cloakrooms and common rooms when they are preparing for or having a break from work. Regrettably the facilities provided are often substandard, grim or non-existent. It is all too common for a nurse to change into uniform in a cold locker room, queue up for half her short lunch break to buy a plate of unwholesome institutional food, and spend the rest period during the night shift in the ward sister's office, surrounded by filing cabinets and locked cupboards. Penny pinching and a disregard for the everyday experience of people working in demanding health care environments have meant that providing good facilities has not been seen as a priority, let alone the right of every employee.

As with so many aspects of health, safety and welfare at work, many of these needs are covered by explicit regulations or guidelines; the problem is converting them into action. Knowledge of the official minimum will at least give you a base from which to start, and to ensure that the best possible facilities are provided in any upgrading or new building. Nurses working in offices and employed outside the NHS, such as in industry and higher education, should ensure that their employers take account of their particular health needs too. The Health Education Authority initiative Health at Work in the NHS, launched in 1992 to contribute to the government's Health of the Nation policy, focused both on the personal health of staff and on the promotion of healthy workplaces. This, and campaigns such as the 1995 *Nursing Times* Work Well Campaign (see Box 3.1) are examples of recent actions aimed at improving staff facilities and environments. The standards they set should not simply be aspirations but the norm.

Changing rooms

The nurse who has to wear a uniform, but lives outside the hospital or clinic and is not permitted (or not supposed) to wear it off the premises, may spend a couple of hours a week in the changing room. Minimum standards may be inferred from the Factories Act, and are set out in the Workplace (Health, Safety and Welfare) Regulations 1992, which became effective for new workplaces from January 1993 and for all workplaces from January 1996. For example the regulations specify that employers must provide 'suitable and sufficient' accommodation – convenient to workplaces – for workers' own clothing not worn during working hours and for 'special clothing worn at work but not taken home'. These should be in the changing rooms, not a separate room.

Accommodation should be clean, warm, dry and well-ventilated, and 'so far as is reasonably practicable' include clothes drying facilities and suitable rest facilities for pregnant women or new mothers. You might consider whether your changing room is near your place of work, with a shower, private changing cubicle, secure personal locker, entrance area for wet outdoor clothes and plenty of space for each person. If the answer to any of these is no, you could have a case for pressing for upgrading. You should

---

Box 3.1 *Work Well – creating a friendly environment for nurse and patient*

Nursing Times' six-month Work Well campaign in 1995 set out 'a range of achievable changes you can make to the environment in which you work, from the colour of the paint on the walls in your ward or community unit . . . to the way your shifts are organised and the effects this has on your care'. The magazine 'adopted' Patience Two Ward at Nottingham City Hospital, not because it had a particularly poor environment, 'but because it is typical of the many units that nurses work in throughout the UK. It is a large hospital made up of modern and Victorian buildings. . .. Old, dilapidated equipment, furnishings and fittings that have constantly been repaired rather than replaced, and a building layout that is hard on nurses' legs and patients' patience all help create a working environment which could be demoralising and detrimental to the physical and mental well-being of staff and patients alike'.

Six months before the current staff moved in, Patience Two was used as a substitute for wards awaiting their new location. Consequently those passing through had not been too concerned about what it looked like or how they should look after it:

> 'We had high hopes when we moved up here, but what we've done is move from a dump to a tip' (Annette Robinson, ward manager).

> 'A lick of paint wouldn't go amiss in some places, but even that gets political when you compare it to bed losses' (Vicky Hughes, staff nurse) (Reid, 1995).

---

inform your safety rep of your concerns, and discover if she/he and your managers are aware of the deficiencies.

Toilets and washrooms should have clean, running hot and cold or warm water, soap and clean towels or hot air driers, accessible and adequate fixtures such as mirrors and shelves, and should be easy to get to. By law there should be at least one toilet for every five employees of each sex, two for between six and 25, and an extra one for each additional 25, up to 100. These detailed guidelines are worth looking at as a benchmark (see the References section at the end of this section).

Ward or clinic cloakrooms

The HSE and DoH say there should be a small cloakroom near the clinical area with a toilet and washbasin, hanging spaces for coats and cloaks and small personal lockers for each member of staff to secure their valuables while on duty. Yet the lack of such facilities in many places leads to nurses sneaking off to use the patients' toilets, while the arrangements for hiding handbags and purses are as varied as they are ingenious. Theft is endemic in the NHS, as in most large organisations, but there is often a failure to provide staff with secure facilities to avoid tempting the thief – this is especially the case for students, agency nurses and others on temporary placements.

Common rooms

Too many workplaces lack a comfortable and accessible room in which to relax during breaks. Too often nurses have to grab a quick cup of coffee in someone else's office or spend the night break in the patients' dayroom, or in the ward itself, because there is nowhere else to go. As a result they are often interrupted by other health staff, patients and visitors, which does not allow them to return from their break feeling refreshed and rested.

Staff restaurants

Mealtimes are often little more than a scrum in the attempt to remove apron, find bag, reach the canteen, queue up for dinner, eat it and rush back to the ward within 30 minutes – not conducive to calm or good digestion. Good digestion is also hampered by the type of food usually available – stew and chips or a soggy salad being a common option, although many trusts have

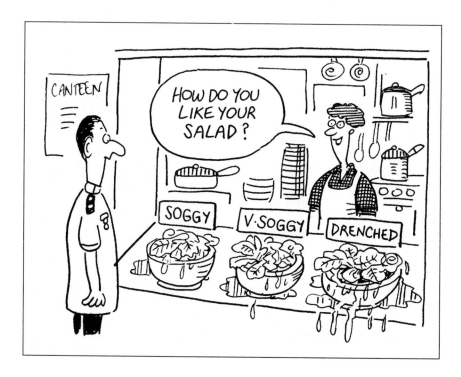

made efforts to introduce better catering. Some employers realise that health promotion begins at home and provide carefully balanced, nutritious and attractive food, but they are still in the minority. Budgetary constraints in trusts and the contracting-out of catering have led to a reduction in some out-of-hours meal services, with evening and night staff able to choose only from inadequately restocked vending machines. There is no excuse for failing to provide comprehensive meal facilities for staff at all times. It remains a disciplinary offence to eat from patients' meal trolleys, though without good staff facilities the temptation to do so is great.

References, further reading, contact organisations and resources on facilities

CIBSE (1986) *CIBSE Guide*. The Institute produces a number of useful guides connected with work environments. London: Chartered Institute of Building Service Engineers.

HSC (1992) *The Workplace (Health, Safety and Welfare) Regulations*. Sudbury: Health and Safety Commission.

HSE (1992) *Workplace health, safety and welfare*, Workplace (Health, Safety and Welfare) Regulations ACoP and guidance, L24. Sudbury: Health and Safety Commision.

LRD (1995) *Office health and safety*. Labour Research Department (booklet). London.

Reid, T. (1995) 'Improving work conditions', *Nursing Times*, vol. 91 no. 24 (14 June), pp. 26–30.

TUC (1997) *Hazards at Work. TUC Guide to Health and Safety*. London: Trades Union Congress. See Chapter 5, 'The working environment and welfare', pp. 55–78.

Unison (1992) *The Workplace Health, Safety and Welfare Regulations 1992*. Unison guide ref no. 0919. London: Unison.

Lighting

Light is such a familiar feature of our environment that we rarely stop to consider whether it is adequate for our needs. Yet the quality of lighting in the workplace is a key factor, and like many other potential hazards it is amenable to many measures for improvement. Good illumination is indispensable to good nursing and to the safety of both nurses and patients, in all areas of the hospital or clinic. Whether you are writing reports, reading drug charts, doing a procedure or helping someone to the toilet at night, you need to be able to see what you are doing.

Poor lighting leads not only to mistakes and lower efficiency but also to poor health. As well as falls and other injuries, working in the gloom or glare (poor lighting may also be too bright!) has been reported as the cause of headaches, eye strain and other health problems. Many workplaces today are entirely lit by fluorescent light, which is increasingly popular with employers because it is cheaper, but there is disturbing evidence of associated ill-health. Unlike standard electric lighting, the spectral emission from fluorescent light extends into the ultraviolet end of the spectrum, and has been implicated in photosensitivity leading to a kind of allergy, and skin trauma similar to sunburn.

Modern building design sometimes favours environments with little or no natural light, while old buildings are often dark and obscured from daylight by other buildings nearby. In general a mixture of artificial and natural light is best for workers and clients; natural light is more soothing and everyone likes to be able to see out of a window. Special attention must be paid to lighting in health care premises at night – while the patients need restful sleep, in an unfamiliar place they also need careful lighting if they have to get up, which must also comply with fire and safety legislation. Night nurses need good bedside lighting and clear light at their desk or station: recent research suggest that short exposure to appropriate bright light in their breaks may reduce the disruption to their circadian rhythms (Costa *et al.*, 1995). Well-lit corridors and exterior lighting in hospital or clinic grounds are important for security.

Solving the problems

The Factory Inspectorate has pinpointed cost-cutting as 'a disquieting cause of unsatisfactory lighting', and this is clearly relevant to health care settings. The Factories Act emphasises that lighting should be 'sufficient and suitable', whether natural or artificial, and employers should not try to make savings at the expense of nurses' and patients' wellbeing. Statutory rules and the recommendations produced by the Lighting Division of the Chartered Institution of Building Service Engineers and others can provide a baseline for pressure on managers to improve lighting.

If management is unwilling to act, it is useful to obtain a lighting survey. This may be carried out by the health and safety inspector; the local electricity company or the CIBSE Lighting Division may also offer advice. If all else fails you can use a camera light meter as a rough guide. The results may give you some useful facts to support comments and complaints from staff.

Many lighting problems can be solved by good design and better equipment, which today may actually save money because it is produced with due regard for energy conservation. The choice of colour for walls, ceilings and paintwork also has an effect. For the night nurse's desk it is possible to obtain a lamp which sheds a good light without disturbing nearby patients, and good 'watch lighting' is available for bedside care. Where the lighting is too bright, such as in a theatre where white walls enhance the glare, special shades can help. Photoelectric switches, sensitive to light, can achieve the right balance between natural and artificial light. Nurses who have any input into renovations or designs for new buildings – and safety representatives, who have the right to be involved – should raise these points.

Finally, as protection in case other measures fail but not as a substitute for them, nurses should ensure that they care for themselves. Recommendations include:

- Resting your eyes in natural light after being in artificial light for a long period, so go outside during your break if possible.
- Resting your eye muscles after close work on reports, assignments and so on, by looking out of the window or into the distance at least every quarter of an hour.

Action to prevent eyestrain is vital for people who work with computers. These are now an almost universal piece of ward or surgery equipment, and the risks they carry have been widely publicised. The TUC guidelines on work with VDUs suggest that after each hour of work there should be a 15-minute break, following continued evidence that many workers experience eyestrain and related problems. Recent research by Eichenbaum (1996) notes that 10–15 per cent of people presenting for routine eye examinations complain of computer-related headaches and eye strain.

The nurse is unlikely to sit in front of a VDU for hours unless she is using a computer for research, writing or data processing. She should be aware of the possible hazards of the use of computers, however. Apart from eye trouble, higher rates of miscarriage, stillbirth and fetal malformation possibly attributable to low-level radiation from VDUs have been discussed. The latest information from the Health and Safety Executive implies that these fears are groundless, but it is best to err on the side of safety, especially by having frequent short breaks from VDU work. Under the Health and Safety (Display Screen Equipment) Regulations 1992, employers must analyse work stations, assess and reduce risks, and ensure that the minimum recommended requirements are met, together with adequate health and safety training. Employees covered by the regulations can ask their employer to provide and pay for eye and sight tests.

References, further reading, contact organisations and resources on lighting

CIBSE (1994) *Code for Interior Lighting.* London: Chartered Institute of Building Service Engineers.

Costa, G., Gaffuri, E., Ghirlanda, G., Minors, D.S., Waterhouse, J.M. (1995) 'Psychophysical conditions and hormonal secretion in nurses on a rapidly rotating shift schedule and exposed to bright light during night work', Work and Stress, vol. 9, no. 2/3 (April–September), pp. 148–157

Craig, M. (1981) *The Office Workers' Survival Handbook.* London: British Society for Social Responsibility in Science.

Eichenbaum, J. W. (1996) 'Computers and eyestrain', *Journal of Ophthalmic Nursing & Technology*, vol. 15 no. 1 (January), pp. 23–6.

HSE (1987) *Lighting at Work*, HS(G)38. Sudbury: Health and Safety Executive.

HSE (1996) *Working with VDUs*, IND(G)36(L) C 1750. Sudbury: Health and Safety Executive.

LRD (1991) *VDUs and Health and Safety*. London: Labour Research Department.

Polglase, J. (1995) 'Seeing the emergency exit in its proper light', *Occupational Safety and Health*, vol. 64, no. 3 (March), pp. 82–5.

TUC (1997) *Hazards at Work: TUC Guide to Health and Safety*. London: Trades Union Congress. See Chapter 5, pp. 61–5; also Chapter 25, 'Display screen equipment', pp. 235–40. This guide is thorough in going through standards of light measurement and how to survey your workplace lighting provision.

Unison (1994) *The Workplace Health, Safety and Welfare Regulations*, Unison guide ref. no. 0919. London: Unison.

Unison (1994) *Display Screen Equipment Regulations*, Unison guide ref. no. 0920. London: Unison.

The Lighting Industry Federation, Swan House, 207 Balham High Street, London SW17 7BQ.

Temperature and ventilation

Working in a hot and stuffy atmosphere is not only unpleasant, it can also be bad for your health. The nurse faces particular problems because her needs may conflict with those of the patient; most hospitals tend to be very warm for the patients' benefit (although the temperature can plummet at night) but the nurse may find such heat oppressive. The law says the temperature should be at least 16 degrees Celsius for most types of work, or at least 13 degrees Celsius for work involving 'severe physical effort'. A thermometer need not be visible in every room, but should be available for checking if the temperature feels uncomfortable (Workplace etc. Regulations 1992, section 7, and Section 2 of the Management of the Health and Safety Regulations 1992). Studies suggest a preferred level of around 18 degrees for hospital wards and 20 degrees for offices, canteens and dining rooms.

In hot weather female nurses often don't wear tights or stockings, but this is likely to require official approval. Once again there is little in the way of statutory guidance, though the Approved Code of Practice for the Workplace Regulations suggests that other factors be considered, such as the insulation of hot pipes, provision of an air cooling plant, shading of windows, siting of workstations away from hot areas, and the provision and use of fans and increased ventilation in hot weather. Good design and windows which can actually be opened are important. In cold weather nurses may similarly encounter official rigidity, for example being forbidden to wear cardigans on duty.

How warm you feel depends not only on the temperature itself, but on the type of work you are doing, on the humidity and on the air flow, through ventilation or draughts. The ventilation of public buildings is often controlled alongside temperature. Growing awareness of conditions such as humidifier fever and Legionnaires' disease spread via air-conditioning has alerted people to the safety issues, although action usually comes after the event. There are two main types of ventilation relevant to health care premises: general and exhaust. General ventilation should be a total air-cleaning system designed to distribute fresh air throughout the building at a comfortable temperature and humidity, while exhaust ventilation is designed to remove hazardous fumes and the like.

The health hazards of poor systems may be hard to pin down, but they have been documented in a number of workplaces. Where the air is too dry and the air conditioning is not humidified, the lack of moisture dries up mucous membranes, leading to sore throats and respiratory problems. The TUC suggests that the level of humidity indoors should be between 40 per cent and 75 per cent, but warns against the potential health hazards of humidified air. Humidifier fever often appears to be a feverish cold or virus infection, but is actually an unpleasant disease resembling farmer's lung, which is caused by amoebae breeding in the water reservoirs of air-conditioning systems. The ducts become contaminated and the spores spread, finally being sprayed out into the atmosphere. If there is an unusually high incidence of this type of illness, it may be worth having the system checked and overhauled; it is also important that some windows can be opened, though in modern buildings they are often sealed. Safety reps should be involved in the assessment of designs for new or replacement systems. Regulation 6 of the Workplace etc. Regulations 1992 states that in enclosed workplaces, employers must provide 'effective and suitable' ventilation to supply a 'sufficient quantity' of fresh or purified air.

There is a trend towards using ioniser air-conditioning systems which may emit ozone to make the air fresher. However even small amounts of ozone can irritate the mucous membranes, while cheap systems have been found to give out hazardous levels of the gas; if you are worried you should ascertain what kind of system is being used. Expert advice is available from the British Institute of Heating and Ventilation Engineers and the Chartered Institute of Building Services Engineers.

References and resources on temperature

HSC (1992) *The Workplace (Health, Safety and Welfare) Regulations 1992*. Sudbury: Health and Safety Commission.

HSC (1992) *The Workplace (Health, Safety and Welfare) Regulations 1992*, Approved Code of Practice (ACoP) L24. Sudbury: Health and Safety Commission.

HSE (1992) *Ventilation of the Workplace*, EH22. Sudbury: Health and Safety Executive.

TUC (1997) *Hazards at Work: TUC Guide to Health and Safety*. London: Trades Union Congress. See Chapter 5, pp. 56–61.

Unison (1994) *The Workplace (Health, Safety and Welfare) Regulations 1992*, Unison guide no. 0919. London: Unison.

Williams, N. (1993) 'Working in a hot environment', *Occupational Health*, vol. 45, no. 8 (August), pp. 275–7.

Noise

Noise – defined by the Concise Oxford Dictionary simply as 'loud or undesired sound' – can cause stress, fatigue, loss of concentration, hypertension and insomnia when it is prolonged or excessive in the workplace. Although the nurse is not exposed to the continual din of heavy machinery or the industrial processes which cause occupational deafness, noise at work can nevertheless be an irritant, disrupting not only the patients' peace but also the nurse's ability to do her work calmly and carefully.

There are clear regulations on noise in the workplace, deriving from Section 6 of the Health and Safety at Work Act, and more specifically from the Noise at Work Regulations 1989 and the associated Code of Practice. The code of practice produced by the HSE gives mandatory limits (known now as Action Levels or ALs) above which employees should not be exposed. The first AL for continuous noise is 85 decibels (dB), which is roughly equivalent to the sound of a heavy lorry passing at seven metres and is rarely relevant to health care premises. The regulations place the second AL, the limit above which ear protection is compulsory, at 90dB, so recognition of the problem is precise.

The employer has a duty to ensure the health, safety and welfare of all employees and therefore to make the workplace as pleasant as possible, and the HSE suggests an action plan for employers in assessing noise. Employees are obliged to use ear protection in 'ear protection zones', use any equipment supplied by the employer under the regulations and report any defects. Manufacturers must supply data from noise tests.

Temporary noise such as building work is difficult to control, but it may be possible to confine the worst effects to particular times of day when the ward or department is noisy anyway – avoiding patients' rest periods or visiting time, for example – or to times when the place is empty if it is not an in-patient area. Ask your manager, steward or safety rep to intervene.

Permanent noise may require more persistent action since its reduction may entail expense. If the noise is very loud, management, or failing that the unions, may commission a noise survey from external consultants who can advise on preventive measures. Some of the steps taken in industry may be appropriate: routine maintenance of machinery or equipment which is excessively noisy because of worn-out parts or lack of lubrication; resiting of noisy machinery to somewhere less obtrusive; installing insulation and soundproofing; and checking the noise levels of different makes of equipment before purchase.

Traffic is often a problem, especially in summer when the windows are open. Double glazing and insulation may help, as well as notices in the street reminding passers-by to be quiet. In extreme cases it may be possible to secure the rerouting of traffic to avoid in-patient buildings, or to redesign the ward layout. This may also be relevant when the ward is close to the kitchens or other sources of frequent noise. While noise is obviously not the only factor involved in choosing the best design, it should be taken into account.

Some practical measures are simply common sense. Quiet footwear, separate rooms for very ill confused patients, and just being aware of the need to talk and move quietly at particular times can all help, as can carpeting to absorb sound. The loud, intrusive telephone which is always ringing – all too familiar in a busy ward – may be quietened down to a gentler tone, or even better, a ward receptionist employed to answer it. Radios and televisions may be annoying to staff and patients alike, so headphones should be used. Patients' call buzzers should be audible without being intrusive. Mobile telephones should be turned off in clinical areas: not only are they intrusive, but they may interfere with clinical equipment such as electronic pumps and monitoring devices. All these measures can help create an atmosphere which helps the nurse's peace of mind as well as the patient's.

References, further reading, contact organisations and resources on noise

Dias, B. (1992) 'Things that go bump. . .', *Nursing Times,* vol. 88, no. 38 (16 September), pp. 36–8.

HMSO (1989) *The Noise at Work Regulations 1989.* London: HMSO.

HSE (1995) *Noise at Work: a guide for employees.* IND(G)99(L)Rev. Sudbury: Health and Safety Executive.

HSE (1995) *Introducing the Noise at Work Regulations,* IND(G)75(L). Sudbury: Health and Safety Executive.

Payling, K. J. (1994) 'A hazard we can no longer ignore: effects of excessive noise on well being'. *Professional Nurse,* vol. 9, no. 6 (March), pp. 420–1.

TUC (1997) *Hazards at Work: TUC Guide to health and safety.* London: Trades Union Congress. See Chapter 12, 'Noise', pp. 131–138.

Association of Noise Consultants, 6 Trap Road, Guilden Morden, near Royston, Hertfordshire SG8 0JE. Tel.: 01763 852 958.

Institute of Acoustics, PO Box 320, St Albans, Hertfordshire AL1 1PZ. Tel.: 01727 848 195.

Royal National Institute for Deaf People, London area: tel. 0171 916 4144; Manchester: tel. 0161 242 2316; Glasgow: tel. 0141 332 0343.

Tinnitus Helpline, tel: 0345 090210.

Conclusion

Nurses often seem to have very little control over their environment, whether in the hospital ward, accident and emergency unit, out-patient clinic, health centre, classroom, office or even car. Yet when the environmental hazards discussed here arise, from the mildly irritating to the life-threatening, they can affect the health and well-being of all. All the more reason, then, for nurses to insist on the establishment, monitoring and review of standards and rationales for environments of practice and care. These standards can generally be based on existing laws and approved codes of practice, which means they should be reviewed and updated according to any changes.

4   Stress

Stress is a common topic today – the subject of innumerable magazine articles and television programmes – but how often is the prevention of unnecessary stress seen as the legitimate concern of a safety representative, or indeed as the responsibility of a health services manager?

'Health and safety at work' is a phrase which immediately makes us think of physical hazards such as slippery floors, sharps or cytotoxic drugs rather than the less tangible but potentially equally harmful risks of working in a job which is demanding emotionally. Moreover the occasionally inevitable stresses of such work are exacerbated by poor conditions, domestic commitments, shift work and many other factors.

Stress is in fact a major occupational hazard, and is responsible for more time off work than accidents – an estimated 37 million working days a year. The bodily changes which occur in response to stressful conditions can cause all sorts of problems if the conditions have to be endured continuously, rather than in a brief episode, when the changes are essential to effective functioning. The problems caused are not only the obvious ones such as headaches or depression; heart disease, asthma, diabetes, dermatitis, peptic ulcers and many other 'physical' illnesses have been linked with stress.

There is now a large amount of research and a large body of knowledge on work and stress. Most of the literature, in nursing and other fields, places the emphasis on telling people how to cope, after giving a description of the physiological mechanisms involved. What the experts often fail to do is to challenge the idea that stress is a fact of life – accepting the status quo rather than separating out the inevitable, even desirable stressors from those which should be eliminated. In fact many stressors in our working lives could be prevented. Many are the direct result of the failure of employers to regard the health and welfare of their staff as a top priority, as illustrated in major surveys of nurses' morale (for example Seccombe and Smith, 1997; Gulland, 1997).

Nursing has been characterised as stressful, the stress attributable both to the hazards of nursing and to associated psychosocial factors. In 1984 Morton-Cooper described the working environment of nurses as 'optimum for manufacturing stress . . . an enclosed atmosphere, time pressure, excessive noise or undue quiet, sudden swings from intense to mundane tasks, no second chance, unpleasant sights and sounds, and standing for long hours' (quoted in Borrill et al., 1996).

These stressors can lead to mental health problems. Over a quarter of NHS trust staff are reported as having probable mental health problems –

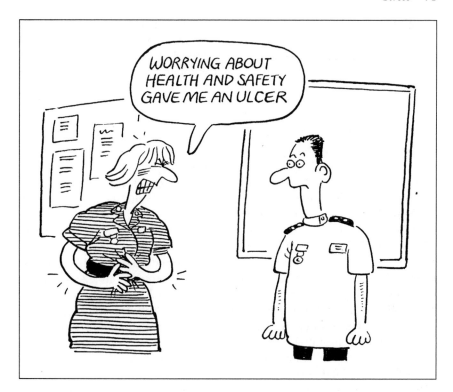

this is especially marked in senior nurses and staff nurses; extra unpaid hours and higher levels of patient need are associated with poorer mental health; staff mental health is better in trusts with greater cooperation, communication and performance monitoring; and those who use staff counselling have notable improvements in mental health (Borrill, 1996).

The irony has often been noted that health services employers, despite their commitment to improving people's health, are no better at protecting their staff than many others. When NHS resources are inadequate, staff are expected to make sacrifices such as working even harder or forgoing large pay rises so that patients do not suffer. Nurses in particular, with their professional ethic of dedication and service before self, are so used to papering over the cracks at immense personal cost that many of them still feel guilty at the notion of fighting for themselves; and so the vicious circle of exploitation continues.

The fact that stress is at least on the agenda, though, is a healthy sign that nurses are being more open about the problems they experience. We are starting to acknowledge that there is no dishonour in airing our difficulties and turning to each other for support. When such discussion is permitted and encouraged, before long people start to investigate the causes of stress and ask whether they are preventable, and then begin to see that stress need not always be a fact of life. Working closely with people who are suffering will always be central to nursing and will always be distressing at times, but an enormous amount can be done to ensure that the nurse is supported, and to remove many of the stressors which oppress her today. Learning how to manage stress is important but it is not enough; tackling its causes is also crucial.

How stress is defined

The enormous volume of literature on stress explores all sorts of dimensions, ranging from physical measurement of the body's chemical changes through to social psychology and psychiatry. Mostly we use the word 'stress' to describe an unpleasant feeling of too much pressure and a subsequent inability to cope, although the experts are careful to distinguish between 'stress' – the response of the body to any demand made on it – and 'distress' – the associated harmful effects when stress is in excess of the optimum. They also point out that prolonged lack of stimulation can be stressful to some people; boredom can also be bad for you. Figure 4.1 summarises the distinctions between stress, stimulation and rest. Bond (1986) gives a useful working definition of stress: 'the experience of unpleasant over- or under-stimulation, as defined by the individual in question, that actually or potentially leads to ill health'.

Physiologically we respond to potential stress with chemical changes which prepare our bodies for the ensuing 'fight or flight', but damage results if the changes happen continuously rather than in one short incident, and if the 'fight or flight' for which we are prepared never actually happens. The

Figure 4.1 *Distinguishing between stress, stimulation and rest* (reproduced with permission from Bond, M. *Stress and Self-Awareness: A Guide for Nurses*. London: Heinemann Nursing, 1986.)

	↓ **A lot of pressure**	↓ **Little or no pressure**
	STIMULATION	**REST**
Pleasant ⟶	interested excited	peaceful calm
	OVERSTIMULATION	**UNDERSTIMULATION**
Unpleasant = stress ⟶	anxious irritable	bored frustrated

whole process is a complex set of interlocking psychological and physiological phenomena which is not fully understood by scientists. What concerns us here, though, is not so much the psychophysiology as what stress means to nurses day to day.

We all know what the feeling is, and we can all recognise that some degree of stress is necessary or even enjoyable in some situations; in emergencies, for example, our performance is improved by the sharpness of the physiological and mental response generated by the body's internal mechanisms. Stress can be positive in its effects, and this so-called 'eustress' can be an exciting, life-enhancing force. But when we talk of stress in nursing we aren't thinking of those feelings, but of the wearing, debilitating experience of unrelieved pressure through overstimulation, or of the grinding dullness of understimulation, or a rapid seesaw between the two (Figure 4.2).

In some respects the term 'stress' is so wide-ranging as to be almost meaningless, and this contributes to the difficulty encountered when trying to pin down its causes. Absenteeism in nursing, wastage, sickness rates and increased drug, alcohol and tobacco abuse have all been named as responses to stress, but linking cause and effect directly is a problem in view of the multiple factors and individuals involved – although there is a commonly accepted perception of stress as one important facet of all those trends. Much of the evidence about the extent of stress in nursing is in any case difficult to measure and much of it is qualitative; there is no shortage of it, and it can be found in any nursing magazine or everyday canteen conversation.

Figure 4.2 *Adaptation of the human function curve* (reproduced with permission from Bond, M. *Stress and Self-Awareness: A Guide for Nurses.* London: Heinemann Nursing, 1986.)

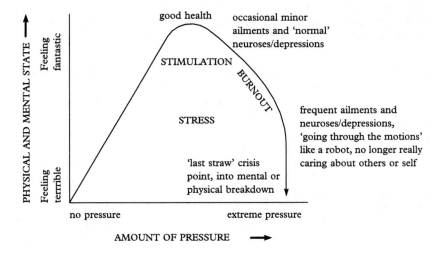

One junior sister's experience on an acute medical/elderly unit is typical:

> We don't talk about things that bother us on this ward. The main
> concerns are shortages of staff, a shortage of resources and so on. We all
> carry it around but we don't share it. I feel fairly dysfunctional as a
> person, as a nurse and as a manager. . . . I go home and get angry, but
> then the waterworks start and I feel sad. And I feel guilty that I'm no
> longer doing a job I was good at (Kennedy and Grey, 1997).

The fact that such heartfelt outbursts are common demonstrates the widespread existence of stress in nursing. There should be great cause for concern
about an occupation where the drop-out rate in training reaches 40 per cent
in some places; where many qualified practitioners leave and never return;
and where more people every year appear before professional conduct
committees for incidents arising from drug or alcohol abuse. The anecdotal
evidence is too strong for us ignore the misery being suffered by people who
are themselves expected to help others.

An examination of the factors which are at least in part responsible for
putting pressure on nurses may help us to highlight and tackle the
preventable causes of distress. In many ways, stress exemplifies the most
serious problems of nursing today, and lessons should be learned from it.

One way of classifying the wide range of issues implicated in nurses' stress is
to consider separately those which are broadly social questions affecting
people in all kinds of jobs, such as racism or lack of child care; those which
are primarily the employer's responsibility, such as pay and working conditions; and, finally, those which are closely concerned with nursing itself, both
the nature of the work and the culture and values of the profession.

References on the extent of stress in nursing

Borrill, C., Wall, T., West, M. *et al.* (1996) *Mental Health of the NHS Workforce.*
    Institute of Work Psychology, University of Sheffield, and Department of
    Psychology, University of Leeds.
Gulland, A. (1997) 'Stress and low pay cited as NT poll reveals poor nurse
    morale', *Nursing Times*, vol. 93, no. 5 (29 January), p.6.
Kennedy, P. and Grey, N. (1997) 'High pressure areas', *Nursing Times*, vol. 93,
    no. 29 (16 July), pp. 26–30.
Seccombe, I. and Smith, G. (1997) *Taking Part: registered nurses and the labour
    market in 1997*, Studies report 338. London: Royal College of Nursing/
    Institute for Employment.

Societal stressors

Many of the causes of stress in nursing are not, of course, specific to the job,
but are common in society as a whole. Although the culture of nursing still

encourages a defensive refusal to admit to feeling stress, nurses are no more immune than anyone else. They too can become mentally or physically ill, or try to cope with stress by turning to alcohol or drugs. Nine out of ten nurses are female, and the particular stresses experienced by all working women are an important factor in the life of the average nurse. Despite improvements in the position of women, and acknowledgement of the need for equality shown in measures such as the Equal Pay Act and the Sex Discrimination Act, most women shoulder the lion's share of day-to-day domestic responsibility on top of their employment. The dual role of having one paid and one unpaid job often results in physical and mental strain. Working part time or taking a break from work to care for young children (41 per cent of NHS nurses, according to Seccombe and Smith, 1996) or dependent relatives (16 per cent) can adversely affect career prospects, job satisfaction and conditions of work.

Domestic labour

Most women still take it for granted that it is their role to run the household and ensure that partners and families are fed, clothed and cared for. Shopping in lunch breaks and doing housework or cooking a meal after a tiring shift are such common features of women's lives that it is often regarded as a 'natural' division of labour. How many women can assume that their male partners will think about buying a loaf of bread, let alone preparing the supper when they come from work? Underlying this inequality there is an assumption that women's work is less important or arduous than men's, and that it's only done for pocket money anyway. Yet more and more women who are wives, partners and mothers are choosing to work outside the home and many are forced to for financial reasons, especially those with partners who are unemployed, or those who are lone mothers (12 per cent of all families).

Child care

It is still assumed that the care of children, like housework, is primarily the woman's responsibility, even when both partners work full time. It is usually the woman who gives up her job when the children are small, returns to work part time and has to take time off when a child is ill or needs to go to the dentist. And the NHS, like most other employers, in effect punishes women by regarding children as their problem. Instead of having shifts, facilities, holidays and attitudes tailored to the family's needs, the woman is made to feel like a square peg in a round hole as she juggles with these often conflicting demands.

The UK's notorious lack of child care provision is simply the most glaring example of our society's failure to regard children as a collective responsibility rather than an individual problem. Only 55 per cent of parents place their children in day nurseries, although surveys show an overwhelming demand for them (Waters, 1997). The NHS depends heavily on female labour, yet a recent study has reported that only 33 per cent of nurses have access to workplace nursery or creche facilities, and only 5 per cent are able to use them (Seccombe and Smith, 1996). Some of these function only during office hours, which is no use for nurses working unsocial shifts.

The Labour government's commitment to family-friendly social policies provides support for such initiatives as the Swedish approach – Timecare, piloted in 11 trusts in 1997 – where staff choose their working hours to fit their family commitments. This brings a greater element of choice (Millar, 1997). However the cost of child care is often too high: research by the Day Care Trust shows that UK parents must pay 90 per cent of the costs themselves, which for a nurse with two children and a salary of £15 000 could amount to 40 per cent of her income (Waters, 1997). And employers appear ready to open child care facilities in times of staff shortage, only to abandon them when unemployment rises.

Caring for dependants

Millions of women and a lesser number of men perform the role of unpaid carer for sick or disabled relatives or neighbours. Like child care, this is often undertaken on top of their jobs and household work; time off from the ward or clinic is rarely time for relaxation and recharging the batteries, and the pleasures of spending time with an elderly parent or disabled child are lost in the rush to get everything done. This hidden welfare state, though, is barely acknowledged by employers and little is done to support the carer financially, emotionally or socially.

Three quarters of all nurses marry and have a break in their professional career, usually when they have children. The issues raised here are therefore of major relevance both to the individual nurse and to her employing authority – but almost no attention is paid to them. The repeated demands of the TUC and health service unions have made little headway in the NHS. Of course the problems are complex, especially at a time of scarce resources, but continuing to ignore them is prolonging a major cause of stress on nurses.

Sexual harassment

Sexual harassment is not trivial – it's primarily an exercise of power and position to bully members of the opposite sex (usually, though not exclusively, men harassing women). Nearly all women have at some time experienced sexual harassment, ranging from wolf-whistles from a building site or bottom-pinching by a male doctor to persistent sexual advances or rape. The subject is often treated as a joke, but most women find it distressing and offensive. There isn't much research, but what there is suggests that many nurses are harassed sexually, with psychological and physical health effects. The tabloid image of the nurse as a sexy young thing in black suspenders makes her particularly susceptible to such approaches, at work and elsewhere.

It is hard for female nurses to tackle harassing male patients, who see sexual innuendo as bound up in the nurse's role, and are anxious to assert their machismo in the face of hospital-induced dependency. Senior nurses may also exploit their position by harassment of more junior staff, as recent professional conduct cases demonstrate. The trade union UNISON, which has campaigned against sexual harassment, says its members hesitate to report it for a number of reasons: the don't think they will be believed, they fear the publicity or they think they will be punished or ridiculed. Recently a nurse who reported an indecent assault by a doctor was abused by her nursing colleagues for causing trouble – she should have grinned and borne it.

In the late 1980s courageous women firefighters fought a successful tribunal case against male colleagues who sexually humiliated them, but cases such as that of senior police officer Alison Halford, whose path to promotion was blocked by men who made damaging allegations about her personal life, show how far there is still to go.

Other causes of nurses' stress also stem from society's attitudes. Discrimination against people who are black, homosexual, disabled or in some other way seen as different from 'the norm' causes much distress, and creates emotional and practical obstacles to job satisfaction, career development and self-esteem.

Racism

The UK health services have always relied heavily on black people and others from ethnic minorities, both British citizens and those who were encouraged to migrate to the UK to solve its labour crises. Yet like most other UK organisations, the NHS is institutionally racist and black nurses report many abuses, including verbal insults, blocked promotion and other sources of stress (see Box 4.1).

Box 4.1   *The double-glazed ceiling*

One black woman's experience in the NHS is typical of many. 'After 22 years as a nurse, midwife, health visitor, health promotion officer and nurse tutor, Neslyn Watson-Druee quit the NHS in 1989 because she was told that as an intelligent black woman she was intimidating and had no chance of promotion.'

Source: Porter, 1997.

The London Association of Community Relations Councils, in its 1985 survey of health authorities' equal opportunities practices, found widespread racism, reflected in 'the volume of suspicion and complaint, increasingly supported by evidence, that health authorities discriminate against black people'. The racism might have been direct and deliberate, but more often it was indirect and unconscious, 'frequently the result of the unthinking operation of a system which discriminates against ethnic minority groups' (LACRC, 1985).

There is nothing to suggest that matters have improved since then: a number of studies show that racial discrimination and inequality in nursing is still widespread. Research by the King's Fund (1990, 1991), for example, found the following:

- African-Caribbean nurses are concentrated in enrolled nurse grades.
- A lack of equal access to training and career development.
- Underrepresentation of African-Caribbean nurses in senior grades.
- Underrepresentation African-Caribbean applicants for first level courses.
- African-Caribbean nurses are leaving the NHS in disproportionate numbers.
- African-Caribbean applicants are disproportionately unsuccessful.
- The number of African-Caribbean applicants for training is declining.

This last point has been clearly articulated:

> My grandchildren don't want to be pushed to the back of the queue like I was; young people nowadays won't tolerate bad manners and being treated unfairly. They want to know that they can make it to the top, be rewarded for hard work and won't always be expected to do the dirty jobs nobody else wants to do (Mensah, 1997).

Nurses from African-Caribbean, Asian and other ethnic groups are often subjected to racial harassment by their colleagues, patients and relatives, and may be told by their managers 'not to be too sensitive' or that 'people of that 'older' generation are bound to be prejudiced'. These are intolerable statements, and nurses who suffer racial harassment ought to get firm support from their employers and managers. The situation is being challenged by the unions, and by individuals bringing racial discrimination cases to industrial tribunals and clinical grading appeals. Monitoring of recruitment, career progression and access to training is being adopted. However it's not hard to conclude that if you are not white, you are almost certainly disadvantaged in the health services.

Homophobia

The fear of homosexuality, which leads to discrimination against men and women who are gay, is as widespread in nursing as it is in society as a whole.

The attitudes towards AIDS reported in and fostered by sections of the media have revealed the true extent of this ignorant and damaging prejudice. Nurses who are open about their sexual orientation have found themselves the subject of abuse or unpleasant gossip, while others have been moved off children's wards because they are gay.

References and resources on societal stressors

Cortis, J.D. and Rinomhota, A.S. (1996) 'The future of ethnic minority nurses in the NHS', *Journal of Nursing Management*, vol. 4, no. 6 (November), pp. 359–66.

King's Fund (1990) *Racial Equality: The Nursing Profession*, Occasional Paper no. 6. London: King's Fund Equal Opportunities Task Force.

King's Fund (1991) *Racial Equality in the NHS*, Equal Opportunities Task Force final report. London: King's Fund.

LRD (1994) *Tackling Harassment at Work*. London: Labour Research Department.

LACRC (1985) *In a Critical Condition: a survey of equal opportunities in employment in London's health authorities*. London: London Association of Community Relations Councils.

Mensah, J. (1997). 'Positive action', *Nursing Standard*, vol. 12, no. 10 (26 November), pp. 22–3.

Millar, B. (1997) 'Working the family–friendly shift', *Nursing Times*, vol. 93, no. 41 (8 October), p. 15.

Nursing and Midwifery Staffs Negotiating Council Staff Side (1992) *Action towards equality for nursing staff, midwives and health visitors*. London: NMNC Staff Side.

Payne, D. (1995) 'Unequal treatment. . .', *Nursing Times*, vol. 91, no. 46 (15 November), pp.16–17.

Policy Studies Institute (1995) *Nursing in a Multi-Ethnic NHS*. London: Policy Studies Institute.

Porter, R. (1997) 'The double-glazed ceiling'. *Nursing Times*, vol. 93, no. 17 (23 April), p. 17.

Seccombe, I. and Smith, G. (1996) *In the Balance: registered nurse supply and demand, 1996*, Studies Report 315. Brighton: Royal College of Nursing/ Institute for Employment.

Waters, J. (1997) 'Child care: the missing link', *Nursing Times*, vol. 93, no. 41 (8 October), pp. 14–15.

Employer-induced stressors

Workers in the NHS face all the stressors induced by society as a whole, as we have seen, but they also have to cope with extra problems related to their status as employees of an underfunded public service. Nurses are mostly employed by NHS trusts, who decide how to spend their own budgets and therefore have considerable influence over staff well-being, yet the amount of money available for improving pay and conditions depends largely on how much the government allocates – a political decision made at the highest level.

NHS staff, including many nurses, are among the lowest paid of all workers. Unlike many others, though, NHS staff once enjoyed the full benefits of collective bargaining through the Whitley Councils, where staff and management representatives negotiated not just pay but also a huge and complicated agreement on conditions of service, ranging from productivity bonuses to compassionate leave. The Conservatives removed many of Whitley's powers, devolving them to NHS trusts, the Pay Review Body and the annual pay rounds, but it still plays a valued role in protecting employees' rights and welfare. The post-1989 NHS reforms introduced nurses to the insecurity of short-term contracts, casualisation, the competitive market culture, and an attempt to introduce local pay rates and local bargaining. This was resisted successfully by the unions, though not without some nurses being forced into accepting local terms and conditions. These changes increased staff stress, together with the strain of annually treating increasing numbers of patients under the continued government demand for 'efficiency savings'.

Most of the stressors outlined in this section are preventable, and the NHS trade unions are a vital source of support and action (Seccombe and Smith, 1996).

Workload

A recent survey of nurses at sister/charge nurse level and above found that workload is the major cause of occupational stress (RCN, 1997a), and there is no shortage of other evidence to demonstrate the traumatic effect of shortages or misallocation of precious resources. Yet while excess workload is almost universally acknowledged as a problem, there is a kind of reality gap when it comes to acknowledging pressures on the individual nurse. Senior nurses, themselves under stress, often try to contain the distress by forcing nurses to 'cope', rather than by taking more decisive collective action to force employers and the government to intervene.

The pressures of workload can be classified into three main groups: the number of staff, type of staff and physical resources. The actual number of pairs of hands is often what nurses have in mind when they talk about excessive workloads – there are simply not enough people to do the work. The nurse has to choose between conflicting priorities among her patients, with physical tasks tending to take precedence over psychological or emotional work. She has to cut corners and deliver care in ways which go against what she has been taught and which reduce her sense of satisfaction, and may even cause her physical harm. Recent Swedish research, for example, suggests that nurses are at higher risk of back and neck injuries when under stress (Josephson *et al.*, 1997).

Second, there is the question of the type of staff employed. Proper workforce planning will not solve all the problems of understaffing, but much more can be done by managers to ensure that the workers in each care area have talents, qualifications and attributes which are appropriate both to the patients' needs and to the balance of the staff team. Employing more support workers, for instance, could help relieve the sheer volume of work, but is no substitute for qualified nurses; careful attention must be paid to the skill and grade mix of the nursing team.

Good workforce planning addresses not only the mix of staff but also the way they are deployed. Today there is an unfortunate tendency to regard good planning as making the maximum use of each person's labour without any regard for individual needs and circumstances. Moving nurses from one ward to another because of fluctuating workloads, or changing their shifts at very short notice, may on the surface be the most 'efficient' use of staff but it is ultimately destructive; it ignores the nurse's need to work in a well-established team, to build up good relationships with patients, and to use the troughs in workload for less pressing tasks such as teaching. In the long run, it is probably inefficient as well as stress-inducing.

Finally, insufficient and poor-quality physical resources are also workload stressors, imposing additional demands on nurses (RCN, 1997a; Seccombe and Smith, 1997). Beds which cannot be adjusted for height, badly designed bathrooms and dingy dayrooms are potential hazards to physical health, but they are also examples of another major contributor to nurses' stress, since they impede the ability to work well.

Shiftwork

The hours of work are another source of stress. Nurses do a great deal of unacknowledged and unpaid overtime, cutting short their breaks and leaving late because there is still work to be done. The Factories Act states that employees should not work more than a four-and-a half-hour stretch without a 30-minute break, but in practice the nurse's concern for her patients often leads her to forgo her rights. Sometimes she has little choice, as moral blackmail is exerted to keep her working.

The odd timing and variation of shifts can also be shattering. They are an inescapable facet of providing a 24-hour service, but much could be done to soften the effects – for example by avoiding ten-day stretches without a break, or the eleven-hour night shift, which as well as being unpalatable to most staff tends to reduce their efficiency. The familiar pattern of a late shift followed by an early start the next day can be exhausting too, especially if the journey home is long and transport poor; some nurses report sleeping difficulties when they have no time to unwind before going to bed in preparation for an early start.

There have been many valuable recent studies of nurses' shift-work (Barton *et al.*, 1995; Buchan, 1995; Healy, 1997; Humm, 1996; Millar, 1997), providing much corroborative evidence for nurses who want accepted patterns altered in favour of healthier options: the 'earlies–lates–nights–days off' rotation pattern, for example, with at least 12 hours between shifts, appears the least disruptive (RCN, 1997b). Studies of night duty highlight how the body's normal circadian rhythm is disrupted by reversing day and night activity (Costa *et al.*, 1995). The initial process of adaptation leaves the body's functions out of synch, a likely cause of fatigue and malaise. Rotating night shifts prevent nurses from adapting fully and their faculties are dulled; adjustment is poorer when the shift exceeds eight hours. Physical problems include hyperacidity, constipation, loss of appetite, insomnia and a greater susceptibility to disease.

The social and psychological consequences of shift work can be as stressful as the physical ones. A study of groups of healthy student nurses' experience of night duty found increased irritability, hypersensitivity to criticism and heightened feelings of hopelessness in nearly three quarters of the respondents (Healy, 1997). Working unsocial hours restricts leisure activity and the opportunity to see friends, and may exacerbate the difficulties of caring for children and other dependants outlined in the previous section. The lack of nurseries, for example, forces some women to become night nurses so that they can care for their children during the day, snatching a little sleep before returning to work.

Home/work conflicts

The conflict generated by having to do two jobs, one at home and one at work, is faced by millions of women, and nurses are no exception. Domestic commitments may inhibit career prospects in nursing, but the NHS as an employer fails to acknowledge its responsibility; it relies on the labour of women, very often as part timers, but makes little effort to organise working hours, holidays, facilities or in-service training to support the employee.

Attitudes towards maternity and paternity leave, compassionate leave and the timing of holidays are good examples. Nurses are protected by their legal rights and some by the improvements secured by the Whitley Councils, but they are largely defenceless against an employer who regards their personal needs and wishes as subordinate to the demands of the organisation. Clearly compromise is sometimes necessary, but nurses often have no say in decisions which affect their lives. Moral blackmail is often exerted to prevent them from taking compassionate leave, or to persuade them to take their holiday at undesirable times.

Pay and conditions

Finally, poor working conditions and low pay contribute to stress. Both are linked to resources; the less the amount of money made available for health care, the less there is to improve wages and working conditions. Low pay leads some people to work overtime for extra cash, or to moonlight by doing agency work on top of full-time employment. How can people working such long hours give good care or recharge their batteries? Nurses' earnings have remained below the national average for non-manual workers, and nearly two-thirds of nurses believe they would earn more money for less effort outside nursing (Seccombe and Smith, 1996).

A recent continuing study has confirmed the continued fall in nurses' morale and looked at the links between stress, mental health and morale (RCN, 1997a). Morale was explored through 'attitude statement' surveys on perceptions of pay, job satisfaction, career prospects and future intentions. Pay satisfaction had declined: in 1992, 45 per cent of respondents agreed they could be paid more for less effort outside nursing; by 1996, 62 per cent agreed. Job satisfaction was an increasingly important factor. Ill-health, injury and redundancy accounted for nearly a third of NHS job changes in those surveyed. In 1993, 25 per cent agreed 'I would leave nursing if I could'; in 1996, 38 per cent agreed. Four out of five would not recommend nursing as a career, and 82 per cent were dissatisfied with their workload. Only 16 per cent agreed with the statement 'Nursing will continue to offer me a secure future' (Seccombe and Smith, 1996).

The lack of capital investment in the NHS means that many nurses work in decrepit, substandard surroundings, and some have to live in them too. Managers and teachers and may be crowded into small offices with inadequate clerical help or equipment, while practitioners change in over-crowded cloakrooms and eat in dingy cafeterias. Poor working conditions contribute to the sense of being undervalued as a person and of having no control over your work, which leads to high stress and low morale.

References and resources on employer-induced stressors

Barton, J., Spelten, E., Totterdell, P., Smith, L. and Folkard, S. (1995) 'Is there an optimum number of night shifts? Relationship between sleep, health and well-being'. *Work and Stress*, vol. 9, nos 2/3 (April–September), pp. 109–23.

Buchan, J. (1995) 'Shifting the pattern of nurses' work', *Nursing Standard*, vol. 9, no. 45 (2 August), p. 29.

Costa, G., Gaffuri, E., Ghirlanda, G., Minors, D. and Waterhouse, J. (1995) 'Psychosocial conditions and hormonal secretion in nurses on a rapidly rotating shift schedule and exposed to bright light during shift work'. *Work and Stress*, vol. 9, nos 2/3 (April–September), pp. 148–57.

Healy, D. (1997) 'Blues in the night', *Nursing Times*, vol. 93, no. 15 (9 April), pp. 26–8.

Humm, C. (1996) 'A shift in time', *Nursing Standard*, vol. 10, no. 38 (12 June), pp. 22–4.

Josephson, M., Lagerstrøm, M., Hagberg, M. and Hjelm, E. (1997) 'Musculoskeletal symptoms and job strain among nursing personnel', *Occupational and Environmental Medicine*, vol. 54, no. 9, pp. 681–5.

Millar, B. (1997) 'Working the family-friendly shift', *Nursing Times*, vol. 93, no. 41 (8 October), p. 15.

RCN (1997a) 'Stress and morale in nursing', Employment Brief 12/97. London: Royal College of Nursing.

RCN (1997b) 'Shifting the balance: Towards best practice in shift working and patient care', Health and Safety at Work leaflet no. 6, re-order No. 000 733. London: Royal College of Nursing.

Seccombe, I. and Smith, G. (1996) 'In the Balance: registered nurse supply and demand, 1996', Studies Report 315. London: Royal College of Nursing/ Institute for Employment.

Professional stressors

On top of the stressors faced by most other health service staff, nurses must also deal with the problems inherent in the nature and current organisation of nursing work. Emotionally and psychologically, nursing is a difficult job at the best of times; nurses confront serious illness, death and disability every day, as well as the fear and pain felt by every patient. They have to deal with distressed relatives and friends, and to cope with their own sense of loss and pain. Over time they become accustomed to the feelings, sights, sounds and smells, but they do not necessarily learn how to handle them constructively, either for themselves or for others. If they do learn to do so, it is often through their own efforts rather than those of the system, which offers too little preparation, education and support.

The job itself is bound to cause stress. But this is compounded by how the nursing culture has tried to suppress the expression of emotion, its lack of attention to the emotional and psychological needs of practitioners, its educational shortcomings and its hierarchical organisation – all this at a time when the demands on nurses, from their employers and from the profession, are growing almost daily. Innovative research on nurse–patient interaction suggests that the degree of improvement in attention to nurses' emotional and spiritual needs varies within and between workplaces, and is related to changes in political decisions on the role of nursing in health care (Savage, 1995).

A third strand is the perfectionism nurses bring to their work. Research suggests that recruits arrive with a commitment to the pursuit of high, often unattainable standards – described as the 'angel syndrome' by Hingley and colleagues. It may be one of the reasons why people choose nursing in the first place. Thereafter the syndrome is reinforced by senior nurses, whose expectations of juniors are similarly high; chastisement for 'mistakes' is much more likely than praise, and a refusal to accept unreasonable demands is regarded as unprofessional troublemaking or inability to cope. Nurses' expectations of themselves, and the mismatch between these and others' expectations, have been identified as a leading cause of stress.

Individual development

Studies on stress in nursing point to staff development as a tool to minimise stress, although many nurses still receive few opportunities to develop themselves professionally and personally. The lack of attention paid to the needs of the individual nurse in areas such as child care and compassionate leave is also noticeable in the area of professional development, despite the clarity of the statutory requirements laid down by the UKCC. In the past, nursing's traditional ethic of vocational self-sacrifice often went along with an undervaluing of the occupational needs of each person; the modern equivalent – overzealous demands for 'professional commitment' – can be just as damaging. Passivity and underdevelopment leading to long-term apathy is known to be stressful, as is the person's feeling that they do not matter.

Role preparation

The well-documented shortcomings which were evident in pre-Project 2000 nursing education remain sadly true for many in post-basic education and development. At each stage of promotion – to staff nurse, sister or a senior post – or when their work changes, nurses complain of inadequate preparation leading to insecurity about performance and expectations, and cite this as a leading reason for leaving the NHS (Seccombe and Smith, 1997). Being thrown in at the deep end is unfair on the nurse as well as the patient. Linked with this is the growing complexity of nursing work, increased workloads and the demands of mentoring undergraduate nursing students. The recent growth of clinical supervision, however, appears to provide valuable support for clinical staff.

Technical changes in medicine require nurses to keep up to date while the quest to improve nursing care is creating many new demands. Theoretical models, the nursing process and research are important tools and make nurses more aware of the broad knowledge base they need for effective practice. Yet the time and skills needed to acquire that knowledge are hard to obtain when resources are scarce and nursing is not seen as a high priority. The more we learn, the more we realise what we don't know, but we are still trained to appear as if we know it all, and to deny uncertainty or ignorance – a position which is contrary to the UKCC Code of Professional Conduct, and unacceptable in the context of PREP requirements for continued professional development.

Nurses also need support and preparation that is relevant to the field in which they work. Intensive care is often regarded as stressful, but caring for the elderly or people with mental health problems, for example, may be just as stressful in a different way.

Professional autonomy

The search for more professional autonomy, both collective and individual, is widely supported, but the concomitant need to develop support mechanisms is mentioned far less often. Professionalism holds out the promise of more power, yet nurses are still largely powerless in relation to doctors and general managers. Nurses are being encouraged to develop a sense of individual accountability for what they do, not least through the UKCC Code of Professional Conduct; they also need assurance that the responsibility this entails will be buttressed by greater professional protection.

The UKCC's advisory Scope of Professional Practice document urges managers and professional leaders to base local policies and procedures on the principles of the Code and Scope documents, but clinical nurses rightly wish to see such statements matched with supportive actions. They need to be certain that senior nurses support their right to act on their own judgment when they are pressurised by doctors or managers. This is especially important with the extended roles that many nurses now take on in advanced and specialist nursing practice, and in carrying out medical tasks in the wake of government policy to reduce junior doctors' hours. Many nurses welcome the increase in their individual autonomy but they also need adequate education and collegial support, as well as higher indemnity insurance cover, in recognition of the increased likelihood of being held legally accountable in carrying out new work. Individual professional autonomy is in many ways incompatible with hierarchical organisation, and so far insufficient attention has been paid to the profession's collective responsibility to its members.

Nursing students, at the bottom of the pile, suffer particular problems which deserve special attention, including lack of adequate preparation and poor mentor support. Students and newly qualified degree, diploma and Project 2000 graduates are often thrown in at the deep end and are expected to shoulder awesome responsibilities without sufficient support. This abrupt switching of roles, together with the suspicion or even hostility they may encounter from pre-Project 2000 nurses, is an added source of stress on top of other problems such as debts from the years when they were expected to subsist on small student bursaries or grants. The overhaul of nursing education was meant to relieve the pressure on student nurses by taking them out of the labour force and giving them supernumerary status; while it has achieved some improvements, it has also brought new, unexpected sources of stress.

A culture of continuous change

All these factors are linked with far-reaching health and social changes which are transforming the role of nurses – and others – almost beyond recognition. The introduction of general management in the 1980s and the NHS reforms of the 1990s provide glaring examples of poor management of change, but there are many other examples internal to nursing of unwelcome policies being imposed from the top down, the introduction of the nursing process being the most notorious. In the 1990s some managers referred casually to a 'culture of continuous change', but often failed to recognise that change is stressful in itself and needs to be carefully managed.

References and resources on professional stressors

Bond, M. (1986) *Stress and Self Awareness: A Guide for Nurses*, London: Heinemann Nursing.

Hingley, P. and Marks, R. (1991) *The Costs of Stress and the Costs and Benefits of Stress Management*. London: National Association for Staff Support/Royal College of Nursing.

Menzies, I. (1960) *A Case Study in the Functioning of Social Systems as a Defence against Anxiety*. London: Tavistock Institute of Human Relations.

Morton-Cooper, A. (1984) 'The end of the rope', *Nursing Mirror*, vol. 159, no. 19 (5 December), pp. 16–19.

RCN (1997) 'Stress and Morale in Nursing', Employment Brief 12/97. London: RCN Employment Information and Research Unit, Royal College of Nursing.

Salvage, J. (1985) *The Politics of Nursing*. London: Heinemann.

Savage, J. (1995) *Nursing Intimacy*. London: Scutari Press.

UKCC (1992a) *Code of Professional Conduct*. London: United Kingdom Central Council for Nursing, Midwifery and Health Visiting.

UKCC (1992b) *The Scope of Professional Practice*. London: UKCC.

UKCC (1996) *Guidelines for Professional Practice*. London: UKCC.

UKCC (1997) *Scope in Practice*. London: UKCC.

Action on stress

Some of the factors that put nurses under unnecessary stress are not unique to the NHS: they are endemic in society. The search for solutions must therefore concentrate partly on broad social change – which means political action at local and national level using every possible channel. In this section we look at possible action on stress, in particular counselling, peer group support and the collaborative approach of clinical supervision.

Comments such as 'If you don't like the heat, get out of the kitchen' were once a familiar response to discussions of stress in nursing. It is appropriate that those who do not like nursing should leave, but it is also important to take care to recruit people who know what to expect and can be taught how to cope. A better mix of recruits, including more men and older people, could help, with more careful exploration of people's motivation for entering nursing. The 'reality shock' of life on the wards could be eased by better preparation, such as improved liaison with schools to help recruits make a more informed career choice.

Blaming the individual for succumbing to stress is, however, unacceptable. We must look at why so many nurses seem to have trouble coping, and at the personal cost to those who survive. If the system is such that only the toughest survive intact, and many others are damaged on the way, then we should act to change the system itself, rather than expecting the victim to knuckle under, retire hurt or leave altogether.

The stressors identified here as societal, employer-induced and professional are linked in many ways, and the possible solutions are similarly

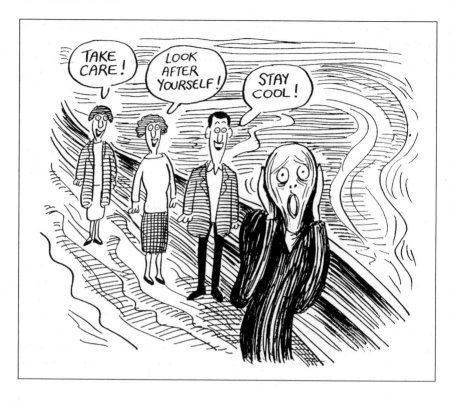

intertwined. Some, such as fighting for more nurseries, are more concrete, while others, such as the nature of the nursing culture, are less tangible; all, however, need to be tackled on a variety of fronts, ranging from the political to the personal.

Stress is costly, but it can be managed. In 1992 the National Association for Staff Support produced an innovative document on the causes of stress and the benefits of stress management, to provide staff with evidence to back up their requests for support services (Hingley and Marks, 1991). It identifies costs to the individual, the organisation, the nation and the NHS, assesses the costs and benefits of stress management, and subdivides costs into the cost of not having adequate staff support and the cost of providing support services.

After discussing stress in similar terms to those in this chapter, Hingley and Marks reached several conclusions: much stress is preventable, so stress management is cost-effective. Costings should include direct expenditure on planning and prevention; expenditure related to later losses, and the cost of treatment and rehabilitation. Indirect elements include loss of expertise and the cost of rebuilding procedures and the team. Monitoring staff sickness levels is suggested as a measure of the success of counselling and other staff support. In the USA, say the authors, Employee Assistance Programmes have had significant results: half the companies offering counselling have shown better individual performance and productivity, absenteeism and staff turnover have been reduced and employer–employee relationships improved. The incidence of disciplinary hearings has been reduced by 'early counselling', and workplace accidents and recurring problems such as alcoholism) have also declined.

The personal response

Many of the strategies for coping effectively with stress can be undertaken by the nurse on her own. *Stress and Self-Awareness: A Guide for Nurses*, by Meg Bond (1986), outlines a variety of useful techniques, with practical exercises, suggestions, reading lists and addresses. Sharing problems and feelings, constructive criticism, positive feedback, learning confidence and assertive behaviour, relaxation training, biofeedback and meditation are all helpful – nurses can choose whichever they find most congenial.

Ask your employer or nursing studies department to run relaxation classes, stress workshops or assertiveness training – some enlightened ones are already doing so. If your request is not met, you may look for local authority or other evening classes – check your local paper. Trade unions and professional organisations also put on their own courses. You could work through open learning materials on your own or with friends and colleagues; packs have been developed specifically on nursing and stress (for example *Nursing Times* Open Learning: see 'Resources').

Counselling

The word 'counselling' is often loosely used as a synonym for an intimate talk where advice is given. This is inevitably part of the nurse's role, in relation both to patients and to more junior staff, and it can often be valuable; again, the more skilled the nurse is, the more effective her or his intervention. However true counselling should not be confused with other legitimate aspects of the managerial role such as staff appraisal, performance review, and informal warnings; the manager must be clear which function she or he is discharging. Discussion about performance may benefit from specific counselling techniques, but it is not counselling and should not be confused with it.

True counselling, which is concerned not with the requirements of the organisation but with the client's well-being, is impossible in the manager–employer relationship. Nurses who are unable to cope with stress despite support from colleagues will often benefit from seeing a professional counsellor who is, and is seen to be, independent of the management hierarchy. This is the most frequent form of stress management intervention (Hingley and Marks, 1991), but few health authorities make such a service available, and despite widespread recognition of the need, growth has been slow. In 1972 the creation of a comprehensive counselling service was said to be an 'urgent top priority' (Briggs 1972), few people took that message to heart. Pressure for better facilities to be offered within and outside the organisation should be exerted by stewards, safety reps, teachers and managers.

Peer group support

All nurses can help reduce stress in their place of work by encouraging open discussion and expression of feelings. Often one person with the courage to speak up enables everyone else to say what they feel; the simple knowledge that you are not alone in your feelings is reassuring. More formally, sisters and teaching staff can hold regular meetings where feelings can be aired. Leading such a discussion is more constructive if the facilitator has relevant skills, developed through further education and independent reading. A skilled outsider can be invited to lead the discussion. Separate groups for junior and senior staff to air their feelings may encourage greater openness. From these discussions, nurses might move on to ask their managers to promote critical incident analysis and introduce clinical supervision.

Clinical supervision

Clinical supervision has been defined as 'an exchange between practising professionals to enable the development of professional skills, an opportunity to sustain and develop professional practice' (Howarth and Faugier, 1994). All nurses should, by right, have access to regular clinical supervision; Johns (1993) suggests that it should be part of their employment contract.

Stress in nursing is accentuated by feelings of low self-esteem, isolation and lack of support. Traditionally, nurses have talked about patients with their colleagues, but have not had a confidential and safe environment to deal with personal and professional stress. Clinical supervision can provide such an environment – approximately 75 per cent of experiences shared in supervision may be stress-related (Johns, 1993). Although some argue that clinical supervision should focus solely on clinical practice rather than personal and professional issues, in reality these overlap and should not be excluded. Nurse managers and nurses alike should be clear that clinical supervision ought not be a management disciplinary tool; if it becomes that, it is bound to fail.

Bishop (1998) identifies the key issues of clinical supervision as protected time, confidentiality, research-based practice, shared expertise and staff empowerment. Trust nurse executives have recommended that clinical supervision should be developed and evaluated throughout the NHS (Department of Health, 1994). The UKCC set out six key statements on it to 'allow more effective professional development' (UKCC, 1996):

- Clinical supervision supports practice, enabling practitioners to maintain and promote standards of care.

- It is a practice-focused professional relationship involving a practitioner reflecting on practice guided by a skilled supervisor.
- The process . . . should be developed by practitioners and managers according to local circumstances (with agreement on the purpose and benefits of supervision, and comprehensive ground rules on issues of confidentiality, how subjects are raised discussed and recorded).
- Every practitioner should have access to clinical supervision, with realistic supervisor–practitioner ratios.
- Preparation for supervision can be made in-house or through external programmes, with incorporation of the principles and relevance of clinical supervision in pre- and post-registration education.
- Locally developed evaluation is necessary to develop knowledge of the benefits and outcomes.

The functions of clinical supervision

Clinical supervision is seen by some as being 'formative', 'normative' and 'restorative' – that is, helping individual development, providing a monitor of professional performance and a chance to unload stress and recharge (Proctor, 1992). Individual development may be assisted by the guidance and questions of skilled and knowledgeable supervisors (probably experienced practitioners) in the course of supervision sessions. Some nurses, especially those unaccustomed to discussing their work, find frameworks useful, such as reflective models which suggest key issues; as they become more experienced or comfortable with supervision, frameworks might become less important.

Using clinical supervision to monitor professional performance is more problematic, especially when a nurse's clinical supervisor is her manager. While it is inevitable that professional and management issues overlap, it could undermine nurses' confidence in clinical supervision if it merges with or seems to be a substitute for performance review (Northcott, 1996). The value of clinical supervision as an arena for unloading stress and recharging should not be underestimated. Exponents of clinical supervision such as Bishop, Butterworth, Faugier and Johns see this 'restorative' function as central, provided it moves from negative moaning to supportive help in alleviating stress (Butterworth, 1996; Bishop, 1998).

When it fulfils these three functions, clinical supervision is immensely liberating for nurses, enabling them to stand back and look at clinical practice and their relationships with patients and colleagues. With competent supervision they can see their successes, be challenged to work through problems and rehearse alternative ways of dealing with issues, as those who have experienced clinical supervision explain. 'A more senior nurse was making unfair remarks about my off-duty rota to me, which I dealt with at the time', said one nurse. 'She was also complaining in my absence that she couldn't find this policy or that policy and accused me of discarding them.

. . . I felt she must have a grievance to be so picky . . . my clinical supervisor and I looked at how I handled the first episode, what else I could have done, and why this nurse might be appearing picky and hostile and what I should do about it.' Another nurse reported: 'A chance to talk about myself and my weaknesses in an environment that encouraged honesty with no criticism but honest feedback helped me very much. I am a much better nurse for the humanity and interest I received through supervision' (both quoted in Butterworth *et al.*, 1997).

The potential impact on nurses

Clinical supervision is still in its relative infancy in UK health care, but there is a vast and expanding literature on it (see the References at the end of this section). Its interest in the context of this book lies in its effectiveness as a means of combating stress. An evaluation of the benefits (Butterworth *et al.*, 1997) found that among the group who received supervision there was a decrease in emotional exhaustion and stress, which was also the case with the control group after they began to receive supervision. Although the feel-good factor is unlikely to be accepted by managers as an adequate rationale for introducing clinical supervision, for staff it may well be central.

References and further reading on clinical supervision

Bishop, V. (ed.) (1998) *Clinical Supervision in Practice. Some questions, answers and guidelines.* Basingstoke: Macmillan *NT Research.*

Briggs, A. (1972) *Report of the Committee on Nursing.* London: HMSO.

Butterworth, T. and Faugier, J. (1994) *Clinical Supervision in Nursing, Midwifery and Health Visiting.* Manchester: University of Manchester.

Butterworth, T. (1996) 'Primary attempts at research-based evaluation of clinical supervision', *NT Research*, vol. 1, no. 2 (March–April), pp. 96–101

Butterworth, T., Bishop, V., Carson, J., Clements, A., Jeacock, J. and White, E. (1997) *It is good to talk. An evaluation study of Clinical Supervision and Mentorship in England and Scotland.* University of Manchester.

Department of Health (1994) *Clinical Supervision: A Report of the Trust Nurse Executives' Workshops.* London: HMSO.

Fowler, J. (1996) 'The organisation of clinical supervision within the nursing profession: a review of the literature', *Journal of Advanced Nursing*, vol. 23 (March), pp. 471–8.

Johns, C. (1993) 'Professional supervision', *Journal of Nursing Management*, vol. 1, no. 1 (January), pp. 9–18.

Northcott, N. (1996) 'Supervise to grow', *Nursing Management*, vol. 2, no. 10 (March), pp. 18–19.

Porter, N. (1997) 'Clinical supervision: the art of being supervised', *Nursing Standard*, vol. 11, no. 45 (30 July) pp. 44–5.

Proctor, B. (1992) 'Maps and models of supervision', in Hawkins, P. and Shohet, R. (eds), *Supervision in the Helping Professions.* Milton Keynes: Open University Press.

UKCC (1996) *Position statement on clinical supervision for nursing and health visiting.* London: UKCC.

Education and training

At both basic and post-basic level, the education and socialisation of nurses plays an important part in determining how creatively they will deal with stress. Confirmation that expressing feelings is permitted and discussion of and practice in stress management techniques should be key aspects of the curriculum, not just confined to a token session but raised where relevant throughout the course. Qualified staff and teachers are influential role models, and the way they tackle the issues is crucial; there is a great need for continuing education to enable those trained to hold different values to rethink them.

The education and training of nurses – both the overt curriculum and its hidden agenda – contribute much to the overall culture of the profession: its values, ethics, behaviour and so on. Innovative nursing research has opened up a discussion on traditionally hidden aspects of nursing, such as studies of the nurse–patient relationship (Savage, 1995), the emotional labour of nurses (Smith, 1992) and the issue of the body in nursing (Lawler, 1991). The difficult task of transforming the nursing culture to one which is more open, supportive and honest cannot be achieved by the educators alone, even with the help of sisters and charge nurses. Every nurse contributes to the culture, and those in leadership positions have a particular responsibility to reshape attitudes.

Networking is one way of achieving this. Formal and informal networks and channels can offer support, contacts and communication, and there are numerous opportunities for nurses to network to improve personal confidence and increase campaigning opportunities.

Conclusion

We have seen that the stressors in nursing spring from many causes, some social, some occupational and some professional, and that they cannot simply be ascribed to personality. Managing stress, and preventing it, is therefore partly a matter of broad social change – which means political action at the local and the national level using every possible channel, including pressure groups, MPs, counsellors and trade unions. Much can be done in health services to tackle the problems and increase awareness, especially by safety reps, stewards and managers. Where policies on social issues such as racism, sexual orientation and sexism do not exist, they should be developed; where they do, more effort should be put into implementing them. A collective approach which emphasises stress prevention is essential to complement pragmatic individual strategies for stress management.

References and further reading on dealing with stress, and changing the nursing culture

Bond, M. (1986) *Stress and Self-Awareness: A Guide for Nurses*. London: Heinemann Nursing.

Hingley, P. and Marks, R. (1991) 'The Costs of Stress and the Benefits of Stress Management', Occasional Paper no. 5. Woking: National Association for Staff Support.

Lawler, J. (1991) *Behind the Screens. Nursing, Somology and the Problem of the Body*. Melbourne: Churchill Livingstone.

Salvage, J. (1985) *The Politics of Nursing*. London: Heinemann.

Savage, J. (1995) *Nursing Intimacy. An Ethnographic Approach to Nurse–Patient Interaction*. London: Scutari.

Smith, P. (1992) *The Emotional Labour of Nursing: how nurses care*. London: Macmillan.

Resource

Emap Healthcare Open Learning, Greater London House, Hampstead Road, London NW1 7EJ. Tel.: 0171 874 0600.

5   Violence and bullying

Violence in health services is a major problem. But it is not confined to patients or relatives abusing or attacking staff. More and more instances are coming to light of staff being bullied by managers or colleagues. This chapter discusses these issues and offers suggestions on how nurses can deal with them.

Violence

Work-related violence is defined by the Health and Safety Executive as 'any incident in which a person working in the healthcare sector is verbally abused, threatened or assaulted by a patient or member of the public in circumstances relating to his or her employment' (Health Services Advisory Committee, 1997). Nurses are in the front line, whether in the accident and emergency department, the psychiatric ward, visiting patients in their homes or travelling home alone after a late shift. Violence to staff can come from many different sources: from an aggressive patient or relative; attacks from intruders inside hospitals or nurses' homes; sexual harassment (verbal or physical) of a nurse in uniform outside hospital premises; and verbal or physical abuse of nurses visiting patients in the community.

Violence to health workers is increasing – in some areas at an alarming rate. For years, low priority was given to combating violence in the NHS; little action or further research followed the 1987 HSAC pamphlet *Violence to Staff in the Health Services* until the 1997 HSAC guidance (quoted above) and new studies by trade unions. Recent examples of violence include a nurse in Portsmouth who was slashed across the eyebrow, a pregnant A & E consultant who was kicked in the stomach, death threats, head-butting and punching. In response to the growing number of incidents, the Leicester Royal Infirmary maternity unit set up a direct police line and other hospitals have taken similarly dramatic steps.

The problem is not unique to the NHS, as more than 350,000 people a year are subject to violent attacks at work and many more go unreported (TUC, 1997). But NHS staff are particularly open to risk: hospital premises need to be open 24 hours a day, and large buildings with several entrances present a security problem and are particularly susceptible to theft and vandalism. Hospital grounds are large and often badly lit, and staff may have to walk long distances between buildings. Nurses may be treating patients who are under the influence of drugs, alcohol, psychosis or simply fear, which can increase aggression. Community nurses visiting patients in their homes are vulnerable to verbal and physical abuse and harassment, and have no back-up support. The NHS and nursing employ a high proportion of women, who are more vulnerable to attack.

Despite long-term union pressure, violence to health care staff has only recently been taken seriously as a health and safety issue. Few health authorities document reports of violence to their staff and there are no comprehensive statistics on violent assaults or criminal incidents on NHS premises. According to Sue Parkyn Smith, chair of the HSAC, the HSE served 10 notices on trusts in 1997 because of poor protection of staff (Gulland, 1997b). In 1992 the NHS Executive set up the National Association of Healthcare Security to improve security through information exchange, and in 1993 the National Association of Health Authorities and Trusts produced a security manual and audiovisual package – but few trusts bought it; security is still regarded as a cost, not a benefit (Elson, 1997).

The legal framework

After the election of the Labour government in 1997, Secretary of State for Health Frank Dobson made a number of public statements condemning violence against health service staff and promising tougher sentences in assault cases. In addition to the new HSAC guidlines, better enforcement of the existing legislation would help to tackle the problem. For example the removal of crown immunity in 1987 devolved responsibility for security to NHS trusts. The following pieces of legislation deal with employers' responsibilities for their employees' safety, including the risk of violence.

Health and Safety at Work Act 1974

This Act requires employers to establish safe systems of work, clearly including action against violence. The *Management of the Health and Safety at Work Regulations 1992* elaborate this through the risk assessment process – remove the risk at source and introduce comprehensive prevention policies to control unavoidable risks.

The Safety Representatives and Safety Committee Regulations 1977 and the Health and Safety (Consultation with Employees) Regulations 1996

These require employers to inform and consult employees about health and safety issues, directly and through trade unions or employee representatives.

The Reporting of Injuries, Diseases and Dangerous Occurrences Regulations 1995 (RIDDOR)

RIDDOR was amended in 1996 to include a requirement for employers to report to the HSE any instances of serious physical violence resulting in injury at work or arising from work (though some unions would like all violent incidents to be reportable, see for example Unison, 1997b).

The scale of the problem

Health care staff are at greater risk of work-related violence than the general population. The 1995 British Crime Survey revealed that 762 doctors per 10,000 and 580 nurses per 10,000, had experienced violence at work, compared with a general sample of 251 per 10,000. In a Unison survey 55 per cent of staff said they has been subjected to violence during the previous two years (Unison, 1997a), while a 1997 survey conducted with the *Nursing Times* and reported on BBC TV's 'Here and Now' stated that nearly half the nurses working in accident and emergency departments had been assaulted by patients and nearly all had been verbally abused.

Accident and emergency departments present an obvious risk: patients may be disoriented by the influence of disinhibiting drugs such as alcohol, or hallucinatory agents such as LSD or solvents, crack cocaine or ecstasy. They may suffer from undiagnosed or poorly monitored mental health problems, or have physical symptoms which trigger uncharacteristic responses to stress in unfamiliar surroundings. A&E patients may be suffering great stress, are possibly in pain, and nay be frightened about their condition and the treatment they may have to undergo. They may have been kept waiting for a long time, allowing frustration and aggression to build up. They may be in casualty following a fight, so will already be feeling violent and aggressive. They may have been brought in by groups of friends who want to hang around until they are treated. As studies on violence in A&E show, the potential for violence from a group is even greater: people want to show off to their peers, and the responsibility for their actions is shared by others, reducing individual shame and guilt. They are more likely to express their boredom and frustration in aggression (Walsh, 1986; Cembrowicz and Shepherd, 1992).

Violence is not confined to A&E and psychiatric units but can occur in any hospital department, or anywhere in the community. Nurses on the general ward or maternity unit may be less prepared for an assault and not equipped to deal with it. Handling violent incidents is much more likely to be covered in psychiatric nurse training and post-registration A&E nursing courses than in general nursing education.

How managers should protect staff

The primary responsibility for dealing with violence to staff lies fairly and squarely with employers, who can reduce the chances of it ever happening and help nurses deal with it in the safest and most effective way possible. Although ultimately it is nurses who face the violence, their ability to contain it is limited.

Risk assessment

The TUC (1997) comments that too many employer policies are merely procedures informing their workers what to do after violence has happened, instead of following the HSAC's risk assessment guidance, as follows.

1. *Identify the problem – look for hazards.*   Each trust should have a committee that is responsible for monitoring violence to staff. It should include health and safety and union representatives as well as management. A formal reporting system should be set up to find out where the incidents are occurring, how often, whether any part of the day or night is a particular problem, and whether the incident could have been prevented, for example with better security, more staff or better lighting. The existence of the committee should be well publicised to encourage staff to report incidents, making clear the potential benefits of the scheme in terms of improved staff safety. Even apparently trivial incidents should be included, such as verbal abuse and threats.

2. *Identify who might be harmed and how.*   The HSAC suggests that 'at risk' groups of employees should be identified. As well as permanent staff, these might include bank and agency staff, ancillary staff, and those who might visit high-risk areas.

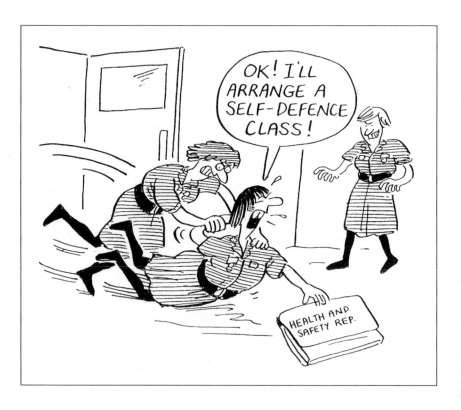

3. *Risk evaluation: are more precautions needed?* Avoidance of risks is the most effective precaution. Changes in working practices, organisation, information, training, incident reporting and responses, and staff support should be considered in an attempt to minimise the risk of violence and its effects.

4. *Record the results of risk assessments.* The results of risk assessments should be recorded and made available to managers, staff and union/staff representatives to enable them to review and revise them when necessary.

5. *Review and revise risk assessments.* Policy review should be integral to health and safety monitoring, in response to new information, any further incidents or accident statistics.

Buildings security

There is a wide range of sophisticated security equipment on the market, including video monitoring equipment and alarm systems. An analysis of the problem may convince some employers that these are necessary, but they may balk at the cost. Cheaper methods include using only one central entrance at night; installing effective locks on doors and windows, especially in nurses' homes; improving lighting in hospital corridors and grounds; and better maintenance of lighting.

Personal security

This should include alarm buttons in casualty departments and mental health and learning disability units, wired to ring in other departments and security desks, and personal alarms for community staff. If staff are having problems getting home after late shifts it may be possible, in consultation with bus companies, to alter bus schedules.

Staffing levels

There should be an adequate number of security staff patrolling the grounds, posted at entrances and available as back-up if staff are in difficulties. Community staff should work in pairs whenever possible, particularly in inner-city areas. Nurses in high-risk settings such as mental health and learning disability units should not be left alone without recourse to immediate help.

Environment

Long waits in casualty departments increase frustration and can trigger aggression. Casualty waiting areas should be made as pleasant as possible, with toys for children, up-to-date magazines, music and television to relieve boredom. There should be plenty of notices warning patients about how long they may have to wait, frequently updated information on the current waiting time, and sufficient clerical and triage staff to cope with fluctuations. The Patient's Charter has brought new standards, and these are to be welcomed, but it has also raised patients' expectations, potentially raising frustration levels if they are not met. Staff changing rooms should be in a busy, central part of the hospital, not down an ill-lit corridor or in another building. Care should be taken when planning departments to avoid unnecessary staff isolation.

Training

Training in how to deal with violent incidents is necessary for all nurses, not just those working in obviously high-risk areas. Nurses who are encouraged to believe they are self-defence experts may end up being even more seriously injured, for example by trying to restrain a patient instead of seeking help. Training in self-defence techniques is important, but learning how to prevent the situation from reaching that point – recognising that a potentially violent situation is developing, and containing and defusing the violence – is even more valuable. Useful de-escalation or defusing skills are described by Paterson *et al.* (1997). Self-defence should be used only as a last resort.

The HSAC recommends that staff are given training in the causes of violence; recognition of warning signs, interpersonal skills, and management strategies for dealing with violence at work.

Protecting yourself

Personal security

Use your health and safety rep to negotiate for more security and security back-up staff in hospitals and hospital residences, and for personal alarms for community nurses and other at-risk groups. Ask for in-service training to deal with violence, and self-defence classes. Report to your health and safety rep (and line manager) any staffing levels that could put your personal security at risk. This includes the withdrawal of security or portering staff. Try to avoid walking through the hospital grounds alone at night. Report broken lights to the works department.

Dealing with violence

Learn to recognise the potential for violence. A group of noisy or aggressive youths coming into casualty, for example, or a patient becoming verbally agitated or restless, gripping the side of his or her chair or talking loudly, may become physically aggressive. Your response can do a lot to defuse such situations:

- Treat potentially violent patients as responsible adults, even if they are not behaving that way. Address them by name. Explain what is going on. Ask permission for any procedure you are about to perform. Deal with the immediate issue, not the person's attitude.
- Keep your voice down. Loud noises can stimulate aggression and will pass on aggressive cues to the patients. Keep cool. Listen to their responses and seek solutions in them.
- Avoid a confrontational pose – stand sideways to those concerned, with your arms by your side, not folded. Don't look them straight in the eye; keep your gaze slightly lowered.
- Stand just out of arm's length: so that you are not invading their personal space and cannot be grabbed. Step back if you feel angry, and leave if you suspect violence is imminent. The best form of defence may be retreat: '[the HSE] advocate breakaway techniques with which [nurses] can protect themselves without hurting anyone' (Gulland, 1997b).
- Develop team protocols and strategies for dealing with violence in order to maximise consistency.
- If working in the community:
  - ensure someone knows where you are;
  - be aware of the nature of local environments, such as high-risk areas for crime, drugs and violence;
  - use safety equipment such as attack alarms and mobile phones;
  - follow management policies and report any violent incidents;
  - avoid night visits unless absolutely necessary;
  - avoid being alone in the GP surgery or health centre.

Unison's guidelines on violence emphasise that staff should feel certain their needs are taken into account, know what to do in the event of a violent incident, and feel confident that any call for help will be answered promptly. 'There is no magic recipe or guarantee of safety even if you follow all the rules . . . self-awareness will limit the risks' (RCN, 1994a).

Reporting violent incidents

Any violent incident should be recorded. It will improve your chances of compensation for any injury and it will help management identify how the incident could have been avoided. The record should include the following:

- Date, time and place of the incident.
- Whether it was a patient or relative.
- If it was a patient, his or her name, sex and age.
- A brief description of the incident.
- Details of action necessary and taken after the incident.
- Assessment of the offender's medical condition.
- Whether drugs or alcohol were involved.
- Any other contributory factors.

Compensation for injury

Patients are rarely prosecuted for assaulting staff and it is up to the individual rather than the health authority to bring an action. It is possible to claim compensation from the Criminal Injuries Compensation Authority (CICA) if you are injured as a result of violent crime; applications can be made to the CICA up to a year after the incident. Injury benefit is payable to the nurse or his/her spouse as a result of being injured in the course of his/her duties if earning ability is reduced by at least 10 per cent, if the nurse is on sick leave with reduced pay as a result of the injury or if the nurse dies as a result of the injury.

Good practice: setting up a violence hotline

Occupational health and safety staff in Frenchay Healthcare NHS Trust, when collating accident and dangerous occurrences data for their quarterly accident report, noted a trend of increasing physical abuse. Further research identified that not only nursing staff but also clerical and ancillary staff were affected. A working party proposed a three-phase approach:

1. Managers would undertake risk assessment to consider how working practices and the environment could be improved.
2. Training packages would be provided by the trust.
3. Occupational health advisers would provide a support network offering counselling and debriefing.

So the Violence Hotline was born and each member of staff was provided with a 'credit card' of information. The concept is simple: if staff have been bullied, threatened or attacked, they or a colleague can contact the 24-hour hotline. During working hours this call is followed up by occupational health staff, often working with the trust counsellor. Out of hours, an alternative message offers immediate support and promise of follow-up the next working day. Statistical evidence from accident reports shows that this three-phase approach has reduced violence to staff by patients and members of the public, while staff tell occupational health advisers they feel much more supported in their work environments.

Contact Frenchay Healthcare NHS Trust, Frenchay Hospital, Frenchay Park Road, Bristol BS16 1LE. See also the report *Occupational Health Nursing: contributing to healthier workplaces*.

Source: English National Board, 1998.

References and further reading on violence

Bibby, P. (1995) *Personal Safety for Health Care Workers.* Aldershot: Arena.

Brennan, W. (1997) 'Pressure points', *Nursing Times,* vol. 93, no. 43 (22 October), pp. 29–32.

Cembrowicz, S.P. and Shepherd, J. P. (1992) 'Violence in the Accident and Emergency Department', *Medicine, Science and the Law,* vol. 32, pp. 118–22.

Elson, L. (1997) 'Hospital Watch', *Nursing Standard,* vol. 11, no. 26 (19 March), pp. 26–7.

English National Board and Department of Health (1998) *Occupational Health Nursing: contributing to a healthier workplace.* London: DoH and ENB.

Gulland, A. (1997b) 'Safety first', *Nursing Times,* vol. 93, no. 50 (10 December), p. 18.

Health Services Advisory Committee (1987) *Violence to Staff in the Health Services.* London: HMSO.

HSAC (1997) *Violence and aggression to staff in health services: guidance on assessment and management.* Sudbury: Health and Safety Commission.

HSE (1987) *Violence to Staff. A Basis for Assessment and Prevention.* London: HMSO.

HSE (1997) *Violence at Work: A Guide for Employers* IND(G)69L (Rev). Sudbury: Health and Safety Executive.

Kidd, B and Stalk, C. (1995) *Management of Violence and Aggression in Health Care.* London: Royal College of Psychiatrists.

Labour Research Department (1997) *Stress, Bullying and Violence – a trade union guide.* London: LRD.

Paterson, B., Leadbetter, D. and McComish, A. (1997) 'De-escalation in the management of aggression and violence', *Nursing Times,* vol. 93, no. 36 (3 September), pp. 58–60.

RCN (1993) *Approaching with care: violence at work,* RCN Nursing Update Learning Unit 038, supplement to *Nursing Standard,* vol. 7, no. 52 (15 September).

RCN (1994a) *Violence and Community Nursing Staff: Advice for Nurses,* re-order no 000 383. London: RCN Labour Relations Department.

RCN (1994b) *Violence and Community Nursing Staff: A Royal College of Nursing Survey,* re-order no.000 381. London: RCN Labour Relations Department.

RCN (1994c) *Violence and Community Nursing Staff: Advice for Managers,* re-order no 000 382. London: RCN Labour Relations Department.

Shepherd, J. (ed.) (1994) *Violence in Health Care.* Oxford: Oxford Medical Publications.

TUC (1997) *Hazards at Work: TUC Guide to Health and Safety.* London: Trades Union Congress. See Chapter 28, 'Violence', pp. 251–5.

Unison (1997a) *Violence at Work – A guide to risk prevention,* pamphlet 1201. London: Unison.

Unison (1997b) *Violence at Work – A guide to risk prevention for Unison branches, stewards and safety representatives,* stock no. 1346. London: Unison.

Unison (1997c) *Violence at Work,* Health Staff Survey. London: Unison.

Walsh, M. (1986) 'On the frontline', *Nursing Times,* vol. 82 no. 37 (10 September), pp. 55–56.

Warren, J. and Beadsmore, A. (1997) 'Preventing violence on mental health wards', *Nursing Times,* vol. 93, no. 34 (20 August), pp. 47–8.

Bullying

Sticks and stones may break my bones, but names will never hurt me, we were told as children – but unfortunately it isn't strictly true. Workplace bullying has become more prominent in the competitive atmosphere of health services in the 1990s. An MSF survey in 1995 found that 72 per cent of the employers surveyed had no policy for tackling bullying, though 29 per cent of the employees thought that bullying had worsened in their workplace over the previous five years (Spiers, 1995). When the TUC opened a telephone helpline for bullied workers in 1997, it received 1771 calls on the first day alone.

Bullying, like violence, is unacceptable. It should be resisted and the bullies held to account in all circumstances. Employers have a duty to protect the health and safety of their employees, and bullying or tolerating bullying behaviour constitutes a failure on their part. This section looks at the incidence of workplace bullying, its causes and ways to combat it.

Bullying may be defined as 'misuse or abuse of power; behaviour which is persistent, offensive, malicious or intimidating; or an unfair use of penal sanctions' (Cox, 1997). It can take many forms, such as:

- Shouting at a colleague or patient.
- Criticising a colleague in front of others.
- Undermining staff by replacing their responsibilities with menial tasks.
- Withholding information deliberately in order to affect a colleague's performance.
- Humiliating or ridiculing someone.
- Setting impossible objectives (RCN, 1997a).

Continuous change and reorganisation have characterised health services in the 1990s, and the style has been set from the top by some senior managers who are under pressure to achieve and insecure about their own positions. Some managers have been promoted without management skills training, which may make them afraid to admit their limitations. In the circumstances, their anxiety may provoke poor judgment, reactive behaviour and panic disciplinary overreaction (Long, 1996).

A 1996 Unison survey showed that two-thirds of its members had experienced or witnessed bullying, in 83 per cent of cases by a manager. Perhaps the hierarchical structure of nursing encourages bullying, and nurses seem reluctant to speak out against bullies for fear of victimisation – which perpetuates the culture of harassment. Most health service unions have now developed antibullying policies and support their members in tackling the bullies.

Four types of bully have been identified by workplace health guru Cary Cooper. Pathological bullies will persecute and torment any victim they can find. Situational bullies are people who threaten subordinates when they are under pressure. A third group, role-playing bullies, think they must act in certain ways, often the result of autocratic management style and 'institutionalised bullying'. Punishing bullies believe you get the best out of staff by punishment rather than reward.

Ironically, it may be the innovative and competent nurse who is bullied; bullying is a symptom of insecurity, even in a powerful manager, who may manipulate and belittle others. This is difficult to combat in isolation. Nurses are not always supportive of each other, so a bully's victim may feel isolated and demoralised.

New legislation such as the Protection from Harassment Act 1997 will make harassment a criminal offence. In extreme cases recourse to the law may be necessary, and preferable to trying to bear the anguish, depression and stress of being bullied. Unfortunately many managers do not take bullying seriously and turn complaints back on the victim – saying they can't take a joke, or if they can't cope, they should leave. Given the misuse of power that is central to bullying, it's not surprising that many nurses are too afraid to complain.

If you are the victim of a bully:

- Remember that bullying is not only wrong, but illegal.
- Enlist the support of your union.
- Keep records of specific incidents.
- Contact an antibullying advice group (see 'Contact organisations' at the end of this section).
- Give your employer written statements of bullying incidents, and offer sample policies on antiharassment to supplement existing workplace policies.
- Suggest the creation of an antibullying, antiharassment network in your workplace, with a designated coordinator and link members, and a 'no blame' disciplinary policy.
- Go as high as it takes to get the bullying taken seriously.

In extreme cases:

- Consider grievance procedures.
- Consider civil court action for personal injury, and action against your employer for breach of employment contract.
- If you have left work because of the pressure, consult your union about a constructive dismissal claim.
- Use the Protection from Harassment Act 1997, when it becomes operative.

Equal opportunities

Women, as well as nurses from ethnic minorities, are more likely to be harassed or bullied, so antibullying policies should be implemented in conjunction with antiracist and equal opportunities policies (Cox, 1997).

Where there is evidence of sexual or racial harassment, the Sex Discrimination Act 1975 and/or the Race Relations Act 1976 should be used in arguing that the employer has failed to do everything possible to prevent bullying. Successful case precedents suggest that this is a useful approach. Yet bullying would be largely eliminated if the following three points were observed:

- Employers should ensure that their equal opportunities policy is given more than lip-service, and is monitored continuously.
- Equal opportunities policies should include specific reference to bullying, making its unacceptability clear.
- Employees should be made aware of this active discouragement of bullying, and asked to bring incidents to management's attention.

Examples of good practice

'Contact officers'

An antiharassment policy was launched at University Hospital Birmingham NHS Trust in 1996, with 'contact officers' in the personnel department, later supplemented by nurses, managers and ancillary staff, to provide support for staff who are bullied and to try to halt the bullying before further sanctions such as disciplinary procedures are required. A contact officer listens to nurses who want to talk about their experiences, and offers confidential advice and guidance (important if your manager is the bully).

Staff support adviser Kate MacArthur hopes the policy 'will be a wake-up call to managers who do not realise that what they think is a tough management style is tantamount to bullying.' The trust is attempting a 'no blame' disciplinary policy.

Anti-harassment policy

In South Birmingham Mental Health NHS Trust the staff support service has drawn up an antiharassment policy, with the director of staff's support and eight nurses providing counselling and support, including work to eliminate bullying and harassment. 'There's been a change in culture since we launched an anti-harassment policy. . ... We've been raising awareness about what harassment is and telling people what kind of behaviour is acceptable and what is not. . . . Everything is becoming more open here', says Karen Lockhart, trust director of staff support. Lyn Witheridge, the trust's chief executive, describes her own experience of being bullied: 'I felt completely isolated and humiliated but I didn't realise I was being bullied. I thought: "I'm an adult, how can I be bullied?" Workplace bullying is insidious and if nothing is done, it just goes on and on.'

References and further reading on bullying

Cox, C. (1997) 'Right on your side', *Nursing Standard*, vol. 11, no. 35 (21 May), pp. 25–6

Gulland, A. (1997a) 'Nipping the bully in the bud', *Nursing Times*, vol. 93, no. 25 (18 June), p. 18.

Hancock, C. (1997) 'Keeping bullies at bay', *Nursing Standard*, vol. 11, no. 41 (2 July), p. 20.

Howard, G. (1995) 'Workplace bullying: the legal perspective', *Occupational Health*, vol. 47, no. 11 (November), pp. 378–9.

LRD (1997) *Stress, Bullying and Violence – a trade union action guide*. London: Labour Research Department.

Long, J. (1996) 'Battle of the bullies', *Nursing Management*, vol. 3, no. 6 (October), pp. 10–11.

RCN (1997a) *Nursing a Grievance? An RCN guide to tackling harassment and bullying at work*, re-order No 000 742. London: Royal College of Nursing.

RCN (1997b) *RCN Model policy on harassment and bullying*, re-order No 000 763. London: Royal College of Nursing.

Spiers, C. (1995) 'Strategies for harassment counselling', *Occupational Health*, vol. 47, no. 11 (November), pp. 381–2

Unison (1997) 'Bullying at Work', pamphlet 1281 (London: Unison. Includes a good checklist for assessing management policies, a draft agreement on prevention, a draft bullying survey and a tear-off noticeboard poster.

Contact organisations

Unison, **MSF**, the **Labour Research Department**, the **TUC** and **ACAS** have all produced literature on bullying.

The Andrea Adams Trust (support and information), Shalimar House, 24 Derek Avenue, Hove, East Sussex BN3 4PF.

Campaign against Bullying at Work (CABAW), MSF, 50 Southwark Street, London SE1 1UN.

The Industrial Society's Information Service (advice on bullying at work), tel: 0171 262 2401.

National Association for Staff Support (NASS), 9 Caradon Close, Woking, Surrey GU21 3DU. tel: 01483 771599.

National Harassment Network (information and support), University of Central Lancashire, Preston PR1 2HE. tel: 01772 893 398.

National Workplace Bullying Advice Line, tel: 01235 834 548.

Workplace Bullying, Dept NS, PO Box 77, Wantage, Oxon OX12 8YP.

Whistleblowing

Mention whistleblowing – speaking out publicly against poor standards or working conditions – and many nurses will think of campaigns such as the RCN's 1991 'Whistleblow', or of Graham Pink, the charge nurse who went public about his concern for the standards of care on his elderly care ward, and was disciplined and labelled a troublemaker. Whistleblowing is never easy, and probably never will be – it's initially far more comfortable to keep quiet, pretend nothing untoward is happening and block out uncomfortable feelings about falling standards of care, staff shortages, bullying and harassment. Yet whistleblowing is the most natural instinct of someone who cares enough about their patients and their self-esteem or professional standards to want to do something when things seem wrong.

Whistleblowing is implicitly encouraged in the UKCC Code of Professional Conduct, which states that each registered nurse, midwife and health visitor is accountable for his or her practice, and in exercising professional accountability shall:

- Always act in such a way as to promote and safeguard the well-being and interests of patients/clients.
- Ensure that no action or omission on his/her part or within his/her sphere of influence is detrimental to the condition or safety of patients/clients.
- Have regard to the environment of care and its physical, psychological and social effects on patients/clients, and also to the adequacy of resources, and make known to appropriate persons or authorities any circumstances which could place patients/clients in jeopardy or militate against safe practice.

Dos and don'ts

There is safety in numbers. Graham Pink's approach was courageous, but his was a lone voice, albeit well supported by the press and some of the nursing hierarchy, and shown with the benefit of hindsight to have been vindicated. Most nurses who have spoken their mind at work, even in a small way, will know how the apparently solid support of 'coffee-room grumbles' soon evaporates when the same subject is broached at 'report' or in a team meeting. The rules of whistleblowing, then, are as follows.

Facts

Make sure you have evidence to support your concerns, preferably witnessed and in writing. Consult with colleagues, sympathetic managers, union reps, counselling services, groups such as Freedom to Nurse (see 'Contact organisations') or the UKCC. Maintain patient confidentiality in all statements, public and private.

Support

Make sure you have the support of your colleagues, if you need it, your line manager if possible, and your union steward or safety rep. If your managers dispute your case, you will need all the support you can get.

Strategy

Reflect on what you feel is the central problem, and consider what you think are the possible courses of action and their possible outcomes – what you would like, and what you would settle for.

Official channels

Use official channels in your workplace if at all possible – you must be seen to have tried every avenue, even if you fail.

If all else fails. . .

Then, and only then should you consider going to the press or other media. Again, do your homework first: discuss the issues with your union reps, with press officers if possible, and plan a press statement and possible responses to questions by journalists, even radio or television interviews. Be sure of your facts, and be sure of yourself. To get this far you have to be thick-skinned, well supported and, some would say, above reproach. Your managers and the media may latch on to any misdemeanour or misjudgment of yours, past or present, and use it to undermine your case, even if it is a good one.

Gagging clauses

The need for – and risks of – whistleblowing became more marked in the 1990s, when many trusts inserted so-called gagging clauses in their contracts of employment. These generally required staff to seek managers' approval before making any public comment about their workplace. The clauses were ostensibly introduced to protect patient confidentiality, were sometimes used to protect commercial sensitivity, but usually had the prime motive of avoiding the bad publicity which evidence of poor standards would bring. Contracts with purchasers were at stake, the argument went, so it was better to keep quiet.

As the RCN (1992) points out, patient confidentiality is already safe-guarded by the Code of Professional Conduct, so its inclusion in employment contracts is at best redundant, at worst a dangerous and intimidatory management tactic. In its 1991–2 campaign the RCN set out 10 points for whistleblowers, in response to the defensiveness of NHS management:

1. *Stronger support for the UKCC Code of Professional Conduct.* Employers were encouraged to incorporate the code in employment contracts, though comparatively few did so.
2. *Abolish gagging clauses.* Few trusts did so spontaneously.
3. *Confidential counselling at unit level.* This is rare in the NHS, and has mostly been left to the unions to provide (for more details see Chapter 4, 'Stress').

4. *Training for managers.* Managers should be given training in handling staff concerns, to avoid unnecessary confrontation. This, too, seems to have been neglected.

5. *Agreed protocol for concerned staff.* Each unit should have an agreed protocol for staff concerns to be expressed without fear of reprisal, and with promise of appropriate responses to resolve concerns.

6. *Agreed standards of care.* Some progress has been made on this through widespread standards and audit initiatives and clinical effectiveness schemes, which have provided benchmarks to be used in pressing for adequate resources and safe working conditions.

7. *Stronger community health councils.* The underresourcing and ultimate impotence of CHCs is a continuing cause for regret.

8. *Managers' code of conduct.* Caught between the demands of the UKCC code and those of their managers, many nurses felt cornered. It was argued that managers should also be bound by a professional code.

9. *A national inspectorate for health care.* It was suggested that an inspectorate modelled on that for education would work effectively for health care and act as an independent arbiter.

10. *Legislative protection.* The first nine points of these proposals would make whistleblowing virtually unnecessary, but as an additional safeguard, the RCN wanted freedom to speak out without fear of recrimination guaranteed in law.

These proposals, and similar ones by other health service unions, were not received favourably by the Conservative government. Repeated lobbying of the opposition parties was well directed, and after Labour's election in 1997 the climate of opinion started to change. For example the Department of Health pledged itself to a 'New fairer deal for NHS staff' in a press release issued on 25 September 1997. Health minister Alan Milburn launched a staff-centred human resources strategy with a five-point action plan, prefaced by the outlawing of gagging clauses. He said:

> The health and well-being of staff is central to the health and well-being of the NHS. The interests of staff and the interests of patients are inextricably linked. Treat staff well, and they will treat patients better. . . . For too long the emphasis had been on what we expect from staff without addressing their concerns. . . . Commitment is a two-way street.

The Milburn strategy proposes to promote health at work by stopping avoidable accidents and having proper strategies for avoiding violence; recognise and deal with racism head on; ensure sufficiently flexible staffing policies to make the best use of staff; provide improved standards of food and accommodation for junior doctors on call; and ensure that all staff can speak out without victimisation when necessary.

Conclusion

Violence and bullying, gagging of staff, the need for but high risk of whistleblowing – these are symptoms of the climate in which nurses and other health care staff have worked for many years. It will take more than mavericks such as Graham Pink, whistleblow schemes or even ministerial five-point plans to reduce the risks and hazards, but they are important examples for nurses committed to their profession and their patients.

References and further reading on whistleblowing

Castledine, G. (1993) 'Should nurses tell tales?', *British Journal of Nursing*, vol. 2, no. 10 (27 May), p. 532.

Millar, B. (1997) 'Honesty on trial', *Nursing Times*, vol. 93, no. 35 (27 August), pp. 10–11

Pyne, R. and Hunt, G. (1992) 'Changing code. . .', *Nursing Times*, vol. 88, no. 25 (17 June), pp. 20–2.

RCN (1992) 'Nurses Speak Out – Whistleblow: A Report on the Work of the RCN Whistleblow Schemes, order no. 000 170. London: Royal College of Nursing.

Siddall, A. (1997a) 'How to speak out and keep your job', *Nursing Standard*, vol. 11, no. 51 (10 September), p. 14.

Siddall, A. (1997b) ' Welcoming the whistleblowers', *Nursing Times* vol. 93, no. 40 (1 October), p. 20.

Snell, J. (1997) 'Thinking Pink', *Nursing Times*, vol. 93, no. 32 (6 August), p. 34.

Unison (1997) *Campaigning on Health and Safety: A handbook for Unison safety representatives*, stock no. 1352. London: Unison.

Contact organisations

Freedom to Nurse, PO Box 37, Worksop, Nottinghamshire S80 1ZT.

National Association for Staff Support, 9 Caradon Close, Woking, Surrey GU21 3DU.

RCN Nurseline, 8–10 Crown Hill, Croydon, Surrey CR0 1RZ.

6 *Toxic substances and agents*

Health workers are exposed to a huge range of toxic substances in the drugs, chemicals and gases they work with. The hazards these substances present, particularly their long-term effects, are often incompletely understood even by the manufacturers and scientists. And the people who have to handle them may not think to associate periodic headaches, skin complaints, dizziness or nausea with the workplace.

Toxic chemicals

Every day nurses handle a huge range of chemicals – disinfectants, solvents, cleaning agents – which can have both local and systemic toxic effects. Many of them are so familiar, both at home and at work, that it is difficult to associate them with any adverse symptoms. Little information is ever circulated about potential hazards and how to protect yourself.

Chemicals can be inhaled as dust or vapour, absorbed through the skin, splashed into the eyes or swallowed. Their effects can include:

- occupational dermatitis
- dizziness
- headaches
- breathlessness
- irritability
- nausea and vomiting
- nose and throat irritation
- tiredness
- sleeplessness
- chest trouble
- worsening of asthmatic and eczematous conditions
- reproductive hazards: miscarriage, infertility, congenital abnormalities
- heart, lung and liver disease
- kidney damage
- cancer.

The most common side-effect, particularly among nurses, is occupational dermatitis – a generic term referring to irritation and inflammation of the skin, in varying degrees of severity (sometimes known as contact dermatitis (HSE, 1997). It is the commonest occupational disease in industry and the

---

Box 6.1   *Badly handled*

A health authority which ignored its responsibility to ensure the health of a nurse in an endoscopy unit working with glutaraldehyde was found to have been in breach of the Health and Safety at Work etc. Act. Bristol and Weston Health Authority was fined £1000 plus costs.

---

greatest single cause of prolonged sickness absence. The HSE estimates that around 84,000 people a year contract it, at a cost of up to £20 million a year. Nurses are at risk because of frequent hand washing and exposure to a range of skin irritants, including drugs, disinfectants, cleaning agents, and latex gloves. It is so common among nurses that most regard it as an occupational hazard and simply put up with it (but see Box 6.1). How often have you ruefully regarded your chapped and blistered hands, reached for the hand cream and carried on, putting it down to winter weather and 'one of the perks of the job'?

Three groups of substances can cause dermatitis:

Primary skin irritants

These cause direct inflammation of the skin in the area of immediate contact only. They include bleaches and phenolic compounds such as some disinfectants.

Sensitisers

These substances cause a specific allergic response known as sensitisation. Several episodes of exposure are usually required and a person who does become sensitive to a particular substance may do so after years of exposure with no problems. Once sensitised, however, you are likely to remain so, reacting to the particular substance even with minimal contact. The effects may extend beyond the area of direct contact, causing swelling of the lips, eyelids and face, and nausea or vomiting. Sensitising agents include some drugs (notably antibiotics) and antibacterial soaps. Patch testing may be needed to pinpoint the precise substance.

Photosensitizers

These substances may be either irritants or sensitisers but require the stimulus of sunlight or ultraviolet light.

Protection

Under current health and safety legislation, employers are obliged to assess the risks and take actions to prevent toxic effects. The following checklist is a guide to regular monitoring. Don't wait until the accident happens.

Chemicals – action checklist

1. Get information on the substances you deal with. Full information on all chemicals should be provided by the manufacturer and made available by the employing authority. The provision of relevant information is a key part of the employer's responsibilities under the Health and Safety at Work Act, the Management of Health and Safety at Work Regulations 1992, and COSHH. Your health and safety rep should circulate this information. The information you should be provided with includes the chemical name of a substance, its trade name, its known hazards, storage precautions and precautions for its use. Suppliers have specific obligations under the Chemical (Hazard Information and Packaging) Regulations 1995 (HSE 1997).

2. Wherever possible, potential irritants should be replaced with non-harmful substances. Safety reps can negotiate for substitutes. Ethylene oxide, for example, is now considered so dangerous that it should no longer be used at all. Be careful, though, that the substitute isn't just as bad. Formaldehyde is often used as a substitute, and while not as dangerous, it still has some serious side-effects (Table 6.1). Chemical disinfectants are often unnecessary: detergents or heat disinfection can be equally or more effective, and cheaper. Question the use of disinfectants on your ward or unit.

3. As a last resort, protective clothing will reduce skin contact with toxic substances, and masks will provide a certain amount of protection from toxic dust and aerosols. Extra clothing can include gloves, gowns, aprons, eye shields or safety spectacles and boots, according to the nature of the work and level of risk. Latex gloves, worn by sensitised staff, may inflame or actually provoke dermatitis due to an allergic response to the compounds in the latex or a build-up of moisture within the gloves. PVC or silicone gloves can be used instead of latex and the gloves should have cotton linings. Cotton gloves are only useful to handle powders. They provide little protection against liquids.

4. Ventilation. Check that your workplace is adequately ventilated, including mechanical ventilation systems where chemicals are stored, prepared or used in high concentrations.

5. Training. Staff who use known irritants and sensitisers should be trained in handling and safety procedures, including the appropriate use of protective clothing and storage and transport precautions.

6. Report and record any incidences of dermatitis and other skin complaints; their source should be fully investigated and the need for additional protection explored.

7. Skin care. Cover all wounds and abrasions; use a bland soap for hand washing wherever possible, and dry your hands thoroughly. Barrier creams are unlikely to prevent allergic contact dermatitis but can help to

Table 6.1   *Chemicals in common hospital use: their associated hazards*

Chemical	Use	Potential hazards
Phenolic disinfectants Clear: Sudol, Hycolin, Clearsol, Stericol White: Izal	Disinfectant, fumigant	Irritant to eyes, nose, throat; giddiness, nausea, headaches; skin sensitiser. Long term exposure to vapour could cause kidney damage
Hypochlorites Liquids: Chloros, Sterite, Domestos, Septomite, Diversol	Disinfectant, cleaning	Skin irritation; eye and nose irritation
Alcohol	Skin prep, disinfectant	Skin irritation; giddiness, nausea, headaches
Iodine	Skin prep	Skin sensitiser
Formaldehyde (liquid or gas): Formalin	Steriliser, disinfectant	Severe dermatitis and sensitisation; respiratory effects; nose and eye irritation; possible risk of respiratory carcinomas
Ethylene oxide	Steriliser	Severe dermatitis (burns or blisters); irritant to eyes and respiratory tract – can cause conjunctivitis, bronchitis and pneumonia; dizziness, vomiting, abdominal pain; neuropathic effects, e.g. damage to peripheral nerves, paralysis, death if exposed to very high levels; blood disorders – high white cell count, chronic anaemia, leukaemia; possibly carcinogenic; reproductive effects – birth defects, chromosomal damage; highly inflammable, potentially explosive
Glutaraldehyde: e.g. Cidex, Tego-Dor, Fectol	Antiseptic, steriliser	Eye, skin, lung irritation; contact dermatitis; headaches, dizziness, slowed reactions; can cause unconsciousness at high levels; possible liver damage – possibly carcinogenic; blood changes; not explosive but reacts violently with oxidising agents – should be stored alone
Mercury	Thermometers	Severe skin reactions; contact with large quantities may have reproductive effects and can cause immediate anaphylaxis

make skin cleaning easier and less aggressive. Moisturising creams can help to replace the natural skin grease removed by some solvents.

8. Health surveillance. Staff regularly exposed to known irritants should be monitored. This could include blood and urine tests, skin tests and checks on lung, liver and kidney function, depending on the chemicals used and the level of exposure. Staff with a history of skin problems should be made aware of the risk at the beginning of their employment.

9. Accidents. If you splash any chemical in your eye, rinse it immediately and thoroughly with plenty of cold water; if any is swallowed, rinse your mouth with water. The usual advice is also to drink plenty of water. In both cases report the incident and seek medical advice immediately (See 'Contact organisations' at the end of this chapter). Chemicals splashed on the skin should be washed off immediately. If they splash on your clothes or uniform, change before they can soak through to the skin.

Glutaraldehyde

Glutaraldehyde is the liquid chemical disinfectant of choice for heat-sensitive instruments such as flexible endoscopes. It is one of a number of aldehydes, available since the 1960s, and is used by hospitals, dentists, GPs, vets and others for the disinfection and sterilisation of their instruments. A closely related chemical, formaldehyde, is used in many manufacturing processes, for example food, paper, timber products and paints.

Its value as a sterilising agent lies in its broad antimicrobial properties – bactericidal, fungicidal and viricidal; it is also non-corrosive (MDA, 1996). The problem with glutaraldehyde, however, is that it is toxic, bio-irritant and sensitising, having irritant effects on the eyes, skin and respiratory tract. Direct contact results in dermatitis or exacerbates eczema. It vapourises at room temperature, and the vapour may cause rhinitis, asthma or conjunctivitis. It may also result in dizziness, headaches, nausea or skin discolouring (Cowan *et al.*, 1993). Sensitisation produces further allergic reactions and sometimes a total loss of tolerance to chemicals (O'Connor, 1997a).

The HSE lowered the occupational exposure standard of 0.2 parts per million in 1997, recommending a new maximum exposure level of 0.05 parts per million, in line with European and US standards.

Risk assessment

Glutaraldehyde use is covered by the COSHH regulations, requiring a risk assessment and either alternatives to or limits on the risks of its continued use. Suggested ways of reducing risk include the following:

*   A written safety policy on glutaraldehyde.
*   Use of automated washers with a lower potential for skin contact from splashing. Effective sealing is necessary, to avoid increased exposure to vapour.

- Always keep lids on troughs, waste bins and buckets, to help maintain low levels of exposure.
- Suitable local exhaust ventilation.
- Regular monitoring of air samples (see Box 6.2).

Protection

Glutaraldehyde should be stored in a cool, dry environment, in order to minimise vapourisation. Personal protective measures when handling the chemical include wearing a plastic apron and possibly a gown, face mask or goggles, respiratory protection and long gloves.

Health surveillance of people exposed to glutaraldehyde should include pre-employment medical checks for a history of asthma or allergic responses.

Box 6.2 *Innovative practice*

The Inverclyde Royal NHS Trust wished to upgrade its cold disinfection equipment, which used glutaraldehyde. Although personal protective equipment was provided and used, there were complaints about the smell and fumes, as well as eye irritation and breathing problems. The areas were normally ventilated by the supply/extract system in use in the hospital. Significant exposures occurred when endoscopes were being put into trays, syringed to remove air and subsequently removed from the trays and rinsed in water; and also when there was a requirement to disinfect the equipment and to drain depleted glutaraldehyde solution.

Exposure to glutaraldehyde was experienced by those operating the equipment, those nearby and potentially by the person using the endoscope if correct rinsing was not undertaken. Atmospheric monitoring of the sluice and procedure room was considered the only way to establish a baseline of exposure levels, and personal monitoring and background concentration readings were undertaken.

The most significant exposure was during the disposal of used solutions and the disinfection/removal of endoscopes from the tray, with subsequent washing. Significant levels were found 20 minutes after contact with glutaraldehyde in the sluice, so early return to the sluice after disinfecting endoscopes was in itself hazardous.

Economics and design led to the selection of a fully contained, automatic system with fan-assisted removal of any residual fumes. The machine has now been operating successfully for 18 months and within that time has provided a consistent service and maintained the required air standard.

Source: HSAC, 1997.

Any occurrence of occupational asthma or contact dermatitis should be reported and investigated.

Alternatives to glutaraldehyde include peracetic acid and chlorine dioxide. Peracetic acid is less irritant than glutaraldehyde and does not present a respiratory hazard. It contains hydrogen peroxide and acetic acid, however, which are in themselves hazardous. It can corrode copper alloys and damage component parts of endoscope washers (Cowan, 1997). Its actions are bactericidal, fungicidal, viricidal and tuberculocidal. It may also have a more rapid action than glutaraldehyde. Peracetic acid is more expensive than glutaraldehyde, but the cost may be off-set by its advantages.

Chlorine dioxide has a similar range of actions to peracetic acid and is claimed by manufacturers to be non-toxic and non-corrosive. Clinical studies, however, have shown that strong, unpleasant chlorine and chlorine dioxide fumes are given off during its preparation and use (Babb and Bradley, 1995).

In conclusion, glutaraldehyde, like all toxic substances and agents, should be treated with care, and whenever possible the safest possible substances used. COSHH regulations and risk assessment should be uppermost in the mind of all staff when working with hazardous substances.

Latex

During the 1990s it has become obvious that latex products present a major health risk. In part, this may be an unexpected by-product of the increased use of gloves in clinical procedures to protect against viruses such as HIV and hepatitis B in blood and other body fluids, and as a precaution when handling toxic substances such as cytotoxic drugs, but that is not the whole story.

A vast range of medical products contain latex (Moore, 1994), including adhesive tape, ambu-bags, bulb syringes, colostomy pouches, condom-type continence aids, elasticated bandages, electrode pads, enema tubing, fluid-warming blankets, gloves (sterile and non-sterile), haemodialysis equipment, incubators, syringes, protective sheets, stethoscope tubing, stomach and gastrointestinal tubes, tourniquets, urinary catheters and wound drains.

There are no accurate figures for the number of nurses affected by latex allergy in the UK, but estimates of its prevalence range from 2.9 per cent to 17.6 per cent (Thompson, 1997). A recent study of 8000 UK health service staff found that 43 per cent of respondents had irritation and type IV sensitivity to latex (Box 6.3) and 10 per cent had type I (Bennett, 1997). There has been extensive reporting and research into the problem in the USA, and around 1000 cases of allergic or anaphylactic reactions (including 15 deaths) have been reported to the Food and Drug Administration. The *Nursing Times'* 1994 campaign to raise awareness of the issue had such a large response from nurses that it continued for over a year (Booth, 1994, 1995; Thomas, 1994).

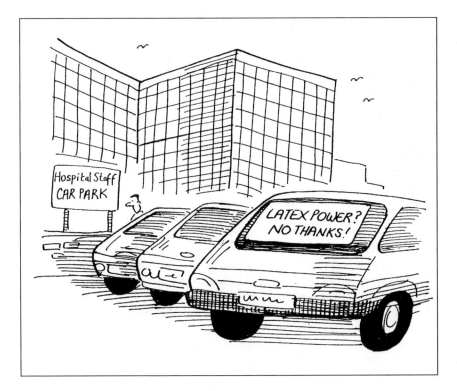

Box 6.3 *Types of hypersensitivity*

There are four types of hypersensitivity reaction (the Gell and Coombs classification), though these reactions may overlap:

Type I is triggered by antigens which penetrate the skin, the respiratory tract or the gastrointestinal tract.

Type II produces reactions on the cell surfaces of antibodies and antigens, such as that which follows an incompatible blood transfusion.

Type III occurs with antigen/antibody responses in the tissues, resulting in cell damage such as febrile conditions, vasculitis and inflamed joints.

Type IV: delayed hypersensitivity. Unlike other hypersensitivity reactions, this is not accompanied by antibody formation; instead, sensitised T-lymphocytes and macrophages respond to the allergen, resulting in tissue damage. It is also known as 'cell-mediated' hypersensitivity.

Allergy and hypersensitivity

An allergy is an abnormal physiological response to any substance normally considered harmless, such as pollen or grass, which are termed allergens. Reaction to a substance may be immediate, but subsides once contact with the allergen is removed. An allergy is generally a localised (non-systemic) histamine reaction, such as occurs with eczema, asthma, hay fever or food allergies.

Hypersensitivity is described as 'an immunological reaction resulting in tissue damage rather than repair or recovery' (Thompson *et al.*, 1994). It occurs after previous contact with an allergen, and is literally an excessive sensitivity to a substance, with local and systemic symptoms, which range from mild eczema to life-threatening anaphylactic shock.

In the case of latex allergy, or more accurately, latex hypersensitivity, it is thought that the corn starch powder which is added to gloves to make them easier to put on may draw the 'extractable proteins' of latex from the gloves, allowing them to be inhaled as atmospheric dust. If you become sensitised to latex you should avoid all latex products.

Symptoms can be mild, experienced as an itchy rash, or gross, including respiratory problems such as wheezing, shortness of breath and anaphylaxis. With latex, hypersensitivity is of type I and type IV (see Box 6.3). It may be weeks or years before a hypersensitive response is experienced, but it is irreversible.

Latex sensitivity type I is known as immediate hypersensitivity. Immunoglobulin E (IgE) antibodies are produced upon exposure to the allergen. Symptoms appear quickly, between five and 30 minutes after exposure, and may include wheal and flare reactions, skin reddening and wheezing. There is also a risk of anaphylactic shock, cardiac arrhythmias or arrest and death. For some individuals, just close proximity to latex produces a reaction and the need to avoid latex will mean a job change or even early retirement. Once the latex is removed from contact, the symptoms usually disappear within two hours.

Latex sensitivity type IV is known as delayed or cell-mediated hypersensitivity. This is the most common type of latex allergy, occurring when T-lymphages and macrophages are activated by the allergen – usually chemical additives used in the manufacture of latex products and found on the surface of latex – producing tissue damage. This does not necessarily appear rapidly – it may be six to 48 hours after exposure – and produces a contact dermatitis (not to be confused with irritant contact dermatitis), skin reddening (erythema), skin cracking and blistering, pruritis, oedema and eczema on the fingers, palms, and forearms.

Diagnosis can be made most accurately by a skin prick test, or less accurately by a radio-allergosorbent test (RAST) or an enzyme-linked immunosorbent test (ELISA).

Action

Many employers have drawn up practice guidelines, screening tools and education programmes for staff and patients in order to minimise the risk of latex sensitisation. In the USA, the American Association of Nurse Anaesthetists has suggested the definition of 'latex-free environments', many hospitals have drawn up latex protocols, and some nurses have filed lawsuits because of respiratory disease allegedly caused by latex exposure. In 1993 the Food and Drug Administration ruled that a prominent warning should be placed on all medical devices containing latex. In the UK, the MDA has published guidance on latex sensitisation, which is available for all health care employers (see 'Contact organisations' at the end of this section).

Action checklist

1. The EU Personal Protective Equipment Regulations 1992 legally require employers to provide safe equipment. Make sure your employer has a policy on latex sensitisation, with a commitment to providing latex-free or low allergenic products to anyone who requires them.
2. Anyone affected by latex hypersensitivity should be covered by the Disability Discrimination Act, which requires that if people acquire disabilities through work, 'reasonable adjustment' of the workplace must be made. The RCN is supporting some prematurely retired nurses with latex sensitivity in filing civil claims for negligence against employers (Waters, 1997).
3. All nurses should be offered screening and sensitivity testing.
4. The extractable protein levels on all gloves should be marked (no test for this exists yet, but a European Standard is being developed, which it is hoped will be usable when the EU Medical Devices Directive is adopted in 1998).
5. Health services supplies departments should refuse to buy products which exceed the maximum acceptable level of extractable proteins, once this has been set.
6. Make your practice as safe as possible:

   - be aware of latex risks;
   - avoid using latex gloves whenever possible;
   - if this is unavoidable, for example when non–latex gloves are too restrictive, avoid using powdered latex gloves;
   - report any irritation to the skin after contact or suspected contact with latex;
   - wash hands thoroughly after glove use;
   - review workplace policies on glove use.

References, further reading and resources on toxic chemicals

AANA (1993) 'American Association of Nurse Anesthetists Latex Allergy Protocol'. *Journal of American Association of Nurse Anesthetists*, vol. 61, no. 3, pp. 223–4

Abbott, L. (1995) 'The use and effects of glutaraldehyde: a review', *Occupational Health*, vol. 47, no. 7 (June), pp. 238–9.

Babb, J. R. and Bradley, C. R. (1995) 'A review of glutaraldehyde alternatives'. *British Journal of Theatre Nursing*, vol. 5, no. 7 (October), pp. 20–4.

Bennett, D. (1997) 'Throw down the gauntlet', *Nursing Times*, vol. 93, no. 46 (12 November), pp. 14–15.

Booth, B. (1994) 'Sensitivity test', *Nursing Times*, vol. 90, no. 36 (7 September), pp. 30–2.

Booth, B. (1995) 'Hand in glove', *Nursing Times*, vol. 91, no. 4 (25 January), pp. 22–3.

Booth, B. (1996) 'Latex allergy: a growing problem in health care', *Professional Nurse*, vol. 11, no. 5 (February), pp. 316–19.

Bullard, J. (1991) 'Use and abuse of glutaraldehyde', *Nursing Times*, vol. 87, no. 38 (18 September) pp. 70–1.

Cole, A. (1997) 'Gloves: the pros and cons'. *Nursing Times*, vol. 93, no. 6 (5 February), pp. 44–6.

Cowan, T. (1997) 'Sterilising solutions for heat sensitive instruments', *Professional Nurse*, vol. 13, no. 1 (October), pp. 55–8.

Cowan, R. E., Manning, A. P., Aycliffe, G. A. J. *et al.* (1993) 'Aldehyde disinfectants and health in endoscopy units'. *Gut*, vol. 34 (November), pp. 1641–5.

Cullen, J. (1996) 'Avoiding chemical poisoning'. *Kai Tiaki: Nursing New Zealand*, vol. 2, no. 7 (August), pp. 20–1.

Friend, B. (1994) 'Occupational hazard . . . respiratory sensitisers at work' *Nursing Times*, vol. 90, no. 50 (14 December), pp. 20–1.

HSAC (1997) *Risk Assessment at Work: Practical examples in the NHS*. ISBN 0 7521 0941 3. London: Health Services Advisory Committee, Health and Safety Commission.

HSE (1991) *Health surveillance of occupational skin disease*, MS24; *Medical aspects of occupational asthma*, MS25. Sudbury: Health and Safety Executive.

HSE (1996) *Approved guide to the classification and labelling of substances dangerous for supply CHIP 97 – Chemicals (Hazard Information and Packaging)*, L100. Sudbury: Health and Safety Executive.

HSE (1997) *ACOP Control of Substances Hazardous to Health Regulations 1994*, L5. Sudbury: Health and Safety Executive.

Jeanes, A. (1997) 'Know How – Latex sensitisation'. *Nursing Times*, vol. 93, no. 40 (1 October), pp. 54–5.

Medical Devices Agency (1996) 'Decontamination of Endoscopes', Device Bulletin 9607. London: MDA.

Menzies, D. (1995) 'Glutaraldehyde – controlling the risk to health', *British Journal of Theatre Nursing* vol. 4, no. 11 (February), pp. 13-15.

Moore, A. (1994) 'Latex-allergy: implications for patients, health care workers and NHS suppliers', *Bandolier Special Bulletin for NHS Supplies* (July), pp. 1–12.

Nightingale, K. (1996) 'Risk – what risk?', *British Journal of Theatre Nursing*, vol. 6, no. 1 (April), p. 29.

O'Connor, T. (1997a) 'Poisoned careers'. *Kai Tiaki: Nursing New Zealand,* vol. 3, no. 11 (December–January), pp. 16–17.

O'Connor, T. (1997b) 'Glutaraldehyde dangers'. *Kai Tiaki: Nursing New Zealand,* vol. 3 no. 11 (December–January), p.18.

Pennell, D. (1995) 'Chemical caution', *Kai Tiaki: Nursing New Zealand,* vol. 1, no. 10 (November), p. 22.

RCN (1994) *Safety Representatives' Manual.* London: Royal College of Nursing, Labour Relations Department.

Thomas, L. (1994) 'Glove story', *Nursing Times,* vol. 90, no. 36 (7 September), 33–5.

Thompson, G. (1997) 'Ways of avoiding latex allergy', *Community Nurse,* vol. 3, no. 2 (March), pp. 33–4.

Thompson, G., Ruane-Morris, M. and Lawton, S. (1994) 'Lines of defence', *Nursing Times,* vol. 90, no. 41 (12 October), pp. 48–1.

TUC (1997) *Hazards at Work: TUC Guide to Health and Safety.* London: Trade Union Congress.

Waters, J. (1997) 'Latex gloves: still a serious occupational hazard', *Nursing Times,* vol. 93, no. 25 (18 June), pp. 56–8.

Contact organisations

Poison Information Centres (open day and night):

Belfast:	01232 240 503
Birmingham:	0121 554 3801
Cardiff:	01222 709 901
Dublin:	Dublin 379 964 or 379 966
Edinburgh:	0131 229 2477
Leeds:	0113 243 0715 or 292 3547
London:	0171 635 9191 or 0171 955 5095
Newcastle:	0191 232 5131

The British National Formulary (BNF) has a section on the emergency treatment of poisons.

Latex Allergy Information Service, 176 Roosevelt Avenue, Torrington, CT 06790, USA.

MDA guidance: *Latex Sensitisation in the Health Care Setting* – available free to NHS employers from the Department of Health, PO Box 410, Wetherby, Yorkshire LS23 7EL, or from the Medical Devices Agency, Ordering Department Room 1207, Hannibal House, Elephant and Castle, London SE1 6TQ.

The National Latex Allergy Support Group, 37 Little Acorns, Bishop's Cleeve, Cheltenham, Gloucs, GL5 24Y.

Waste anaesthetic gases

Several surveys and animal experiments have established that even low levels of waste anaesthetic gases can have severe reproductive effects on both men and women. They have also been linked with cancer and liver disease. The area where there has been more research than any other is into the search for a suspected link with reproductive activity (AAOHN, 1995; Foley, 1993; Guirguis *et al.*, 1990), particularly spontaneous abortion, which is shown to occur with significantly greater frequency in women exposed to anaesthetic gases. Ether, which is virtually unused now, has long-recognised carcinogenic properties. But other commonly used gases such as nitrous oxide, halothane, pentathane, triluene, ethane and cyclopropane have been identified as potentially harmful, particularly to anaesthetists, theatre nurses and theatre technicians who face continuous low-level exposure. Health workers exposed to nitrous oxide, for which UK control limits only commenced in 1994, were recently shown to have early bone marrow damage – a potential hazard to midwives, dental nurses and all theatre staff.

The risks

Reproductive effects

In women, these include reduced fertility and increased incidence of spontaneous abortion. There is also evidence of a link with congenital abnormalities, including spina bifida, microcephaly, hydrocephaly, cleft lip and palate, and cardiac abnormalities. In men, there is evidence of reduced sperm count and mobility, and damaged sperm.

Carcinogenic effects

Evidence of excess cancer occurrence has been found in female hospital staff, concentrated among anaesthetists and theatre staff, including nurses.

Effects on the liver

Gross liver effects have regularly been noted in patients given anaesthesia, arousing concern as to the effects on theatre staff of long-term, low-level exposure.

Nervous effects

Headache, fatigue, irritability and loss of sleep.

Protection

Anaesthetic gases can escape into the working environment from a variety of sources: when the anaesthetist actually administers the gas; from leakages in faulty equipment; and from the patient's breath, particularly in the post-operative recovery period.

Ventilation

In 1977 the US National Institute of Occupational Safety and Health declared there was no safe level of exposure to waste anaesthetic gases. Adequate ventilation of theatre premises is the most important preventive measure, including scavenging systems to collect waste gases and ventilation systems to renew the air regularly. Anaesthetic equipment should be regularly checked for leaks and closed-system anaesthesia used wherever possible.

In the UK, the 1994 Occupational Exposure Standards (OES) for anaesthetic agents were set at 100 parts per million (ppm) for nitrous oxide, 50 ppm for enflurane and isoflurane, and 10 ppm for halothane, all over an eight-hour period. Guidelines on staying within these limits were issued by the Health Services Advisory Committee (HSAC) in 1996, requiring the installation of active rather than passive scavenging systems in all operating theatres. This is expensive: it cost £80,000 for the Southampton General hospital NHS Trust to install such a system in 13 operating theatres (Green, 1996; JNM, 1996).

Monitoring

Regular checks for contamination of the atmosphere in operating suites should be carried out and the results made known to health and safety reps and staff.

Equipment maintenance

Regular maintenance of equipment is vital, including machines, valves, seals and containers, and scavenging and ventilation equipment.

Nursing procedures

Avoid getting too close to the patient's face post-operatively: anaesthetic gases have been detected on patients' breath up to ten days later.

Pregnancy

If you are pregnant, avoid working in theatres – request a transfer to a non-exposed area without loss of pay or seniority, citing the Management of the Health and Safety at Work Act Regulations 1992, which in 1994 incorporated the EU Pregnant Workers Directive, requiring risk assessment of reproductive hazards, redeployment or suspension on full pay for new or expectant mothers (see Chapter 2, 'The legal framework', and Chapter 9, 'Reproductive hazards', for further details).

References and resources on waste anaesthetic gases

AAOHN (1995) 'Reproductive hazards: an overview of exposure to health care workers', *AAOHN Journal*, vol. 43, no. 12 (December), pp. 614–21.

Cooper, N. G. (1994) 'The measurement of anaesthetic gases – legal requirement'. *British Journal of Theatre Nursing*, vol. 3, no. 10 (January), pp. 29–30.

Foley, K. (1993) 'Update for nurse anaesthetists – occupational exposure to trace anaesthetics'. (American Association of Nurse Anaesthetists). *AANA Journal*, vol. 61, no. 4 (August), pp. 405–12.

Green, S. (1996) 'Nitrous oxide – A potential hazard', *British Journal of Theatre Nursing*, vol. 6, no. 6 (September), pp. 27–33.

Guirguis, S. S. *et al.*, (1990) 'Health effects associated with exposure to anaesthetic gases in Ontario hospital personnel', *British Journal of Industrial Medicine*, vol. 46 (July), pp. 490–7.

HSE (1996) *Occupational Exposure Limits*, EH40. Sudbury: Health and Safety Executive.

Journal of Nursing Management (1996) 'New guidance on controlling exposure of health services staff to anaesthetic agents', JNM, vol. 4, pp. 179–82.

Johnston, J. (1993) 'Nitrous oxide: your health, not theirs', *British Journal of Theatre Nursing*, vol. 3, no. 6 (September), pp. 29–30.

RCN (1995) 'Hazards for Pregnant Nurses: An A–Z Guide, Health and Safety at Work leaflet no. 4, reorder no 000 496. London: Royal College of Nursing.

Williams, N. (1993) 'Reproductive hazards in the work place', *Occupational Health*, vol. 45, no. 11 (November), pp. 368–72.

Drugs

All pharmacology handbooks devote a large section to the (often severe) side-effects of drugs, yet little attention is paid to their possible effects on handlers. The one exception is cytotoxic drugs, which are now increasingly recognised as a particular hazard to staff. These will be examined in detail in the next section. The possible hazards of other drugs are almost always ignored. This is remarkable, as nurses spend a good proportion of their time handling drugs and are exposed to them in a number of ways:

- Direct contact: applying creams and ointments without gloves; solution splashing on skin or eyes.
- Inhalation: mixing the drug in powder form or counting tablets; drugs administered as aerosol sprays; drugs forming an aerosol spray under positive pressure when being mixed.
- Ingestion: deliberately – the temptation of self-medication; or accidentally – directly or indirectly via the hands or splashing into the mouth.

Adverse effects

Skin reactions

The most common effect of handling drugs – skin reactions – can include allergic contact dermatitis, sensitisation or photocontact dermatitis. A person sensitised after exposure to a certain drug may also subsequently be affected by other substances. Antibiotics are the main problem, particularly penicillin, neomycin and streptomycin. Antihistamines such as promethazine, phenothiazines such as chlorpromazine, and the bronchodilator aminophylline can also cause skin problems.

Sensitisation

If you do become sensitised to a particular drug through occupational exposure, there is a danger of a very severe reaction, for example anaphylaxis, if you later receive the drug directly yourself. It is often very difficult to pinpoint exactly the drug to which an individual has become sensitised.

Respiratory effects

Exacerbation of respiratory conditions such as asthma. Asthma can also directly follow sensitisation to a drug.

Carcinogenic or teratogenic effects

Several antibiotics are recognised teratogens, including actinomycin-D, mitomycin-C and streptomycin. Some immunosuppressants, used for example in organ or tissue transplantation, may have carcinogenic or teratogenic effects.

Protection

Find out about the drugs you are handling. The manufacturer is required by law to provide information on the known side effects to both handlers and patients.

- Wash and dry your hands thoroughly after handling drugs. Keep cuts and abrasions covered with a waterproof dressing.
- Never apply topical preparations with your bare hands. Wear gloves or use a spatula. Don't handle tablets.
- Wear full protective clothing when handling cytotoxic drugs and others where indicated.
- Do not squirt solutions into the atmosphere. Expel excess air from a syringe into the empty vial.
- Rinse splashes and spillages immediately with cold water.

Cytotoxic drugs

Despite the known, local toxic effects from contact with cytotoxic drugs and the suspected long-term systemic effects, safety policies for the handling, preparation and administration of these highly toxic substances are random and haphazard, with wide variations.

Evidence of the systemic effects of cytotoxic drugs on handlers is inconclusive and controversial, varying considerably from drug to drug. An investigation of the association between occupational exposure to antineoplastic drugs found that skin contact with drugs brought a statistically significant increase in events such as altered menstrual cycles and ectopic pregnancy (Valanis *et al.*, 1993; Saurel-Cubizolles *et al.*, 1993). Other reported reactions include inflammation of the mucous membrane, skin pigmentation, and corneal ulceration if the eyes are contaminated. Evidence of long-term systemic effects is less conclusive, but many cytotoxic drugs have been shown to have mutagenic and possibly carcinogenic properties (Saurel *et al.*, 1993) and there is increasing evidence that this can affect handlers. Excessive mutagenic activity in the urine of nurses after handling cytotoxic drugs has been demonstrated, for example by Valanis *et al.* (1993), and the carcinogenic risks from cytotoxic drugs has been examined in a comparative study of occupational cancer risks (Hewitt, 1992).

The evidence remains controversial, but as the list of cytotoxic drugs is growing all the time it seems sensible to work on the assumption that all are potentially systemically dangerous to handlers, and to work out safety procedures accordingly.

Routes of contamination

Inhalation

A toxic aerosol or dust, usually generated from the syringe or rubber-topped vial when the solution is drawn up, is probably the greatest risk to handlers. Its danger is often forgotten as it is unseen.

Ingestion

Although possible, this method of contamination is unlikely.

Skin contact

This can have an irritant effect. Some drugs may also be systemically absorbed through the skin.

Protection

Unlike chemicals, there are no 'safe' levels of employee exposure to pharmaceutical products. Guidelines are available from the HSE but many hospitals have no systematic policy or procedure for dealing with cytotoxic drugs, and the level of ignorance of the hazards present is appallingly high.

A survey of nursing and medical staff in the mid 1980s revealed widely variable practices in the preparation and handling of cytotoxic drugs (Goodman, 1985). More recent follow-up research (Goodman, 1997), undertaken to develop chemotherapy guidelines for the RCN, found evidence of continued inconsistent or poor practice:

- A general belief that staff are not at risk and a lack of hazard awareness.
- Poor disposal practices.
- Low awareness of risks from excretions.
- Varied access to and usage of laminar flow equipment.
- Pressure on time leads to personal protective equipment not being used.
- A lack of set or standard procedures when using cytotoxic drugs.
- Few centralised pharmacy services.
- Lack of analysis of data on errors and exposure incidents.
- No specified levels of training or competence.
- Junior doctors are unlikely to have received training in handling cytotoxic drugs but are expected to cover for specialist nursing staff out of hours.

The HSE has withdrawn its previous guidance (MS21, *Precautions for the safe handling of cytotoxic drugs*) and at the time of going to press has no timetable for the introduction of revised guidelines. It is likely, however, that any new national guidelines will be consistent with those of the RCN and the British Occupational Hygiene Society (HSE, 1997).

The following advice is based on Goodman's recent report (1997), so far unpublished. The main principle is that all work with cytotoxic drugs should be based on the assumption that any exposure is potentially hazardous. The aims of the guidelines are therefore to minimise exposure, as no safe threshold for exposure exists, and to ensure the safety of patients, staff and the environment.

Staff education

All staff should have access to information, education and training in the safe handling of cytotoxic drugs and should understand the principles of risk control. Cytotoxic drugs should only be handled by those who understand the principles of safe practice and only professionally qualified and competent practioners should be required to prepare and/or administer these drugs. Education should be regularly updated, with staff able to demonstrate their knowledge of drugs and their effects, as well as appropriate protective measures and good handling techniques.

Employer responsibilities

Full and comprehensive risk assessment, as required by the COSHH regulations, is the employer's most significant responsibility. Local policies and procedures in the handling of cytotoxic drugs will depend primarily on this risk assessment. The employer is responsible for delegating the task of cytotoxic drug handling and other tasks relating to their storage, transport and disposal. All information relating to their use should be communicated to those handling the drugs and practices should be continually monitored and reviewed. The employer must provide staff with access to appropriate protective equipment and waste disposal facilities.

Practitioner responsibilities

Practitioners have the right to refuse to administer any drug if they feel they lack sufficient knowledge, skill and experience in its handling or if the situation is inappropriate. Individual safe practice is not enough, however, to ensure a safe environment. Guidelines for team practices and safety are necessary.

Drug preparation

It is the mixing and preparation of cytotoxic drugs that potentially carries the most significant risk to the handler, through contact or inhalation. All cytotoxic drug preparation should therefore be carried out by trained pharmaceutical staff, either in centralised pharmacies or in controlled facilities in clinical areas. A class II microbiological safety cabinet should be used for this purpose, and checked for defects at least every six months. Warning signs should be posted in cytotoxic drug preparation areas and unauthorised staff should be excluded. There should be clearly posted spillage procedures and all eating and drinking in the area should be banned.

In the absence of a controlled pharmaceutical environment, the purchase of prepared drugs from another pharmacy or commercial source should be considered. Two other situations justify the preparation of drugs outside a controlled environment: drugs with a very short 'shelf life' which may be required out of pharmacy hours; and oncological emergencies which may require the immediate use of cytotoxics which cannot be prepared in advance. In these circumstances, the drugs should ideally be prepared by a trained pharmacist or pharmacy technician. Facilities should be quiet and away from patients. There should be a work-surface protection against spillage – a sterile, absorbent, plastic-backed pad or laminate or a stainless steel surface with lips; a sink, running water and eyewash, waste disposal containers, protective gloves and gowns, facial and respiratory protection, and a spillage pack.

Personal protective equipment (PPE)

The extent of PPE to be used should be determined by local risk assessment.

- Gloves: appropriate disposable gloves should be worn at all times when contact with cytotoxic drugs is likely. High-quality latex gloves are the most comfortable and usually offer the greatest degree of dexerity, although PVC may be substituted, for example in cases of latex allergy. Gloves with little or no powder are preferred, since powder may absorb cytotoxic contamination. Gloves should be changed immediately if damaged or if significant contamination occurs. A new pair should be used for the administration of each dose.
- Eye and face protection: chemical safety goggles or a face shield should be worn during drug preparation if a material is not being handled in an appropriate cabinet or if splashing or airborne dust is a possibility during administration.
- Gowns: cotton gowns offer no barrier to cytotoxic drugs as the solution can simply soak through. Ideally gowns should be disposable and made of low-permeability fabric with a closed front, long sleeves and elastic cuffs, which should be tucked under the gloves. Plastic aprons, with or without armlets, may be an acceptable alternative, following a COSHH risk assessment.
- Respiratory protection: this is required in the absence of an enclosed cabinet or suitable exhaust ventilation. Surgical masks do not protect against aerosol inhalation and a disposable filtering facepiece respirator (FFP2 or FFP3) is recommeded if there is any risk of inhaling solid or liquid particles.

All PPE should bear the European CE marking, which means the item complies with European regulations.

Administration techniques

The administration of cytotoxic drugs should be handled by appropriately trained and competent professionals who are fully aware of the drugs they are handling. Intravenous drug administration should be carried out in a safe environment which allows unhurried, undistracted practice, using approved methods of administration defined by local policies and protocols. The procedure should be stopped if there is any uncertainty about any checks made or if there are any demonstrable side effects or complications.

Oral preparations should be managed using the same 'no touch' principles. Disposable gloves should be worn and tablets should be preferred to solutions, preferably contained in blister or foil packs. The crushing of tablets should avoided, but if it is essential, protective clothing and equipment should be used and pharmaceutical advice sought.

Other routes of administration include intraperitoneal, isolated limb perfusion, intrathecal, intra-arterial, intrapleural, pericardial, subcutaneous and nebulised. The same principles apply as with oral and intravenous administration; specialist pharmacy advice must be sought.

Accidental spillage

Spillage prevention and containment should be aimed at minimising human and environmental exposure. The management of a spill should be based on clear local policies and procedures and on access to appropriate facilities, techniques and protective equipment. Spillage kits should be available in all areas in which cytotoxic drugs are stored, prepared, transported, administered and disposed of. They should contain instructions on handling the spill; protective clothing, including gloves, overshoes, gown and respirator; absorbent pads, a sharps container, a scoop for glass fragments and prelabelled disposal containers.

If a spillage comes into contact with the skin, the affected area should be washed thoroughly with soap and water or other pharmacy recommended solutions. Affected eyes should be washed with copious amounts of water and immediate medical attention sought. The incident should be recorded in the staff and departmental records.

Handling waste and waste disposal

Contaminated material – including bottles, vials, PPE and any other items used to prepare and administer cytotoxic agents – should be disposed of in leakproof, puncture-proof containers, suitably labelled and conforming to local policies and national regulations. To avoid the risk of aerosol spraying, needles and syringes should not be clipped and tubing and giving sets should be disposed of intact.

Sharps boxes should be plastic with absorbent material in the base and tight-fitting lids, which should be sealed when the container is filled to recommended capacity. Waste should be segregated and not allowed to accumulate before incineration.

Monitoring staff health

If staff are to handle cytotoxic drugs regularly, a reference blood sample should be taken and stored at the beginning of employment. Pregnant nurses should avoid exposure to cytotoxic drugs for the whole of their pregnancy – and earlier if a pregnancy is planned. Staff working with cytotoxics should avoid exposure to radiation as there is some evidence of an interactive effect between certain cytotoxics and radiation in patients treated with both, although the significance for occupational exposure is difficult to assess.

All spillages involving skin or eye contact should be recorded in the staff records.

References and further reading on cytotoxic drugs

Goodman, C. (1985) 'Cytotoxic drugs: their handling and use', *Nursing Times*, vol. 81, no. 47 (20 November), pp. 36–8.

Goodman, I. (1997) *National Clinical Guidelines for the Administration of Cytotoxic Chemotherapy*, unpublished. Oxford: RCN Institute.

Hewitt, J. (1992) 'Cancer Risks of nurses: to assess the carinogenic potential of antineoplastic drugs. PhD thesis University of Illnois, Chicago. Health Sciences Centre (CINAHL Abstract).

HSE (1996) *Good Health is Good Business: employer's guide*, MISC045. Sudbury: Health and Safety Executive.

HSE (1997) 'Minutes of the Cytotoxic Drugs Workshop' (14 March). London: Health and Safety Executive.

RCN (1994) *Safety Representatives' Manual*. London: Royal College of Nursing.

Saurel-Cubizolles, M., Job-Spira, N. and Estryn-Behar, M. (1993) 'Ectopic pregnancy and occupational exposure to antineoplastic drugs'. *Lancet*, vol. 341, no. 8854 (8 May), pp. 1169–71.

Valanis, B., Vollmer, W., Labuhn, K. and Glass, A. (1993) 'Acute symptoms associated with antineoplastic drug handling among nurses', *Cancer Nursing*, vol. 16, no. 4 (August), pp. 288–95.

Wiseman, K. and Wachs, J. (1990) 'Policies and practices used for the safe handling of antineoplastic drugs', *AAOHN Journal*, vol. 38, no. 11 (November), pp. 517–23.

Radiation

The hazards of radiation can be neither touched, seen, heard, smelled nor tasted. Nurses are likely to be aware of its damaging potential by observing the effects on patients undergoing radiotherapy, but they may not think of themselves as being at risk.

Disasters such as the explosion at the Chernobyl nuclear power station in 1986 highlighted many of the known health problems caused by radiation. High doses are of course fatal, while acute somatic effects such as burns, cataracts and sterility follow exposure to intermediate doses. No less dramatic, but emerging after a longer interval, are the delayed somatic effects, notably cancer (especially of the bones and breast, and leukaemia) and damage to the fetus. The human reproductive organs are particularly susceptible and radiation can lead to genetic abnormalities, perhaps persisting for generations.

The level of radiation to which nurses are exposed in hospital is on average very low, but the gravity of its effects suggests that all possible care should be taken to protect health workers. X-rays are the most obvious radiation source but others such as radioactive implants, liquids and wastes mean that general wards, laundries, theatres and mortuaries are all areas where staff may need to be especially vigilant.

Sources of radiation

Radiation energy is defined as ionising or non-ionising; the latter does not change the atomic structure of the cell and is not our concern here. Ionising radiation, however, is widely used in medicine both diagnostically and therapeutically. The sorts of rays most widely used in hospitals are X-rays, generated in an electrical machine, while beta and gamma rays are obtained from radioactive substances called radioisotopes. For practical purposes the sources of radiation in hospital can be divided into four groups.

Sealed sources

These are radioactive substances sealed in a coating and housed in solid containers for transport or storage. Some are implanted in patients, for example when treating carcinoma of the cervix, while other small sealed sources are used in laboratories.

Unsealed sources

These are usually in liquid form for use in laboratory tests or injection into patients. Iodine-131 for treatment of cancer of the thyroid is an example.

Wastes

These are used radioactive chemicals, equipment or surface covers that cannot be decontaminated, and radioactive excretions from patients.

Machines

Nuclear medicine employs a variety of machines to emit a purposefully directed beam, but some scattering and leakage of rays is also likely. X-ray sets, scanners, accelerators and electron microscopes come into this category. X-rays account for 90 per cent of hospital radiation

Safety levels

To what extent are nurses and other health workers at risk from radiation? The controversy shows no signs of being settled, although there seems to be broad agreement that the notion of a 'threshold' safety level is no longer acceptable. There is no safe level of radiation, and in view of the lack of consensus it is best to assume, as in so many other health and safety arguments, that exposure – intentional or otherwise – must be kept to an absolute minimum and the strictest safety precautions observed. Because the effects are cumulative, careful monitoring of staff health over extended periods is also essential.

The two crucial measures of radiation are the substance's 'activity' (the amount of radioactive material) and its 'half life' (how quickly it decays). The 'Sievert' indicates the energy received by tissue and therefore the potential damage – an important distinction because some types of radiation are more likely than others to produce adverse biological effects. The Sievert is equivalent to 100 rems, the previous unit of measurement. For women of reproductive capacity, the permitted exposure limit to the abdominal area is 13 milliSieverts (mSv) in a three-month period, and for pregnant women the exposure limit is 10 mSv during the 'declared term of pregnancy'.

The half-life of a radioactive substance is the time it takes for its activity to decay by half – in other words, how quickly it fades. This varies from as little as six hours (technetium 99Tm) to 1600 years (radium), so the substances differ greatly in their potential for damage, a factor that also has implications for medical uses.

Legislation

The Ionising Radiation Regulations 1985 apply everywhere that ionising radiation and radioactive substances are used, and the HSE is the responsible regulatory body. The regulations are currently being reviewed to bring them in line with draft EU regulations and are expected to be in place by 1999 or 2000.

The 1985 regulations require that:

1. Employers ensure that doses are 'as low as is reasonably practicable'. This principle of dose limitation is known as the ALARP. It is supplemented by the international advisory body, the International Commission on Radiological Protection (ICRP) with two riders: the principle of justification – that the benefit of a dose to the patient outweighs the possible detriment to the staff – and the 'as low as reasonably achievable' (ALARA) principle, on the ground that no radiation dose is entirely free from risk.
2. Employers carry out an investigation when a worker's recorded dose exceeds 15 mSv in any one year.
3. If a worker's dose exceeds 30 mSv in any three-month period the HSE must be informed.
4. If any worker receives an annual dose (in any 12-month period) in excess of 50 mSv, the HSE must be notified by the employer or the Approved Dosimetry Service.

The radiation adviser in the Nottingham City Hospital NHS Trust suggests that no person's annual dose should approach 15 mSv, or even 5 mSv, which is the current maximum exposure limit from all sources for the general public. Workers are also obliged to obey any local rules for the use of ionising radiation, and if issued with film badges or other dosimetry equipment they must follow the guidelines for their use.

Staff protection

Official guidelines for protecting workers are contained in the *National Radiological Protection Board Guidance Notes for the Protection of Persons against Ionizing Radiations for Medical and Dental Use*, revised in 1988. The HSE has produced guidance on occupational exposure and dose limitation (see References). In December 1985 all health authorities were ordered to comply with the new statutory Ionising Radiation Regulations and were reminded of their responsibilities, as outlined in the approved code of practice. As with all such legislation, managers, safety reps and others must ensure that compliance is not merely lip service, but an active daily responsibility.

The code of practice makes an important distinction between classified and unclassified workers. Employers must decide which staff should be 'classified' and therefore given regular health checks, personal radiation badges, medical and dose records and detailed training. This should include nurses working permanently in radiotherapy departments as well as others such as radiographers; their annual radiation exposure is recommended to be no greater than 50 mSv a year, although in practice the average doses rarely exceed a lifetime average of 15 mSv a year.

Unclassified workers are those whom the employer can prove to be exposed to less than three-tenths of the recommended dose for classified workers a year. They are not officially entitled to the same protective measures, although employing authorities can (and sometimes do) take steps to ensure that some of the more vulnerable staff are covered. Remember, the guidelines provide minimum standards only.

Action

The action necessary to protect nurses from radiation can be considered in three categories: recognising the hazard, monitoring the hazard, and reducing exposure to the hazard.

Recognition

All sources of radiation, however small, must be labelled with the internationally recognised radiation symbol reproduced on a yellow background. Warnings and instructions should be translated in hospitals where a number of staff and patients speak a different first language. Warning lights outside X-ray rooms and other devices must be kept in working order.

Every nurse is likely to come across radiation at some time and it is essential that everyone undergoes full in-service training – with no loss of pay or time off – in order to learn to recognise the hazards, gain awareness of problems and become familiar with the emergency procedures. Everyone should also be familiar with the local rules – standard working instructions for staff drawn up by the trust or employer in consultation with the radiological protection adviser. These should be prominently displayed and widely discussed, including input from nurses on issues such as the care of radioactive patients.

Monitoring

The simplest method of measuring how much radiation each person has received is through the use of a film badge worn during working hours. The film should be changed and developed monthly; it shows the level of radiation by a blackening of the plate, but this only applies to the part of the body where the badge is fastened. Badges should therefore be worn at the most vulnerable point – usually the gonads.

Steps must be taken to investigate the cause if cumulative exposure is approaching or has exceeded the limit, as shown in the radiological safety officer's records. The staff member should immediately be moved to an area where she or he will not be exposed to further radiation. Undesignated staff who are regularly exposed should press for badges, and everyone should be informed of the results. Remember, though, that the badge gives no protection, and that it only records exposure after the event – which might be too late. Furthermore it does not record the dose to the whole body. In high-risk areas, or if it is recognised that someone may receive a higher than normal exposure, digital direct dosemeters may be worn, which measure in microSieverts (that is, 1000 times smaller than milliSieverts) and can give instant readings and warning of dangerous levels.

Film badges are only a rough guide, and should not be regarded as a substitute for detailed environmental monitoring by management. Careful measuring such as correlation tests using thermoluminescent dosemeters should be conducted annually, and always when new equipment is introduced or old equipment moved. The results should be reported to safety reps.

Reducing exposure

The best protection against radiation is to minimise exposure to it. Distance, shielding and speed are three important principles to remember.

Distance is crucial because the further away you are from the source, the less radiation you will receive in a given time – according to the Inverse Square Law, the dose rate decreases markedly with distance: if the distance is doubled the dose is reduced to a quarter, for example. This is especially important when a mobile X-ray machine is used in a ward, or when nursing radioactive patients. The nurse should not be asked to give physical support to a patient being X-rayed unless it is essential (with a child, for example, the parent can be asked to help). Nurses who are pregnant or hoping to be should never be involved.

Shielding is valuable because materials such as concrete or lead absorb a large proportion of a beam of radiation. Radiotherapy and diagnostic departments are built with protective materials of this kind. Wearing a lead apron or standing behind a mobile shield also reduces exposure, but it is a last resort and should only be used if the procedure is impossible to redesign or replace. Nursing a patient in a lead apron or tunic is cumbersome but the temptation to ignore the protection must be avoided.

The less *time* spent near a source, the less radiation is received, so speed is another vital principle to bear in mind. Treatment and care must be carried out as quickly as efficiency allows.

Other measures can also help to reduce exposure. First, is there an alternative procedure which is safer? Ultrasound is less risky than conventional X-rays, while the Selectron is safer than caesium implants in treating cancer of the cervix. Second, is the procedure really necessary? There is some evidence that diagnostic X-rays are overused, thus exposing patients and staff unnecessarily – either because the procedure is ordered thoughtlessly, or because the equipment may be old and/or faulty, resulting in a need to repeat the process. Lack of resources means that old equipment is not replaced or properly maintained, an issue to be tackled by staff organisations. Finally, care should be taken to rotate staff duties to minimise each person's exposure; for example when nursing radioactive patients in the ward, staff should share the responsibility for direct care.

Action checklist

The following is a source-by-source guide for checking radiation facilities and protection measures (with thanks to the Hospital Hazards Group).

Diagnostic and therapeutic X-ray sets and sealed sources:

1. Does each set have a warning light on the control panel that is visible during operation? Can it function without the warning light? When was it last maintained, and is notice of maintenance posted on the set?
2. Are rooms marked with warning signs? Are areas near X-ray sets adequately protected?
3. Can weak patients be supported by equipment? Are relatives asked to help, and are staff given full instructions?
4. Are staff given film badges or dosemeters, and are these regularly checked and the results made known?
5. Are more X-rays taken than is strictly necessary?

Small sealed sources:

1. Are there prominent notices outlining the emergency procedures to follow when a source is punctured or broken?
2. Are all patients with implants monitored for radiation, and detailed nursing advice issued accordingly?

Unsealed sources:

1. Are all wards, theatres and clinics monitored regularly and systematically? Are records of the results displayed?
2. Have all staff been trained in handling the source, and in emergency procedures?
3. Are all non-urgent nursing procedures avoided with radioactive patients? Is a supply of protective clothing available for emergencies? Is contaminated laundry separated and labelled?
4. Are special facilities provided for the disposal of routine wastes, as well as instructions to all staff about disposing of and avoiding contamination from radioactive urine, faeces, vomit and so on?

Representation:

1. Does your employer have a radiological safety committee, with trade union/professional representatives?
2. Are safety reps given all relevant information, and permitted to inspect records, as is their right?
3. Do you know how to contact the radiological protection officer – the principal source of advice to health authorities?
4. Are the local rules known to all staff and readily available?

References and further reading on radiation

Department of Health and Social Security (1973). *The Safe Use of Ionizing Radiations: A Handbook for Nurses.* Edinburgh: HMSO.

Department of Health (1985) *Health Services Management: Ionising Radiations Regulations 1985,* available from Health Publications Unit, DSS Distribution Centre, Manchester Road, Heywood, Lancs OL10 2PZ.

Hospital Hazards Group (1979) *Radiation Hazards in Hospitals.* London: British Society for Social Responsibility in Science.

HSE (1991) *Additional guidance on the Ionising Radiation Regulations 1985,* L7. Sudbury: Health and Safety Executive.

HSE (1992) *A framework for the restriction of occupational exposure to ionising radiation,* HSG91, Health and Safety Executive Guidance. Sudbury: Health and Safety Executive.

HSE (1993) *Ionising Radiations (Outside Workers) Regulations,* L49(ACoP). Sudbury: Health and Safety Executive.

HSE (1994) *The protection of persons against ionising radiation arising from any work activity,* L58. Sudbury: Health and Safety Executive.

TUC (1997) *Hazards at Work: TUC Guide to Health and Safety.* London: TUC.

Mercury

Have you ever snapped a mercury thermometer or knocked over a sphygmomanometer? What did you do next? Mercury seems such a small hazard that it can be overlooked; in fact it is a significant hazard to nurses, their patients and others in clinical settings. All clinical areas where mercury is present should have the appropriate equipment to deal with mercury spillage.

The potential hazards of accidental mercury spillage are skin reactions, anaphylaxis and reproductive effects.

Spillage

The COSHH regulations require employers to provide workers with information and training to handle mercury spillage safely. Suggested action to deal with spillage:

1. Clear the immediate area of people and open the windows if possible – mercury gives off a potent vapour. If it is a small spill in an open environment, respiratory protective equipment such as disposable respirators are not necessary, but if a large spill occurs in a confined space such equipment should be used. There are commercial kits available to clear small spillages.
2. Put on gloves and a disposable apron, and draw up the spilt mercury into a syringe, making sure you do not inhale or touch it. Do *not* use a brush or broom to collect it.
3. Follow local procedures for the disposal of mercury. This should include the placing of the recovered mercury, and the cleaning materials, in a sealed container, to be disposed of by a competent person from the estates department. Some authorities suggest submerging the contained mercury in a closed jar of water.
4. Record and report the incident to your manager, and to the Occupational Health Department.

Alternatives to mercury thermometers

Many hospitals have tested and chosen other equipment for clinical temperature monitoring and you may want to suggest to your manager that safe alternatives to mercury-containing equipment be considered (see Box 6.4). There are four main alternatives (O'Toole, 1997):

- Single-use: these consist of plastic strips with heat-sensitive chemical markers. They are suitable for oral, axillary or rectal use, but have a limited range (between 35.5 and 40.4 degrees Celsius).
- Digital analogue: these are battery operated, with a thermistor tip. They are suitable for oral, axillary or rectal use, and have a range of 32–42 degrees Celsius.

- Electronic predictor: these are battery operated, usually supplied with disposable covers, and separate probes for oral, axillary or rectal use – an advantage in reducing the risk of contamination and infection. They have a range of 31.6–42.2 degrees in the 'predictor mode', and 26.7–42.2 degrees in the 'monitor mode', but are significantly more expensive than single use or digital analogue devices.
- Infra-red tympanic: these have a probe which is placed in the external auditory canal, and measure the core temperature accurately, with a range of 25–43 degrees. These devices cost between £100 and £400.

Mercury's hazardous nature makes the use of alternative substances attractive to risk management terms. If your workplace changes to non-mercury thermometers, all mercury thermometers should be disposed of by the pharmacy or the COSHH adviser (O'Toole, 1997).

Box 6.4   *Good practice*

The Bridgend and District NHS Trust incident-reporting procedure revealed a high number of incidents over a short time-span involving broken mercury thermometers. The trust had purchased 450 thermometers in the previous 12 months, representing around nine potential exposure incidents per week. Staff awareness of the associated health risks was inadequate and broken thermometers were accepted as normal.

Spillage kits were placed in all areas where mercury thermometers were used, a staff training programme was developed and the pathology department agreed to store used mercury spill kits, which were disposed of periodically by a registered contractor. This controlled the risks adequately, but to eliminate the hazard, alternatives were identified and tested within the trust. Criteria for choosing a replacement included accuracy, safety, ease of use, risk of cross-infection, price (including cost of extras such as batteries and disposables), patient group and robustness.

Source: HSAC, 1997.

References and further reading on mercury

HSAC (1997) *Risk Assessment at Work: Practical examples in the NHS*, Health Services Advisory Committee, ISBN 0 7521 0941 3. London: Health and Safety Commission.

HSE (1996) *Mercury and its inorganic divalent compounds*, EH17. Sudbury: Health and Safety Executive.

O'Toole, S. (1997) 'Clinical observations: Alternatives to mercury thermometers', *Professional Nurse*, vol. 12, no. 11 (August), pp. 783–6.

7 Infection and infection risks

Hospitals and other health care settings are full of germs whose hazards are particularly insidious because they are not visible. Dangers that cannot be seen tend to be ignored, played down or forgotten.

Recent research has shown that over 60,000 in-patients a year (almost 3 per cent) develop hospital-acquired infections (Gould, 1994a; Waters, 1997; Courtenay, 1997). Part of the problem is attributed to large variations in staff knowledge and poor implementation of infection control policies, and new national infection control guidelines and surveillance schemes have been proposed (PHLS, 1997). The development of a national strategy to improve knowledge, raise standards and reduce risk is long overdue.

The risk to patients of a hospital or health care acquired infection is well documented. Yet nurses themselves are particularly at risk from microbiological hazards because they deal intimately with infected patients: with their excretions, secretions, specimens, wounds, dressings and bed linen (see Box 7.1). This risk is too often downplayed, either by nurses themselves or by their managers.

Despite the introduction of universal precautions, potential sources of infection are still too often treated as innocent until proved guilty. Cloudy urine is just cloudy urine until the bacteriological report confirms an infection. Soiled bedpans are piled up during the night to cut down on noise rather than being washed or pulped immediately. Infection control policies can be directed wholly towards protecting the patient, while the health and safety of the nurse is given less emphasis.

Hospitals in particular make ideal breeding grounds for germs. They contaminate creams and ointments and lurk in half-finished solutions or stagnant tap water, flower vases, sinks, toilets, bedpan washers, suction apparatus, ventilators and humidifiers. Used linen is loaded with staphylococci from patients' skin and if the linen is transported loose around the ward or corridors it spreads potentially harmful microbes.

Hospital buildings are notorious for pest infestation – rats, mice, ants, flies, cockroaches, pigeons and even cats, which all carry microbes on their bodies and in their droppings. In old hospitals pests breed in holes and crevices in the fabric of the building, while the design of some new hospitals makes the problem even harder to control, with wide service ducts allowing pests to spread throughout the buildings. Hospital patients are more susceptible to infection as their natural resistance is lowered through illness or drugs. Shared toilet facilities and close proximity to other patients increase the risk of cross-infection and make the working environment for nurses more hazardous.

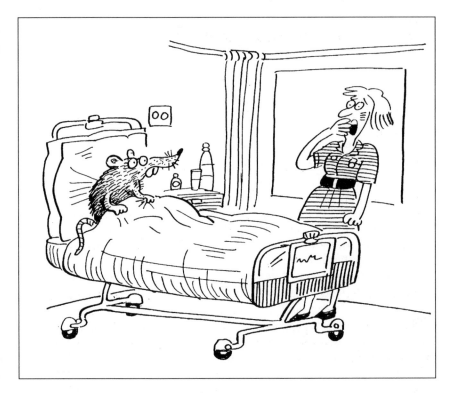

The most common microbiological hazards are bacteria which normally exist harmlessly in the bowel or on the skin but can cause trouble if they penetrate elsewhere. While bacteria are usually susceptible to antibiotics, strains of antibiotic-resistant bacteria such as staphylococci and streptococci have developed, making the control of infection even harder.

Microbiological hazards

Bacteria

Staphylococcus aureus are normally resident in the skin and can cause respiratory infections if inhaled, food poisoning if swallowed or abscesses if they enter an open wound.

Escherichia coli are normally resident in the bowel. They can cause infection of the bladder, and can be spread via toilet door handles and flush levers or by failing to wash hands after dealing with faeces.

Salmonellae are found in raw foods and are spread by insufficiently cooked or heated food, or by allowing cooked and uncooked meats to be stored together or prepared on the same surface. Salmonellae can cause food poisoning or typhoid.

Box 7.1   *The main routes of microbiological infection*

Ingestion – from infected food or soiled hands.
Inoculation – via a contaminated needle, such as hepatitis B or HIV.
Implantation – if an open cut or abrasion is infected.
Inhalation – many micro-organisms are airborne and can survive for
    long periods in dust or on bed linen. Aerosols, from a bedpan
    macerator or a syringe, can carry atomised particles of an organism
    suspended in air, which can be easily inhaled.

Streptococcus are normally resident in the bowel, and can cause acute tonsillitis, otitis media, scarlet fever and septicaemia.

Pseudomonas is found in decaying organic matter, and can cause wound and urinary tract infections.

Proteus, normally resident in the bowel, is also found in decaying organic matter, and can cause wound and urinary tract infections.

Viruses

Viral infections also constitute a hazard to health care staff: the two most serious are hepatitis B and human immunodeficiency virus (HIV), the virus that causes AIDS.

Other viruses are particularly dangerous to pregnant nurses. In diseases such as rubella the virus crosses the placenta, infecting and damaging the growing fetus. Varicella zoster (chicken pox) and herpes simplex can also cause developmental defects, as can cytomegalovirus, while mumps can result in male infertility. Nurses working with children should be particularly aware of these hazards.

Protection

Infection control policies

The development of sound infection control policies and the education of staff are essential to infection control. The policies should be concise, clear and consistent. They should be supported by current research and agreed by clinical leaders and educationists. Infection control guidelines should not lie gathering dust on a shelf but should be accessible to all, including nursing auxiliaries and domestic, portering and clerical staff, as well as nurses and doctors (see Box 7.2).

Most hospitals and trusts now have infection control committees and an infection control nurse who can intervene when policies are not adhered to, collect data on infection outbreaks and staff health, provide information to all staff on potential hazards and receive staff complaints. Some hospitals, such as the Queen's Medical Centre, Nottingham, have link nurses who are the 'eyes and ears of the infection control team on the wards'.

Agreed policies and procedures should always be prominently and legibly displayed in the workplace, protected from wear and tear. They might be expected to include universal infection control precautions (UICPs), described below.

'They all know what they have to do – they just don't do it', says Mike Kelsey, consultant microbiologist at the Whittington Hospital (*Health Service Journal*, 1997). Studies show, however, that while as many as 50 per cent of staff do not adhere to hospital infection control policies, many staff members are unaware of what their hospital or trust policies are. Yet staff are interested in questioning clinical practice, in order to improve it and to avoid infecting themselves and their patients (Gould, 1994a; Ward, 1997a, 1997b; Courtenay, 1997).

Education

One of the biggest problems in infection control education is the inconsistency of theoretical content between various health care settings and between education and practice settings. Microbiology should be taught explicitly in combination with the infection control procedures of clinical environments. Qualified staff should also receive appropriate education to prepare them for supervisory roles in this area (Courtenay, 1997).

Surveillance

The PHLS (1997) recommends that surveillance should be integral to normal health care activity. It calls for 'radical improvement in the content and accessibility of medical and nursing records', and for the feeding back of the results of surveillance in order to increase awareness of infection risks. Wilson (1995) defined surveillance as 'the systematic observation of the occurrence of disease, with analysis and dissemination of the results . . . it enables staff to focus on specific problems, take appropriate action to prevent infections occurring, and by doing so, improve the quality of patient care'.

Universal infection control precautions (UICPs)

UICPs are internationally agreed measures, first used in 1987. It is recommended that all patients be regarded as potentially infectious, and that health care workers routinely use barriers (single-use gloves, plastic aprons, eye/face masks) to avoid risk of contact with blood or body fluids; wash their hands thoroughly before and after patient contact, after removing gloves, and immediately after contact with any blood, body fluids or mucous membranes. Needles should never be resheathed, and all used clinical waste disposal should occur as near its source as possible, according to local policy.

Box 7.2   *Infection control policy in your workplace*

1. Do you have access to an infection control policy in your workplace?
2. Is it concise, clear and consistent?
3. Is it research-based and reviewed and audited regularly by clinical and education staff?
4. Are infection control and microbiology taught in the health care studies department where you are/were a student? Is there a match or a mismatch between theory and practice?
5. Are the nursing and medical records in your workplace designed and used with surveillance of hospital-acquired infection in mind?
6. Does your workplace take part in the Nosocomial Infection National Surveillance Scheme (NINSS)?
7. Could you discuss infection control and audit with the infection control nurses for your workplace, in order to reduce the risks to patients and nurses?

Hand washing

'The basic principles have not changed for 20 or 30 years. You need clean hands, clean equipment and the systems to provide them' (Maureen Johnson, vice chair of the Infection Control Nurses Association, quoted in *Health Service Journal*, 1997).

Hand washing is probably the single most effective way of safeguarding the health of staff and reducing cross-infection, yet many hospitals and clinics have appalling hand-washing facilities. There should be plenty of wash basins, especially near lavatories, with decent soap and proper drying facilities. Disposable paper towels are safest, and research now suggests that liquid soap in wall containers is less likely to become contaminated than individual tablets in dishes (Gould, 1994a, 1994c; Gould and Chamberlain, 1997). Special 'disclosing' liquids such as Glo-Germ may be obtained to monitor staff hand washing techniques, while fluorescent dust can be used to show how rapidly germs can spread (see Box 7.3).

Box 7.3   *When to wash your hands*

- After using the lavatory.
- Before a meal.
- After handling a patient and/or discharge from a patient.
- After handling soiled or infected linen.
- After removing gloves and other protective clothing.

Cleaning

Inadequate or misdirected cleaning can vastly increase the risk of infection. Cleaning equipment such as mop heads (which should be detachable), cloths, sponges, scrubbing brushes and buckets should be washed daily in hot water (at least 65°C) and detergent and stored dry.

The number of bacteria in the air has been shown to double during and after sweeping the floor with a broom. Correctly designed vacuum cleaners with built-in air filters, or oil-impregnated cotton or nylon mops are safer and more effective. Vacuum cleaners should conform to noise limits. Carpets should be vacuumed daily and other floor surfaces dry-mopped and washed with ordinary detergent.

Surfaces above floor level should be vacuumed or damp dusted with water and possibly a detergent. Chemical disinfection is not usually necessary.

Disinfectants are only active when wet and the surface will dry quickly. Cloths should be colour-coded for different areas – sluice, kitchen or patient areas. Spillages involving bacterial infection should be cleaned with a clear soluble phenolic disinfectant. Those involving a viral infection should be covered with paper towels soaked with 1 per cent hypochlorite (for example Milton, Domestos, Presept) and left for 30 minutes. Spilt blood should be treated with chlorine granules before being cleaned up. Disposable gloves and a disposable apron should be worn.

Microbes can gather in water that is left to stand for several days. Any water used for cleaning should be drawn fresh from the tap. The water in flower vases should be changed regularly, and the vases washed and dried before being refilled.

Disinfectants

Disinfection means the removal or destruction of harmful microbes. Although it is usually associated with chemical disinfectants, it can also be achieved through heat or cleaning. Widespread advertising campaigns have convinced many people that chemical disinfection is the only effective method, although there is no evidence to support this.

Chemical disinfectants are expensive and may even be less effective than heat or ordinary detergents. They react differently to different substances, some are inactivated by hard water, or even by the dirt itself, and they may be incompatible with the soap or detergent used. Studies have shown no appreciable difference in the reduction of microbes following floor cleaning with soap and water and with a chemical disinfectant solution.

To work effectively a contact period is necessary. Thus pouring disinfectants down lavatories is less effective than simply flushing. Poured down drains they will do little more than mask a bad smell. The drain should be unblocked and the cause of the smell removed. Never use two disinfectants together. Always make sure you use the right strength solution and do not top up an old solution – always make up a fresh one. Insist that suppliers provide dispensers to avoid spillage of concentrated disinfectants and ensure accurate measuring.

Laundry

Avoid shaking cubicle curtains and bed linen. Bag all linen by the bed and do not transport it loose. Even if it is not infected or visibly soiled it can carry potentially harmful microbes from the patient's skin. Colour-coded bags should be available for used, soiled or infected linen. Infected linen should always be clearly marked and placed in two bags, the inner one with soluble stitching so that laundry workers do not need to handle the contents. Blood- or faeces-stained linen from patients infected with hepatitis B or HIV should be incinerated.

Isolation

There should be a clear hospital policy on when patients should be isolated and when they should be barrier nursed. During a hospital epidemic, or an outbreak of an infection such as MRSA, cohort isolation can be used, in which a whole bay, ward or unit is treated as an isolated area. Nurses must be fully trained in barrier nursing techniques. Whenever a patient is being barrier nursed there should be plenty of warning notices for nurses and all other staff and visitors. The recent incidence of multi-drug-resistant tuber-culosis has brought suggestions that additional precautions such as negative pressure rooms may be necessary.

Protective clothing

Protective clothing forms a key part of the universal precautions against the transmission of infection between patients and between patients and staff. Used properly, protective clothing can play an important role in protecting the nurse against infection from the patient and *vice versa*, and in reducing cross-infection. Conversely it can create a false sense of security and even increase the risk of transferring infection.

Plastic aprons are the most effective barrier against contamination. The ICNA suggests that barrier gowns are rarely justified or offer protection, and that they are more readily penetrated by moisture or bacteria. If cotton tabards are used, the ICNA recommends they be changed at least daily (ICNA, 1994). Some doctors have been reluctant to wear aprons because they associate them with the more menial duties normally undertaken by a nurse!

The risk of acquiring infection through manual contact is almost always dealt with by regular hand washing, but clean or sterile disposable gloves should always be used when the nurse is likely to come into contact with blood or body fluids; for example when handling urinary catheters or endotracheal tubes, carrying out wound care, or taking blood or urine specimens.

Masks, even the full surgical kind, are only partially effective against infective aerosols and small airborne organisms, and droplet infection is more likely to be spread by the handling of masks. Even if the fabric of the mask provides good filtration, this is lost if it does not fit properly. The rationale for their use is to protect the patient from contamination from the staff and *vice versa*, but current research doesn't support wearing them in many situations, unless there is a risk of being splashed in the face with blood or body fluids, or when working close to a patient with a productive cough.

Goggles and safety glasses can protect the eyes from being splashed with blood, for example during trauma situations, some surgical procedures, dental procedures or labour.

The ICNA suggests there is no evidence of benefit from the use of overshoes.

Specimens

Specimens sent for microbiological examination must be enclosed in sealed plastic bags with the laboratory request form kept separate, then placed in durable metal or plastic containers. The aim is to ensure that all specimens, whether or not they have been identified as being infectious, are transported safely.

There should be a consistent and well publicised labelling system for all specimens to warn the staff carrying and receiving them what they are or may be dealing with. Every specimen must be regarded as potentially infectious.

Waste disposal

Waste disposal is regulated by four main pieces of legislation:

1. Environmental Protection Act 1990 – this places a duty of care with those dealing with controlled waste.
2. Waste Management: a Duty of Care 1991 (Approved Code of Practice).
3. Controlled Waste Regulations 1992.
4. Special Waste Regulations 1996 – defines 'special waste'.

Clear policies should be laid down for the categorisation (usually through colour coding) and disposal of waste. They should be made clear to staff in training and orientation sessions and posted throughout hospitals and clinics on posters and notices. To avoid confusion, there should be as few categories as possible.

Community staff should avoid carrying unprotected clinical waste in their own vehicles. The HSE recommends that community-generated clinical waste is packed in approved clinical waste sacks or sharps containers placed in rigid, leakproof containers with tight-fitting or lockable lids. If it is not removed by community staff, it should be collected separately as clinical waste, by arrangement with the local authorities (Gifford, 1997). The Department of Health suggests that 'There should be absolutely no expectation among trusts for district or any other nurses to transport clinical waste' (Martell, 1997).

Monitoring staff health

All nurses should have a pre-employment medical examination. Vaccination against smallpox, poliomyelitis and rubella should be recommended, tuberculin sensitivity tests carried out and BCG vaccinations offered to non-reactors. The Department of Health requires the immune status of staff to be documented and those undertaking clinical procedures involving body fluids (most health workers) to be immunised against hepatitis B, either by the occupational health department or their GP. By law, this must be provided free by the employer.

Staff should be offered regular training in and updated information on protecting themselves against infection. They should be advised when to report symptoms such as an infected wound, diarrhoea or a specific infection, and when to stay away from work.

Pest control

Every hospital should have one member of staff designated as pest control officer, probably a member of the infection control committee. There should be a pest complaints book to encourage staff to report signs of pest infestation. The designs for new hospital buildings should include pest barriers built into service ducts. Litter should be kept to minimum, and waste products, particularly those containing food and other organic materials, should be disposed of promptly.

Enteric infections

In August 1984 an outbreak of salmonella was confirmed at Stanley Royd Hospital in Wakefield, a hospital for elderly mentally ill patients (DHSS, 1986b). Due to a combination of bad conditions, staff shortages, poor management and a failure to call in outside help, the disease swept through the hospital and 49 patients died. The source of the outbreak was eventually traced to infected chicken in the hospital kitchens. A public inquiry laid the blame for the spread of the infection firmly at the door of local management. One beneficial result was the establishment of the post of Consultant in Communicable Disease Control (CCDC), a designated specialist replacing previous local authority post holders.

The Stanley Royd episode was the worst in a long series of similar outbreaks, of which the incidence was far higher in hospitals than any other public facility – restaurants, clubs, hotels, holiday camps, canteens, schools or shops (Stevenson-Bryan, 1995).

There are several reasons why the figures were so much higher in hospitals. Problems in hospital kitchens included old and outdated premises and equipment, ineffective cleaning, inadequate pest control, poor levels of personal hygiene among kitchen staff due to inadequate facilities and lack of training, bad practice in food preparation and the inadequate reheating of frozen food. Thanks to crown immunity, unlike most other public facilities, hospital authorities could not be prosecuted if their kitchens breached the food hygiene recommendations, which many did.

Jolted by the Stanley Royd tragedy, the government finally removed crown immunity from hospital catering in 1986 and hospital catering was brought under the Food Safety Act of 1990. This has forced health authorities and trusts to tackle the problems in hospital kitchens, and although problems undoubtedly still exist, a recent audit of health service catering showed that poor hygiene practices were not widespread. Out of 11 hospitals visited and 25 surveyed, only one 'was serving regenerated food in a way which could be perceived as breaking the cook–chill guidelines' (HMSO, 1994b).

Other factors conspire to make hospitals a likely venue for food poisoning outbreaks. Hospital patients, in a weakened state and with their immune systems depressed, are more likely to succumb to infection; and a common food and water supply, close proximity and shared toilet facilities increase the risk of the infection spreading. If a patient is incontinent, confused or has a low standard of personal hygiene, these risks are multiplied (Mills, 1996).

So nurses face a double hazard – from hospital food and from the risk of infection from patients, particularly through handling excretions and secretions and collecting specimens. How can the risks be minimised?

Nursing care

Isolation

Infection depends on ingestion of the pathogen, usually by indirect contact – through soiled hands, for example. For severe enteric diseases such as cholera, salmonellosis, E coli 157, typhoid or paratyphoid fever, the patient should ideally be nursed in a communicable diseases unit, or at least in a single room. But this is not always practicable, particularly if several patients are affected. If a patient has a high standard of personal hygiene, therefore, he or she could safely be nursed on the open ward, provided rigorously high nursing standards are maintained.

Elderly mentally ill patients should be isolated, however, and so should children. If there is a widespread outbreak of food poisoning it may be practical to turn the whole ward into an isolation unit – so-called cohort isolation. Isolating the patient at least reminds staff of the risk (both to themselves and to other patients through cross-infection) and that special precautions must be taken, although most of these, such as rigorous hand washing, should be practised anyway.

The patient may also require barrier nursing. Hospital policy on when to isolate/barrier nurse infectious patients should be clearly laid down and consistent.

Hand washing

Hand washing after every nursing procedure is probably the single most important and effective preventive measure to protect yourself and reduce the risk of cross-infection (Gould, 1994b, 1994d; Larson, 1995).

Protective clothing

Plastic aprons should be worn for direct contact with the patient and disposed of for incineration after one use. Masks are not necessary. Gloves must be used if there is risk of contact with body fluids; they should be used once only and must not be regarded as a substitute for effective hand washing, which should be carried out after each procedure.

Disposal of waste

Infected urine and faeces can be safely disposed of in the usual way in the sluice, but bedpans and specimens should always be dealt with immediately. Bedpan washers must reach 80°C for at least one minute to destroy the bacteria, and the nurse in charge of the ward should check this daily. Most modern machines have a dial to read the temperature; if they do not, a crude but effective method is to test the outside of the machine during its cycle with your hand. It should be too hot for contact. Do not overload it, or it will not be able to wash the bedpans or urinals properly. Always report any leaks from the machine immediately. Pools left on the floor or leaking into buckets cause gross environmental contamination.

Macerators for dealing with disposable bedpans are just as effective, providing they are used properly. Always leave the lid down for at least one minute after the cycle has finished. They work like spin dryers and if you open the lid too soon you will receive a shower of faecal aerosols straight in your face. Keep an eye on the seals for signs of wear. If they are not intact the huge centrifugal force during the cycle can spray infected aerosols around the room.

Regular maintenance of the machines is vital. A clearly visible record of dates when servicing was carried out should be kept on the machine, and checked by the safety rep.

Linen and bedclothes used by infected patients should be changed daily, or immediately if soiled, and sent to the laundry in double bags. The inner bag should have soluble alginate stitching – this dissolves during the washing cycle so laundry workers do not need to handle the linen directly.

Disposable crockery and cutlery is preferable, but if this is not available, all crockery and cutlery should be washed at 80°C minimum. Dressings and disposable items should be incinerated.

Management responsibilities

Staff screening

If you suffer from diarrhoea or vomiting you should go off sick and report it immediately. If the symptoms persist, stool specimens should be tested for enteric infections. Screening is vital and should be carried out immediately on any staff involved in handling and preparing food. They should be excluded from food handling until at least three negative stool specimens have been collected on three successive days.

Follow-up of infections

Any outbreak of food poisoning in a hospital should be vigorously followed up, including screening all food handlers and testing samples of all meals served during the previous 48 hours.

Kitchen hygiene

Kitchen hygiene in the UK is primarily governed by the Food Safety Act (1990) and the Food Safety (Northern Ireland) Order (1991). The Food Safety Act was amended following the 1993 EU Food Hygiene Directive, which lays down environmental health requirements for the preparation and storage of categories of food, with particular reference to the temperature at which food is stored, cooked and served; and the separation of raw and cooked meat. 'Assured safe catering systems' have been developed for and with caterers to control food safety problems (DoH, 1993, 1994, 1996a).

It is the direct responsibility of trusts to implement the Food Safety Act. Environmental health officers are required to monitor and report on hygiene standards in hospitals but are not obliged to pass on their findings to the NHS Executive (NHSE). The NHSE told the House of Commons Public Accounts Committee that when problems were reported they asked for copies, supported local managers in resolving the problems and 'had a good intelligence system whereby they were generally aware of the more difficult environmental health reports, and that since the removal of Crown immunity everyone in the Health Service . . . took food safety very seriously indeed' (HMSO, 1994a, 1994b).

While capital investment on properly designed kitchen facilities is important and in many areas very necessary, there are measures that trusts can take that would cost very little but are enormously effective in reducing the risk of infection. Kitchen staff must have food handling training and regular briefings on the risks of bad food handling, as well as proper training in effective cleaning techniques which cost no more in time or resources. Regular microbiological sampling of foods should be conducted; prepared food not used within 24 hours should be thrown away; meat can be bought already chopped or minced to cut down the risks inherent in preparation.

If a hospital has an infection control nurse, she should be involved in monitoring food hygiene in hospital kitchens, but she only has the power to advise or persuade. She can make recommendations to the trust management but has no power to enforce standards (Mercier, 1997).

Most hospitals now use central cook–chill facilities, whereby the food for a number of hospitals is prepared centrally and transported chilled direct to the wards, where it should be heated and served immediately, cutting out the middle stage. This method can cut down the hazards of food preparation in substandard conditions, but if the food is not adequately reheated it can be equally dangerous. An infection source in the food preparation area will also be spread more widely through the use of central preparation facilities (Porter, 1997b).

Nurses' involvement in meal distribution has reduced over the past 10 years. The preparation of light meals – usually involving eggs or soup – on the ward for patients who have missed the regular meal has disappeared and most meal distribution in clinical areas is now handled by catering assistants. While nurses' direct involvement in food preparation does allow them to monitor the nutritional intake of their patients, their poor record of adequate handwashing techniques and their propensity to move swiftly from dressing a wound or disposing of bedpans to serving food and carrying trays, would appear to make it logical to restrict the handling of food by nurses unless they have had specific food handling training.

The alternative is to require nurses to undertake local authority food handling courses, which, ironically, ancillary staff are more likely to do at present.

References on microbiological hazards, protection and enteric infections

Courtenay, M. (1997) 'A little knowledge is a dangerous thing', *Nursing Times*, vol. 93, no. 29 (16 July), pp. 76–8.
DHSS (1986b) *The Report of the Committee of Inquiry into an Outbreak of Food Poisoning at Stanley Road Hospital.* London: HMSO.
DoH (1993) *Assured Safe Catering.* London: HMSO.
DoH (1994) *Guidelines the Safe Production of Heat Preserved Foods.* London: HMSO.
DoH (1996a) *A Guide to the General Food Hygiene Regulations.* London: Department of Health.
Gifford, P. (1997) 'Precautions to be taken over clinical waste', Letters, *Nursing Times*, vol. 93, no. 42 (15 October), p. 21.
Gould, D. (1994a) 'Communicating about infection control', *Nursing Standard*, vol. 8, no. 36 (1 June), pp. 30–4.

Gould, D. (1994b) 'Making sense of hand hygiene', *Nursing Times*, vol. 90, no. 30 (27 July), pp. 63–64.

Gould, D. (1994c) The significance of hand-drying in the prevention of infection', *Nursing Times*, vol. 90, no. 47 (23 November), pp. 33–5.

Gould, D. (1994d) 'Nurses' hand decontamination: practice', *Journal of Hospital Infection*, vol. 28 (September), pp. 15–30.

Gould, D. and Chamberlain, A. (1997) 'The use of a ward-based educational teaching package to enhance nurses' compliance with infection control procedures', *Journal of Clinical Nursing*, vol. 6, no. 1 (January), pp. 55–67.

Health Service Journal (1997) 'Special Report: Infection Control', *Health Service Journal* (supplement), vol. 107, no. 5577 (30 October), p. 4.

HMSO (1994a) 'National Health Service: Hospital Catering in England', National Audit Office Report. (London: HMSO).

HMSO (1994b) 'National Health Service: Hospital Catering in England', House of Commons Committee of Public Accounts Report 49, and minutes of evidence given to the Public Accounts Committee, 23 May. London: HMSO.

HSC (1986) *Industrial Advisory Committee Report: Safety in Health Service Laboratories: The Labelling, Transport and Reception of Specimens.* London: HMSO.

HSE (1991a) *Safe Working and the prevention of infection in the mortuary and post mortem room.* London: HMSO.

HSE (1991b) *Safe working and the prevention of infections in clinical laboratories.* London: HMSO.

Infection Control Nurses Association (1994) *Infection Control: A Community Perspective* (compiled by Worsley, M., Ward, K., Privett, S., Parker, L. and Roberts, J.). London: Infection Control Nurses Association.

Institute of Environmental Health Officers and British Pest Control Association (1985) *Hospitals Can Damage Your Health.* London: British Pest Control Association. (Chartered Institute of Environmental Health Officers).

Jukes, D. (1993) *Food Legislation of the UK.* London: Butterworth Heinemann.

Larson, E. (1995) 'APIC Guidelines for hand washing and hand asepsis in health care settings', *American Journal of Infection Control*, vol. 23, no. 4 (August), pp. 251–69.

Martell, R. (1997) 'Clinical waste campaign steps up after court ruling'. *Nursing Times*, vol. 93, no. 35 (27 August), p. 5.

Mercier, C. (1997) *Infection Control: Hospital and community.* Cheltenham: Stanley Thornes.

Mills, I. (1996) 'Not quite good enough to eat', *Nursing Times*, vol. 92, no. 36 (4 September), pp. 72–5.

Nursing Standard (1997a) 'Innovations: "Clean hands"', *Nursing Standard*, vol. 12, no. 4 (15 October), p. 28.

O'Malley, P. (1992) 'Hygiene for handlers', *Occupational Health*, vol. 44, no. 5 (May), pp. 144–6.

PHLS (1997) Hospital-acquired infection: surveillance, policies and practice (Glynn, A., Ward, V., Wilson, J. *et al.*) London: Public Health Laboratory Service.

Porter, R. (1997b) 'Where's the beef?', *Nursing Times*, vol. 93, no. 37 (10 September), p. 16.

Smith, P. (1991) 'Looking into the refrigerator', *Nursing Times*, vol. 87, no. 38 (*Journal of Infection Control*) (18 September), pp. 61–2.

Stevenson-Bryan, B. (1995) 'Food for thought', *Nursing Standard*, vol. 10, no. 1 (AIDS Focus) (27 September), pp. 5–6.

Ward, G. (1995) *Catering Questions and Answers: Food Hygiene*. Kingston upon Thames: Croner Publications.

Ward, V. (1997a) 'Infectious incidents' (News Comment), *Nursing Standard*, vol. 11, no. 35 (21 May), p. 17.

Ward, V. (1997b) 'Auditing infection', *Nursing Times*, vol. 93, no. 29 (16 July), pp. 71–4.

Waters, A. (1997) 'No time to drop the guard', *Nursing Standard*, vol. 11, no. 36 (28 May), p. 16.

Wilson, J. (1995) 'Infection Control: Surveying the risks', RCN Nursing Update, supplement in *Nursing Standard*, vol. 9, no. 15 (4 January).

Wilson, J. and Richardson, J. (1996) 'Keeping MRSA in Perspective', *Nursing Times*, ICNA supplement, vol. 92, no. 19 (8 May), pp. 58–60.

Contact organisations

Institute of Environmental Health Officers, Chadwick Court, 15 Hatfields, London SE1 0DJ.

The Royal Environmental Health Institute of Scotland, Virginia House, 62 Virginia Street, Glasgow G1 1TX.

Methicillin–resistant *Staphylococcus aureus* (MRSA)

If any four letters are likely to induce panic in health care staff, and among the public, MRSA is high on the list. Without denying its increased incidence, and its potential as a major infection risk, such a response to MRSA may stem as much from ignorance as from knowledge of the nature of the pathogen.

MRSA, a worldwide phenomenon, is a Gram-positive human pathogen which is resistant to most antibiotics, including the powerful modified penicillin, methicillin. The organism *Staphylococcus aureus* is part of our normal flora, carried on the skin, particularly in moist areas such as skin folds – the groin, axillae, perineum and in the nasal mucosa. Generally, it is neither harmful nor of benefit to humans, but if it enters broken skin or a hair follicle it becomes pathogenic.

Methicillin was used first in the early 1960s, and methicillin resistance was reported soon after, with infection episodes into the early 1970s. MRSA appeared to have declined by the early 1980s, but then new strains began to appear.

The first epidemic strain, in 1984, was named EMRSA-1 and was traced to north-east London. It spread throughout the UK, causing some hospital deaths, but declined from the mid-1980s and is now rarely found. EMRSA-2 arose in south-east London and is largely confined there. EMRSA-3 also arose in south-east London, in 1987, and spread throughout England, giving rise to small outbreaks of infection ever since – frequently identified in pathology from pressure sores (Griffiths-Jones, 1997a).

Numerous other strains have emerged, for example EMRSA-15 and EMRSA-16, which were discovered in over 40 hospitals in 1993 and in over 80 a year later (CDSC, 1995).

Those vulnerable to MRSA include the following:

- Patients who are in hospital for long periods.
- Patients in small, high-dependency units such as intensive care and coronary care, burns units, transplant units and neonatal and special care baby units.
- People with open wounds, chronic ulcers and lesions.
- Previous recipients of antibiotic therapy and/or invasive procedures such as intravenous therapy. Such people may become 'colonised' with MRSA and, although not harmed themselves, spread it to others.

Spread

MRSA is spread mainly by hand contact, probably from patient to nurse to patient because of nurses' failure to wash their hands thoroughly between patient contact, possibly on clothing or bedding, or, more rarely, by airborne route. The latter is a particular risk for patients in burns units, or those having skin grafts.

Control

The principles of control are to prevent the spread of the organism to unaffected areas and to treat those patients who are infected or colonised. Screening protocols may be used, particularly in hospitals with no known strains of MRSA, to monitor the infection or colonisation status of all previous known carriers, and possibly of all patients admitted to intensive care units, or admitted from other hospitals.

When a patient is suspected of carrying MRSA, he or she should be accommodated in single room isolation if other patients are at risk, until the laboratory results are known. The Department of Health has issued guidelines on MRSA, and most hospitals will have local protocols which the infection control committee has drawn up and educated health care staff about (see Box 7.4).

Treatment varies according to the site of infection, whether the patient is infected or colonised, and patterns of sensitivity. There are intensive topical regimes used for nasal passage and skin decolonisation – currently up to 10 days of the antibiotic mupirocin applied to the nasal passages, with a seven-day course of skin treatment with antiseptics such as chlorhexidine, povidone iodine and triclosan applied to wet skin and rinsed off in a shower or bath (RCN, 1997).

Together with isolation, screening and treatment, the application of basic principles of infection control (universal infection control precautions) are essential. The basic principles are adherence to an audited hospital infection

Box 7.4   *Good practice*

Sheffield City Council's occupational health nurses have a good working relationship with the consultant in communicable disease control. The consultant set up a working group involving the community infection control nurse, the senior occupational health nurse and representatives from residential community care settings, to develop an MRSA policy document for Sheffield. The aims of the policy are to ensure that:

- People are well informed about MRSA.
- The care and support of people with MRSA meets the same high standards as that given to anyone else.
- All services are accessible and non-discriminatory, and their use non-stigmatising.
- No patient is treated disadvantageously because of MRSA status, known or unknown.
- Increased compassion is shown towards people with MRSA, ensuring they receive respect and support.

Source: DoH, 1998.

References on MRSA

CDSC (1995) *Epidemic methicillin resistant Staphylococcus aureus*, Communicable Diseases Report 5:35,1. London: Communicable Diseases Surveillance Centre (Colindale).

DoH (1998) '*Occupational Health Nursing: Contributing to healthier workplaces*'. London: Department of Health (published jointly with the ENB).

Duckworth, G., and Heathcock, R. (1995) 'Report of a Combined Working Party of the British Infection Society. Guidelines on the Control of Methicillin-resistant Staphylococcus aureus in the community'. *Journal of Hospital Infection*, no 31 (5 September), pp. 1–12.

Dunford, C. (1997) 'Special focus: Tissue Viability. Methicillin resistant Staphylococcus aureus', *Nursing Standard*, vol. 11, no. 25 (12 March), pp. 61–2.

Godfrey, R. (1997) 'The bugs they couldn't kill', *Nursing Times*, vol. 93, no. 14 (2 April), pp. 24–7.

Griffiths-Jones, A. (1997a) 'Essential Guide to MRSA'. London: *Nursing Times* .

Lambert, S. (1995) 'Do staff follow guidelines for dealing with MRSA?', *Nursing Times*, vol. 91, no. 44 (1 November), pp. 25–7.

Nursing Standard (1997b) 'MRSA', RCN nursing update, Learning Unit 073 (supplement) *Nursing Standard*, vol. 11, no. 49 (27 August).

Siu, A. (1994) 'Methicillin-resistant Staphylococcus aureus: do we just have to live with it?', *British Journal of Nursing*, vol. 3, no. 15 (11 August) pp. 753–9.

control policy; effective hand-washing techniques; a clean, dry care environment, adequate protective clothing, linen and waste disposal facilities; and strict aseptic techniques for catheter care and wound care (Griffiths-Jones, 1997a).

Nobody with MRSA should be prevented routinely from returning home or to nursing/residential home care, and though ambulance crews should be aware of patients' MRSA status, no special precautions are necessary. Generally, the risk of MRSA spreading is low for people with good general health and intact skin. Staff of residential and nursing homes, GPs and district nurses should be made aware of MRSA risks in order to prevent colonisation or infection of vulnerable patients and clients.

MRSA is one of a number of antibiotic-resistant pathogens, perhaps made worse by the excessive use of antibiotics in general medicine. Control should be aimed at restricting spread, by detection, isolation and treatment. Nurses are not at risk if their health is good and their basic techniques are sound.

Hepatitis

When the AIDS virus and the risk of its spread dominated public concern, it overshadowed similar stories about hepatitis, which still constitutes an enormous risk to staff and other patients, particularly in renal dialysis units. There have been several serious outbreaks, one of the worst being in Edinburgh between June 1969 and August 1970, when 26 dialysis patients and 12 staff members developed clinical hepatitis. Seven patients and four staff died.

The disease has not abated. The increase in drug abuse over the past two decades has contributed to a steady increase in hepatitis B cases and carriers. The risk to health staff has declined, largely because it has been recognised and safety procedures have been laid down and followed. An active hepatitis B vaccine has been available since 1982. Previously the only option was to give hepatitis B immunoglobulin (HBIG) after exposure, which provided only partial protection. Patients in high-risk groups and all those receiving renal dialysis are now screened. Highly infectious patients are isolated and barrier nursed.

But although it is now better controlled, the risk to health care staff is still present. There is also a risk from carriers of the disease who show no symptoms and do not fall into so-called 'at risk' groups. About 5 per cent of cases in the UK are thought to produce a chronic carrier state when the blood remains positive to the hepatitis B surface antigen (the Australian antigen or HBsAg). This state can also result from a subclinical, asymptomatic dose of the disease.

Nurses working in 'higher-risk' areas (Box 7.5), where time and care is taken over infection control, may actually be at less risk than those in the

---

Box 7.5   *Hepatitis: higher-risk areas*

- Renal and liver units.
- Maternity units.
- Infectious diseases and isolation units.
- Accident and emergency departments. Although not officially categorised as a high-risk area, the risk varies according to the carrier rate in the population served and staff working in an inner-city casualty department may legitimately regard themselves as at greater risk.
- Drug dependency clinics.
- Sexually transmitted disease clinics.

---

so-called 'lower-risk' areas. Frequently, patients may not have been identified as carriers. Junior staff may be inexperienced in infection control procedures, and staff may be moved to areas in which they are inexperienced. Nurses are therefore in close and constant contact with blood and body fluids when the presence of the virus is not suspected. Finally, pressure of time due to staff shortages or a medical emergency can cause safety procedures to be skimped. And although a safe and effective vaccine has been available since 1982, until recently it was offered to relatively few nurses. Now, under European law employers are required to offer free hepatitis B vaccination to all workers at risk from infection.

The virus

There are five main types of viral hepatitis: infective hepatitis (A) and serum hepatitis (B), (C), (D) and (E). All are unpleasant diseases and hazardous to nurses, but the second, commonly known as hepatitis B, is the more serious and has a significantly higher mortality rate – up to 30 per cent compared with 0.2 per cent for type A. It can also cause long-term cirrhosis of the liver, or in rare cases, the development of a primary hepatocellular carcinoma.

There are thought to be over 300 million chronic carriers of hepatitis B worldwide and around two million deaths annually (Smith, 1993). While it is still most common in developing countries, over 100,000 new cases of hepatitis B are documented each year in western Europe alone, although the true incidence could be much higher, as in more than half the cases the disease is subclinical and asymptomatic.

Staff working in higher-risk areas are usually (though not always) aware of the hazards, and should be well versed in the procedures for dealing with them. The risk is perhaps greater when the disease is unrecognised or unacknowledged (see Box 7.6). Nurses must therefore be aware of which patients could be carriers of the virus:

- Patients with undiagnosed jaundice or liver disease.
- Drug addicts.
- Prostitutes.
- Male homosexuals.
- People with extensive tattoos.
- People recently arrived from tropical or subtropical countries.
- People with haemophilia and unscreened blood-transfused patients.
- Renal patients.

Hepatitis C is one of the causes of non-A, non-B hepatitis, with about 100 million carriers worldwide. Between 0.5 and 2 per cent of the population of Europe show evidence of hepatitis C (HCV), with higher prevalence among injecting drug users and in people with haemophilia. There is no greater than average prevalence in health care workers (van Damme, 1996).

Modes of transmission

Infective hepatitis (A), the less serious of the five, is spread by the faecal–oral route and often occurs in epidemics. It has an incubation period of between two and six weeks.

Hepatitis B (HBV), a serum hepatitis, is spread, as its name suggests, by contact with blood or blood products – serum, ascitic or pleural fluid and other exudates. It has been isolated in sputum and blood-contaminated urine and faeces. It is transmitted by direct contamination through inoculation, broken skin, mucous membrane or the cornea. Transfer of infective material can also occur via contaminated surfaces, but there is no evidence of

---

Box 7.6 *A nurse's story*

Marie discovered that she had been exposed to the Hepatitis C virus after working as a dental nurse for many years:

> In the course of my work I regularly changed the long needles used for the administration of local, oral anaesthetic to patients. This entailed screwing and unscrewing these units onto the syringe. The plastic casing had to be snapped off new units after they had been attached and old units had to be unscrewed and disposed of.
>
> Occasionally I would scratch myself with a needle during this procedure. The fact that I had two pairs of latex gloves on made no difference; the sharp would slice through them like a knife through butter. I am pretty sure that I was exposed to HCV during one of these episodes.

Source: Dolan and Hughes, 1997.

airborne spread. It has an incubation period of between six weeks and six months.

Hepatitis C (HCV) is blood-borne with similar transmission routes to hepatitis B. Most people infected with HCV are asymptomatic. Its prevalence is unknown, but thought to be around 300,000 to 600,000 in the UK (Dolan and Hughes, 1997). Vaccination against hepatitis B offers some protection. Hepatitis D (HDV) is known as a delta virus, having a virus-like particle called a delta agent (Thompson *et al.*, 1993) and is infective only with hepatitis B. Hepatitis E is an RNA virus (ribonucleic acid, or RNA, is the genetic messenger of which the virus is composed) and is transmitted similarly to hepatitis A, by the faecal–oral route. Young adults appear to be most at risk, with a mortality rate of 20 per cent among pregnant women who are infected. In the UK, infection should be considered in people with hepatitis-type symptoms who have recently visited high-risk areas such as China, India and Mexico (Butler, 1997).

Prevention of spread

The most recent comprehensive government report on hepatitis was produced by the Department of Health's Advisory Committee on Dangerous Pathogens and published in 1995. Specific nursing guidelines – *Introduction to Hepatitis B and Nursing Guidelines for Infection Control* – were produced by the RCN in 1987 and updated in 1997. These documents are a useful reference source, although hospitals, and in particular recognised high-risk areas, should have their own readily available guidelines.

Nursing care

HBsAg positive patients can be nursed on the open ward unless they are bleeding or likely to bleed, or require parenteral procedures such as dialysis. Remember, the main risk of infection arises from contact with blood or blood products and universal precautions apply:

1. Take particular care with needles and sharp instruments.
2. Report any accidents, no matter how minor.
3. Keep cuts and abrasions covered with a waterproof dressing.
4. Wear protective clothing – disposable gloves and aprons for nursing procedures.
5. When cleaning spillages of blood, urine and faeces, wear a plastic apron and gloves. Disinfect the area with paper towels soaked in 1 per cent hypochlorite (leave for 30 minutes if possible).
6. Blood-stained linen and disposable materials, including gloves and aprons, paper tissues, cotton wool and so on, should be sent for incineration – double bagged and labelled 'Hepatitis Risk – for incineration'.
7. Always wash your hands after contact with a patient.

If you do accidentally prick yourself with a contaminated needle, or are contaminated through a cut or through the eyes or mouth, wash the affected area immediately and report the incident in writing to your manager and safety rep. If you haven't previously been immunised, hepatitis B immuno-globulin should be given as soon as possible, preferably within 24 hours. Under European law all employers are now required to offer hepatitis B vaccine free to all clinical staff (van Damme, 1996).

Employer's duties

COSHH and Management of Health and Safety at Work regulations require employers to undertake a number of duties:

- Undertake risk assessment, introduce control measures, inform staff about risks, identify particularly vulnerable people.
- Obtain informed consent for health interventions such as vaccination.
- Protect confidentiality.
- With regard to the Disability Discrimination Act 1995, some legal opinion suggests that it would be unlawful to discriminate against asymptomatic carriers of hepatitis B by refusing to employ them or dismissing them (Howard, 1996).

Vaccination

The only fail-safe precaution against hepatitis B is vaccination. There is currently no vaccine for hepatitis C or E, but the vaccine for hepatitis B also protects against hepatitis D. In the late 1980s and early 1990s the RCN called for all nurses to be offered the vaccine routinely, and threatened to sue any health authority that did not offer it, on the basis that it would be failing to provide a safe working environment. The vaccination was expensive, but the introduction of new varieties has cut the cost dramatically, and trusts have found that cost preferable to lawsuits from staff who have contracted hepatitis as a result of not having been immunised.

But it is not enough simply to offer the vaccine. Its benefits should be actively promoted, and this includes explaining the risks of the virus and the severity and complications of the disease. Doubts about the safety of the vaccine should be discussed – for example concern has been expressed that the vaccine might be an AIDS risk as it is made from the serum of hepatitis B carriers who may in turn be at risk from AIDS. Extensive purification and inactivation processes have been shown to remove this threat. Staff who are given the vaccine must agree to complete the whole course.

References and contact organisations on hepatitis

Butler, M. (1997) 'Hepatitis from A to G', *Practice Nurse*, vol. 14, no. 35 (June), pp. 35–40.

DoH (1995) *Protection Against Blood-borne infections in the Workplace: HIV, Hepatitis*. Advisory Committee on Dangerous Pathogens. London: HMSO.

Dolan, M. and Hughes, N. (1997) 'Hepatitis C: a bloody business', *Nursing Times*, vol. 93, no. 45 (5 November), pp. 71–2.

Griffiths-Jones, A. (199) 'Hepatitis revisisted', *Nursing Times*, vol. 90, no. 46 (16 November), (*Journal of Infection Control*, vol. 21, no. 6), pp. 58, 60, 62.

Howard, G. (1996) 'Hepatitis B and the employer's duty to vaccinate', *Occupational Health*, vol. 48, no. 8 (August), pp. 284–6.

Murrell, A. (1993) 'Unlocking the virus: providing support and treatment for people with hepatitis', *Professional Nurse*, vol. 8, no. 12 (September), pp. 780–3.

NHSME (1993) 'Protecting Health Care Workers and Patients from Hepatitis B', Health Care Guidelines, HSG(93)40. London: NHSME.

Nursing Times (1996) NT Guide to Hepatitis (compiled by Anne Griffiths-Jones in association with the Infection Control Nurses Association). London: Macmillan Magazines.

RCN (1987) *Introduction to Hepatitis B and Nursing Guidelines for Infection Control*. London: Royal College of Nursing (new guidelines were produced late in 1997).

RCN (1997) 'Universal Precautions' (laminated wall chart), re-order 000 264. London: Royal College of Nursing.

Smith, J. (1993) 'Hepatitis C: A major public health problem', *Journal of Advanced Nursing*, vol. 18, no. 3 (March) pp. 503–6.

Society of Occupational Medicine (1986) *The Prevention of Hepatitis B among NHS Staff*, consultative document. London: SOM.

Thompson, J., McFarland, G., Hirsch, J. and Tucker, S. (1993) *Mosby's Clinical Nursing*. St Louis: Mosby.

Van Damme, P. (1996) 'Hepatitis A, B and C occupational hazards', *Occupational Health*, vol. 48, no. 8 (August), pp. 280–3.

Contact organisations

Occupational Health Nurses, Sheffield City Council, Town Hall, Sheffield S1 2HH. Tel.: 0114 2726444.

The British Liver Trust offers information and counselling to people affected by liver disease. Information line, tel.: 01473 276328. Postal address: Ransomes Europark, Ipswich IP3 9QG.

The Hepatitis C Support Network, PO Box 13036, London NW1 3WG.

HIV and AIDS

When publicity and panic about AIDS proliferated, nurses were understandably concerned about the prospect of nursing AIDS patients, and the risk this presented to their own health. The spread of the disease, however, has meant that more and more nurses are now involved with patients who have AIDS or are infected with HIV.

In fact the risk is low, provided basic precautions are taken. The disease can only be spread sexually, perinatally, by inoculation or, probably, by breastfeeding. There is no evidence that social contact presents any risk. At the time of writing there are no recent known cases of transmission of the virus from patients to health care staff. The disease is transmissible rather than infectious. Many of the other infectious diseases that you come into contact with through your work put you far more at risk. For example you are far less likely to be infected with HIV than hepatitis B. Nevertheless, when handling blood and blood products nurses do face a degree of risk, and scrupulous precautions are necessary. Meanwhile nurses are subject to the same scare stories and media hysteria about this disease as every other member of the population, which inevitably increases concern and with it the considerable stress involved in nursing AIDS patients.

The UKCC states that 'refusing to be involved in the care of patients because of their condition . . . is unacceptable' (UKCC, 1996). This should extend to working with nurses who are themselves HIV positive. There have been cases of discrimination in the employment and promotion of HIV-positive and homosexual nurses and appalling personal treatment of them by colleagues and managers. The RCN advises that there is no reason why a nurse carrying HIV antibodies should not carry on working, as long as she or he is clinically healthy. But complete confidentiality, counselling services and tact and sensitivity are needed. There is currently only one support group for nurses carrying the AIDS virus, the Nurses Support Group.

The disease

Acquired Immune Deficiency Syndrome is caused by the human immuno-deficiency virus (HIV), formerly referred to as human T-cell lymphotrophic virus III (HTLV III) or lymphadenopathy associated virus (LAV). The virus, as its name suggests, compromises the body's immune system, leading to the development of opportunistic diseases and infections such as Kaposi's sarcoma (malignant skin lesions), non-Hodgkin's cerebral lymphoma and pneumocystic carinii pneumonia.

The disease was first detected among young homosexual men in New York, Los Angeles and San Francisco in 1979–80 and the first UK death was reported in 1981. Since then it has spread rapidly, first among the homosexual community and then to other people, including intravenous drug users, haemophiliacs, bisexuals and heterosexuals. Although the proportion of reported AIDS cases from male homosexual relationships is far greater than reported cases in male–female relationships in the UK – in 1992, 76 per cent and 16 per cent respectively (HMSO, 1993) – the proportion of non-homosexuals affected is growing. AIDS should be regarded as a health problem affecting all sexually active people outside a monogamous relationship.

In June 1996 a total of 12,976 cases of AIDS had been reported in the UK, with the cumulative total of recognised HIV infections reported at 27,088. The World Health Organization's cumulative world figure was nearly 1.65 million reported HIV cases, though it suggested that the actual figure was probably closer to 8.4 million.

The PHLS is reluctant to estimate the proportion of HIV-positive people who go on to develop AIDS or AIDS-related ill-health, stating that due to the variability of the development of HIV into AIDS, and the methods of collecting statistics (from voluntary reports by clinicians and microbiologists), reported AIDS cases do not give an accurate picture of the current incidence of HIV infection.

Transmission

The virus is primarily blood-borne, although it can also be carried in semen, vaginal secretions and possibly the breast milk of HIV-positive women. Recent findings suggest that breast feeding doubles the rate of HIV transmission (*Nursing Standard*, 1998). Where breast feeding is avoided, about two-thirds of childhood infection occurs in the delivery period (Mofenson, 1997). It has been cultured in saliva, although it is estimated that it would take an injection of about one and a half litres for this to constitute any risk. Blood-contaminated urine and faeces can also carry the virus. Transmission occurs sexually, perinatally or by inoculation. Intravenous drug users contract the virus by using contaminated needles; haemophiliacs and other blood-tranfused patients through infected blood.

All blood donated in the UK since October 1985 has been screened, but haemophiliacs were hit particularly badly as they depend on pooled blood products. Recipients of ordinary blood transfusions are less at risk, as each unit comes from only one donor.

Once the virus has entered the bloodstream, antibodies appear after a variable length of time. There is currently no test for the presence of the virus itself, simply its antibodies, indicating that the body has reacted to the presence of the virus at some stage. It is still not known what proportion of carriers of the virus will go on to develop full-blown AIDS, although the indications are that the virus may lie dormant in the bloodstream for an average of ten years; the projected figures for HIV and AIDS incidence may not be particularly accurate, and new combination drug therapies are currently postponing the development of HIV into AIDS.

Many HIV-infected people currently remain as asymptomatic carriers. A proportion develop persistent generalised lymphadenopathy – swollen, often painful lymph glands in the neck or armpits. Some of these cases develop into AIDS, others – at least so far – have not. Other HIV-positive people develop AIDS-related symptoms such as fatigue, night sweats, weight loss and persistent diarrhoea. These alone do not constitute AIDS; a clinical diagnosis depends on the patient being HIV-antibody positive and having one or more specified opportunistic infections or diseases.

Staff protection

The main risk to health care staff is infection via the accidental inoculation of infected blood or body fluids, which can occur with used sharps or via the mucous membrane or cuts and abrasions in the skin surface, so safe practice – the application of universal precautions – is the best approach. Care must be taken with the blood and body fluids of all patients, not just known AIDS sufferers, because of the growing numbers of HIV-positive but otherwise asymptomatic people.

A good safety reference is the *AIDS Nursing Guidelines* produced by the RCN, a booklet which puts great emphasis on staff protection (RCN, 1994). There are other reference documents, such as the *National AIDS Manual* (1993; Pratt, 1986), and codes of good practice by the BMA, Unison and others. All hospitals, however, should by now have safety policies and procedures, which are well publicised and circulated to all nursing staff. Some departments, such as operating departments and maternity units, will have special needs. These are well covered in the RCN guidelines and are therefore not dealt with in detail here, except to mention them as a point of which to be aware. Again, such departments should by now have drawn up safety procedures for handling AIDS and HIV-positive patients.

Information and staff support

The principle of universal precautions focuses attention on safe practice rather than 'safe patients', and this remains essential. However there have been cases of nursing staff not being notified when a patient is diagnosed as having AIDS, and this is morally and legally indefensible, unsafe and grossly irresponsible. If you suspect this is happening in your unit, inform the health and safety rep immediately. Management must also keep staff informed of developments in research into the knowledge of the disease itself. It should be included in the basic nurse education curriculum and in continuing education courses, with regular updating for all nursing staff (Faugier and Hicken, 1996).

Nurses looking after patients with AIDS may be under considerable stress and will require support from management. They may be afraid of contracting the virus themselves and their patients require intensive and emotionally demanding nursing care. AIDS patients are usually young, possibly dying and in need of great psychological support. The normal difficulties of dealing with the patient's family and friends under such circumstances may be compounded by the stigma attached to the disease. Family and friends may not even be told the patient's diagnosis.

Staff health

Staff suffering from skin conditions such as eczema should not nurse AIDS patients. Cuts and abrasions should be kept covered. The risk to pregnant staff is disputed. Cytomegalovirus, which can harm the developing fetus, has been isolated in the urine of AIDS patients. While the risk is negligible, a pregnant nurse may be allowed to decline to nurse AIDS patients.

Staff screening

Screening health care workers for the presence of the HIV antibody has serious implications. A positive result is likely to have a profound influence on the person's personal life and possibly their professional life too. It raises very real problems with life insurance and mortgage applications. However staff exposed to AIDS patients should be given the opportunity to have a blood serum sample freeze-stored but not tested. If necessary, and only with the person's full knowledge and consent, this baseline sample could be released at a later date and tested with current sera samples.

Nursing care

Isolation

Some hospitals set up complete wards solely for AIDS patients, although most HIV-positive patients may be nursed on the open ward. The RCN advises that the patient should be nursed in a separate room if he or she is:

- Bleeding or likely to bleed.
- Incontinent.
- Post-operative, with wounds.
- Unconscious.
- Suffering from open skin lesions.
- Mentally disturbed or confused.
- Has added infection risks such as pulmonary infection.

Exclusive or disposable crockery and cutlery need be used only if the patient is bleeding from the mouth (for disposal procedures see below). Patients nursed on the open ward can use the ward bathrooms and toilets. If they have open lesions and/or are being nursed in a separate room, they should have their own washing equipment and use a commode.

Protective clothing

This is not necessary for normal social contact, but should be worn when you are likely to be exposed to blood or body fluids, for example when:

- Collecting and handling specimens.
- Handling and disposing of excreta.
- Conducting a venepuncture and administering intravenous drugs.
- Carrying out invasive nursing procedures - IV infusion care, catheterisation and catheter care, wound dressings.
- Handling soiled dressings or bed linen.
- Handling used instruments and sharps.
- Dealing with spillages of body fluids.

Disposable plastic aprons and well-fitting plastic or PVC gloves should be worn, with a face visor or goggles if the splashing of body fluids is likely. Masks (high-filtration type) are only needed if the patient has a pulmonary infection which indicates a mask is required. Cover all cuts and abrasions with a waterproof dressing.

Disposal of waste

Used disposable material, including soiled dressings and pads, should be sealed in the appropriately coloured plastic bag, labelled 'infection hazard' and sent for incineration (see the HSAC guidelines on the 'Safe Disposal of Waste').

If the patient is able to use the toilet, urine and faeces can be flushed away in the usual way. If the patient is using a bedpan or commode, the used bedpan and contents should go either in the bedpan washing machine, which must have a heat cycle of at least 80° C for one minute, or in the bedpan macerator. Keep the lid closed for at least one minute after the cycle ends to allow the aerosols to settle. Deal with all bedpans immediately after use.

Laundry

Linen that is soiled with blood or body fluids should be double bagged, the inner bag water-soluble so laundry staff do not need to open it, and washed at 95°C for at least ten minutes.

Specimens

Wear gloves and disposable plastic aprons to collect specimens. Label containers and request cards with 'infection hazard' and fasten the lids securely. Seal in a special plastic bag with the request card in a separate compartment and transport in a leak-proof autoclavable box. Alert the laboratory and portering staff.

Equipment

Safe sharps disposal and the prevention of needlestick injuries is the most important safety measure:

- Never resheath needles after use.
- Use a screw-capped evacuated blood collection system for venepuncture.
- Do not snap needles off syringes – this creates an aerosol hazard.
- Do not remove scalpel blades with your fingers.
- Discard all sharps into a sharps container which conforms to DoH standards, seal, label 'infection hazard' and send for incineration.
- Dispose of containers regularly – at least daily.

- Wear gloves when handling sharps.
- When shaving patients use a depilatory cream or their own electric razor (no ward should use a communal electric razor on any patient).

Use disposable equipment whenever possible. Reusable equipment that has been exposed to body fluids must be sterilised after use. Autoclavable equipment is returned to CSSD – sharps or breakables in a stout box, other equipment bagged – labelled 'biohazard'.

Non-autoclavable equipment can be sterilised in 2 per cent glutaraldehyde: immerse for a minimum of one hour before routine cleaning and disinfection. Remember glutaraldehyde is an irritant, therefore wear gloves, a mask and eye protection when handling and use in a well ventilated room. Seek local advice on the use of glutaraldehyde or alternatives.

Inoculation accidents

Milk the affected site to encourage bleeding, then wash the wound with soap and water. Report the incident immediately and complete an accident form. Splashes of blood on the skin should be washed off immediately. Splashes of blood in the mouth or eyes should be rinsed with lots of water or saline. New guidelines have been issued to prevent HIV infection following needlestick injuries (DoH, 1997), which the RCN and the Terrence Higgins Trust (an information and advice group for people with HIV and AIDs) both feel should be mandatory (Porter, 1997a).

Spillages

Deal with any spillages of blood or body fluids immediately: pour sodium hypochlorite 1 per cent on paper towels and place over the spillage. Leave for 30 minutes if possible before wiping up, wearing disposable gloves and apron. Dispose of towels, gloves and apron as for infected waste.

Cleaning

Use hot water and detergent for floors, fixtures and fittings, and a cream cleaner for sinks, toilets, showers and baths. Use disposable cloths and discard daily, and detachable mop heads that are laundered daily. Clean contaminated surfaces with 0.1 per cent sodium hypochlorite, unless there is a frank spillage (see above).

Nursing AIDS patients in the community

Most AIDS patients are now nursed at home, and as the new multiple drug regimes are more widely available, this proportion will increase, with patients choosing to stay at home whenever possible and most hospital admissions being short-stay. A recent survey in Edinburgh showed that between 1995 and 1997 there was a 40 per cent decline in hospital admissions of people with HIV and a 40 per cent decline in AIDS-related deaths, and that between 1994 and 1996 the proportion of patients taking antiretroviral therapy increased from 24 per cent to 49 per cent (Macgregor, 1997). Similar trends have led to new thinking in the planning of community services for people with HIV and AIDS, with the emphasis changing from palliative care to the management of chronic illness (Renton, 1996).

If the person is asymptomatic, normal domestic methods of hygiene and waste disposal are adequate. Patients are advised not to share toothbrushes, razors and so on. Soiled items should be burned or machine washed at 95°C for at least ten minutes. If he or she requires more intensive nursing care, it may be necessary to make arrangements with the local authority for the collection of infected waste and laundry. Supplies of protective clothing, disinfectants and disposal bins for sharps should be kept at the patient's home.

References and contact organisations on HIV and AIDS

De Ruyter, P. (1996) *Living with HIV/AIDS. A Practical Guide for Staying Well.* London: Allen Unwin (includes an excellent UK address list pp. 264–7).

DoH (1997) *Guidelines on Post-Exposure Prophylaxis for Health Care Workers Occupationally exposed to HIV.* Available free from the Department of Health. London: Department of Health.

Faugier, J. and Hicken, I. (1996) *AIDS and HIV: The nursing response.* London: Chapman & Hall.

HMSO (1993) 'The Health and Social Care of needs of people with HIV infection and AIDS'. London. Department of Health.

HSAC (1986) 'AIDS. Prevention of Infection in the Health Services'. Health and Safety Commission Fact Sheet. London: HSAC.

Jones, M. (1997) 'The mixed message'. *Nursing Times*, vol. 93, no. 35 (27 August), pp. 22–4.

Macgregor, H. (1997) 'A new way to care', *Nursing Times*, vol. 93, no. 35 (27 August), pp. 25–26.

Mofenson, L. M. (1997) 'Interaction between timing of perinatal HIV infection and design of interventions', *Acta Paediatrica*, vol. 86 (June) Supplement 421, pp. 1–9.

National AIDS Manual (1993) London: NAM Publications.

Nottingham Health Authority (1991) *AIDS policies for control and management of infection.* Nottingham: Nottingham Health Authority.

Nottingham Health Authority (1993) *Infection Control Manual.* Nottingham: Queen's Medical Centre NHS Trust.

Nursing Standard (1998) 'Transmission of HIV from mother to child', Reports, *Nursing Standard*, vol. 12, no. 36 (27 May), pp. 32–3

Porter, R. (1997a) 'Call for mandatory HIV accident rules', *Nursing Times*, vol. 93, no. 28 (9 July), p. 10.

Pratt, R. (1986) *AIDS: A Strategy for Nursing Care.* London: Edward Arnold.

RCN (1994a) *AIDS. Nursing Guidelines.* London: Royal College of Nursing.

RCN (1994b) *Disposal of health care waste in the community.* London: Royal College of Nursing. Re-order No 000 423.

Renton, A., Petrou, S. and Whitaker, L. (Compilers) (1996) *Community Services for people with HIV infection*. London: HMSO.

UKCC (1996) *Guidelines for Professional Practice*. London United Kingdom Central Council for Nursing, Midwifery and Health Visiting (see p. 24: conscientious objection).

Contact organisations

Terrence Higgins Trust offers information on AIDS and help and advice to people with HIV and AIDS. Terrence Higgins Trust, 52–54 Grays Inn Road, London WC1. Tel.: 0171 831 0330.

The English National Board runs courses for nurses: ENB 934 and ENB R51.

ENB Careers Advisory Service, PO Box 2EN, London WIA 2EN. Tel.: 0171 391 6200 or 0171 391 6205 (between 10.00 a.m. and 4.00 p.m. Monday to Friday). Fax: 0171 391 6207. E-mail: enb.careers@easynet.co.uk

Legionnaires' Disease

Legionnaires' Disease was first identified in 1976 at an American Legion convention in a hotel in Pennsylvania. One hundred and fortynine of the delegates, together with 72 other guests, contracted a pneumonia-like illness within a month of staying at the hotel. Their symptoms included coughing, general weakness and signs of fever. Of the 221 people that contracted the disease, 32 died.

The illness was eventually traced to a previously unidentified bacterium, *Legionella pneumophila*. The bug occurs naturally in soil and water and many scientists believe it could be present in most water supplies. But the bacteria multiply rapidly in certain conditions, such as in warm or stagnant water – making cooling towers, air conditioning units, showers, toilet cisterns and humidifiers prime culprits in the spread of the disease. The organisms are transmitted in water droplet form and the main route of infection is by inhalation of contaminated aerosols.

The first identified outbreak of Legionnaires' Disease in Britain occurred at Kingston Hospital, Surrey, in May 1980. Staff and unions at the hospital were furious to learn of the outbreak from their local paper – management and medical staff had been reluctant to publicise it for fear of causing panic. Eleven people were affected and three patients died. Since then there have been several outbreaks, the most serious of which was in Stafford General Hospital in April 1985, when 31 people died and many more were infected. Other outbreaks have been reported in hospitals in Portsmouth, Bristol, Reading, Newbury, Lincoln and Glasgow. Around 100–200 new cases are reported every year, though the actual incidence may be greater.

Although the bacterium has been identified in several public buildings, including the Houses of Parliament, widespread outbreaks have been most common in hospitals. This is partly because many hospitals have ventilation systems that require air to be passed through cooling towers, and partly because ill people are particularly susceptible.

Patients with a depressed immune system whose defences are already weakened, together with the elderly and people suffering from heart, lung or kidney disease, are more likely to be infected by the bacterium and are less well equipped to deal with it. But staff and visitors are also at risk. A relief nurse working in Bristol died from Legionnaires' Disease in 1985, and during the Kingston Hospital outbreak one of the hospital engineers contracted the disease and was seriously ill. Staff screening after the Stafford outbreak revealed that six nurses had been infected by the organism, although only two showed any symptoms and these were mild. The organism is contracted by inhaling a contaminated aerosol and not by contact with an already infected patient, so nurses are at no greater risk than other hospital workers.

So what can be done to reduce or eradicate the risk of further outbreaks? The Government-appointed inquiry into the Stafford outbreak identified design defects in a wet cooling tower as the source of the problem. 'Urgent consideration should be given to replacing any wet cooling tower with an air-cooled system', the Badenoch report said, and all new hospitals should be provided with air-cooled rather than water-cooled systems.

Existing systems, when replacement is impractical, should be inspected regularly and dosed continually with biocides. Good engineering practice in the selection, design, construction and maintenance of water installations will minimise the danger. Regular maintenance and cleaning of air conditioning and ventilation systems will reduce the risk of an outbreak, as will checking plant design to improve the water flow and eliminate the stagnation. The Notification of Cooling Towers and Evaporative Condensers Regulations 1992 require local authority notification of all devices such as cooling towers or evaporative condensers.

Wholesale eradication of the bacteria is only possible through regular inspection (recommended twice-yearly), routine bactericidal treatment with chlorine or biocides, heat control and system redesign. Although the organism thrives in tepid temperatures – between 20°C and 45°C – it is destroyed at temperatures above 55°C. Experts have suggested that heating hot water systems to 60°C for just one hour a day would destroy the bacteria.

Serious management shortcomings in the handling of the outbreak were also highlighted by the Badenoch report:

- There were delays in testing samples from patients.
- The hospital's infection control committee was not told that *Legionella pneumophila* bacteria had been found in the system five months before the outbreak occurred.

- Doctors were struggling to diagnose the disease, not knowing that the water tower had been contaminated with legionella bacteria.
- The biocide used to treat the cooling tower was ineffective.
- A crisis management team should have been set up in the early stages to help control the outbreak.
- All hospitals should have a plan to deal with serious medical emergencies, like those already drawn up for major accidents.

References on Legionnaires' Disease

CIBS (1991) 'Minimising the risk of Legionnaires' Disease', Technical Memoranda TM13. London: Chartered Institute of Building Engineers.

Cowle, R. (1995) 'TB, cure, care and control', *Nursing Times*, vol. 91, no. 38 (20 September), pp. 29–30.

DHSS (1986a) *First Report of the Committee of Inquiry into the Outbreak of Legionnaires' Disease in Strafford in April 1985* (Badenoch report). London: HMSO.

HSE (1993) *The Control of legionellosis (including Legionnaires' disease)*, HS(G)70. Sudbury: Health and Safety Executive.

HSE (1995) *The prevention or control of legionellosis (including Legionnaires' disease)*, Approved Code of Practice (ACOP)8.

McGeary, T. (1997) 'Legionnaires' legacy', *Nursing Times*, vol. 93, no. 3 (15 January), pp. 56–9.

TUC (1997) *Hazards at Work, TUC Guide to Health and Safety*, see especially pp. 127–8. London: TUC.

Tuberculosis

Tuberculosis rates are now increasing again, after a long period of decline from the early 1900s to the late 1980s. In particular, since 1987 its resurgence has been observed among susceptible groups of homeless people, people with HIV and recent immigrants from the Indian sub-continent, with a rise in annual reported cases in the UK from 5000 in 1987 to 6000 in 1995 (Ormerod, 1996). Some areas of inner London have reported rates that are three times higher than the national average (Mangtani *et al.*, 1995; Pearson *et al.*, 1996).

Separating the various causal factors is hard, and the reduction of control measures cannot be ruled out as a contributory factor. When tuberculosis seemed to be declining, from the 1950s to the mid-1980s, resources were reduced for tuberculosis treatment and health care staff became less familiar with the symptoms, delaying diagnosis, treatment and contact tracing (Reichman, 1991; Mangtani *et al.*, 1995).

The Department of Health set up a working group in 1994 to reexamine trends and produce new guidelines on prevention and control. Reports were produced looking at local incidence and the incidence among homeless people, which is particularly significant (DoH, 1996c, 1996d; Griffiths-Jones, 1997b). Another consequence of medical unfamiliarity with TB after its decline up to the 1980s is late diagnosis, and the patient is often already seriously ill or has even died before a diagnosis is made. A person with delayed diagnosis will certainly be more infectious, possibly with TB positive sputum (so-called 'open' pulmonary TB).

Transmission

TB is primarily transmitted by air – following expectoration by patients with open pulmonary TB, for example. Patients with suspected open TB should therefore be isolated until the diagnosis is certain, and if confirmed to have TB they should be isolated for at least the first two weeks of treatment, though they should not need to be barrier nursed unless they harbour multi-drug-resistant organisms (JTC, 1994). Patients with confirmed 'smear negative' or closed tuberculosis are not considered infectious after the first 24 hours of treatment and may be nursed in an open ward, unless there are vulnerable patients such as those on immuno-suppressive therapy. Standard infection control procedures should be followed.

Staff protection

Staff protection against TB should be based on vaccination. All staff should be tested for immunity to TB and given the BCG vaccination if negative or if their immunity is in any doubt. Staff in high-risk groups, such as those in regular contact with known tuberculous patients or known tuberculous materials, should be kept under regular surveillance, either through periodic tuberculin testing or chest X-rays (see Box 7.7). Staff who have had even a single contact with an infectious tuberculous patient should be identified and monitored.

If you do need to be vaccinated, it is important that you are free from any other infections at the time. No other vaccinations should be given in the same arm for at least three months, and no other immunisations at all for three weeks either before or after a BCG vaccination.

Box 7.7 *Compensated for care?*

A former patient and nursing student contracted multi-drug resistant tuberculosis from another patient at the HIV unit of a major London hospital, after sputum collection from an infected patient. The trust paid the nurse a confidential out-of-court settlement.

Source: *Nursing Times*, 22 October 1997, p. 5.

A small reaction to the vaccination is normal, including an area of hardened skin (up to 12mm in diameter) and some temporary disturbance of the axillary lymph glands. A discharging lesion, ulceration or abscesses (usually because the vaccination has been given too deeply) should be reported and treated.

References and further reading on tuberculosis

DoH (1996b) *Guidelines: Infection Control.* London: Department of Health.

DoH (1996c) *The Prevention and Control of Tuberculosis in the United Kingdom: Recommendations for the Prevention and Control at Local level.* Interdepartmental Working Group on Tuberculosis. London. Department of Health.

DoH (1996d) *The Prevention and Control of Tuberculosis in the United Kingdom: Tuberculosis and Homeless People.* Interdepartmental Working Group on Tuberculosis. London: Department of Health.

Joint Tuberculosis Committee of the British Thorax Society (1994) 'Control and prevention of tuberculosis in the UK', *Thorax*, vol. 49, no. 12 (December), pp. 1193–200.

Mangtani, P., Jolley, D., Watson, J. and Rodrigues, L. (1995) 'Socioeconomic deprivation and notification rates for tuberculosis in London', *British Medical Journal*, vol. 310, (15 April), pp. 963–6.

Ormerod, P. (1996) 'TB: detection and treatment', *Hospital Update*, vol. 22, no. 1 (January).

Pearson, A., Hamilton, G. and Healing, T. (1996) 'Summary of a report of the Working Party on Tuberculosis of the London Group of Consultants in Communicable Disease Control', *Journal of Hospital Infection*, vol. 33, no. 3 (July), pp. 165–79.

PHLS (1996) Public Health Laboratory Communicable Disease Report (CDR), no. 6 (17 May), pp. 179–80. London: Public Health Laboratory Service.

RCN (1996) 'A Shadow from the Past', RCN nursing update Learning Unit 067 (supplement), *Nursing Standard*, vol. 11, no. 1 (25 September). London: Royal College of Nursing.

Reichman, L. B. (1991) 'The U-shaped curve of concern', *American Review of Respiratory Diseases*, vol. 144, no. 4, pp. 741–2.

Shaw, T. (1995a) 'Tuberculosis: the history of incidence and treatment'. *Nursing Times*, vol. 91, no. 38 (20 September), pp. 27–9.

Shaw, T. (1995b) 'The resurgence of tuberculosis: current issues for nursing', *Nursing Times*, vol. 91, no. 40 (4 October), pp. 35–7.

Taylor, D., Redfern, L. and Hardy, P. (1996a) 'Tuberculosis: the role of the nurse', Professional Development Unit 35, supplement, *Nursing Times*, vol. 92, no. 43 (23 October).

Taylor, D., Redfern, L. and Hardy, P. (1996b) 'Tuberculosis: professional issues', Professional Development Unit 35, supplement, *Nursing Times*, vol. 92, no. 44 (30 October).

8 Technological hazards

Every day, all nurses use some kind of equipment in the course of their work, from the latest high-technology gadgets to simple chairs, tables and trolleys. All these objects have in common the fact that they can be dangerous to both nurse and patient if they are badly chosen, poorly manufactured or inadequately maintained. Careful regular inspection to ensure that safety standards are upheld is therefore essential, but nurses should also be involved at an earlier stage to make sure that the equipment chosen is appropriate and easy to use.

An increasing number of nurses are now performing advanced or expanded roles, such as inserting peripheral and central intravenous catheters, performing endoscopies and biopsies, acting as surgical assistants and performing minor operations. These roles have exposed nurses to equipment they have never previously worked with; so knowledge and understanding of the actions and potential hazards of equipment has become even more important.

Influencing the design, making an informed choice, taking preventive measures and reporting defects in equipment are all subjects on which nurses should have a say, for they are likely to be using equipment frequently and will therefore be in a position both to assess its standards and to be affected by any shortcomings. Trusts should develop procedures to ensure greater participation by nurses in appraising products and equipment and reporting their defects.

Much of this can be done through the services of the Medical Devices Agency (MDA), the UK 'competent authority' for operating and regulating EU medical devices directives. The roles of the MDA include device evaluation, appraisal and quality assurance of manufacturers, and the monitoring and dissemination of reported hazards and defects associated with particular types of equipment.

The MDA recognises that many nurses are not even aware of its existence and are generally unaware of how valuable the agency is and could be. It is currently looking at ways of ensuring that its reports and notices consistently reach clinical staff and unit budget-holders.

Equipment safety

Product appraisal

The MDA circulates device evaluation reports on around 140 health care products annually, from pathology test devices, infusion pumps and neonatal incubators to defibrillators, mattresses and bed-rails. Clinical nurses should insist that this information is made available to them and not just to technicians or trust purchasing officers.

Purchasers may make informed choices using MDA information, such as device evaluations on specific equipment, or by contacting the agency's nursing and device information advisers (see 'Contact organisations' at the end of this section). Product selection should be based on the following:

- Considering what is required of a particular item, by both nurse and patient.
- Ascertaining what products are available.
- Checking which products have been evaluated and the nature and the results of that research.
- Drawing up a shortlist of the best potential choices.
- Seeking the advice of appropriate experts, for example the fire officer.
- Seeing, handling and using the potential purchases before buying, either for a trial period in the clinical setting or at exhibitions or display centres. Employers should have a policy to ensure adequate local appraisal.

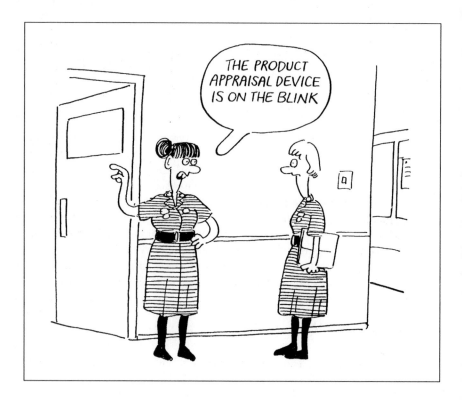

Nurses' purchasing power is increasing and manufacturers are increasingly influenced by nurses' views of their products. Expensive changes to an established design will not of course be undertaken without compelling reasons. Nevertheless, expert nursing opinion could be an important factor in commercial success, especially if it is made public through professional journals. Nurses should cooperate with supplies officers in making their points to regional sales representatives or marketing directors, recording their opinions in writing as well as verbally. They could also have more input to regulatory bodies such as the British Standard advisory panels, and organisations such as the Disabled Living Foundation which work with manufacturers to improve equipment design.

Manufacturer appraisal

Between January 1995 and June 1998 the MDA maintained the voluntary Manufacturer Registration Scheme (MRS), a quality assurance audit of medical device manufacturers. It also published a register of approved companies, in a planned transition period for manufacturers to comply with the medical devices directives. The MRS is being replaced by statutory notified bodies, some of which will be in the UK, and some in other European states. Notified bodies in the UK will be appointed from the private sector by the MDA.

It is apparent from published statements, however, that the MDA is not entirely happy with this arrangement, warning that inexperienced Notified Bodies could apply assessment criteria more appropriate to other industries, and secondly that some notified bodies, motivated by commercial gain, could seek additional business by giving manufacturers an 'easy ride' (MDA, 1995).

Reporting defects

What do you do if you find that equipment is defective? Procedures for this eventuality are now laid down in the Provision and Use of Work Equipment Regulations 1992, and must be based on a dynamic risk assessment policy, not a one-off assessment.

If you suspect the equipment is faulty, do not use it, and report your suspicions immediately. Under the NHS Management Executive notice, 'Reporting adverse incidents and reactions and defective products relating to medical and non-medical equipment and supplies, food, buildings and plant and medicinal products' (HSG[93]13), management is responsible for reporting defects to the Adverse Incident Centre (formerly the National Reporting and Investigation Centre, NATRIC) of the MDA, established in 1994.

During 1996, 4330 device-related incidents were reported to the MDA, of which 43 involved patient fatalities and 45 serious injuries (MDA, 1997). Many reported incidents involving malfunctioning infusion devices: there are more than 400 incidents on the NATRIC database, which includes records from 1983 – and according to the MDA most of these incidents can be attributed to lack of regular checks and maintenance.

Nurses have been injured too: an ITU staff nurse was electrocuted when fluid gathered inside a syringe pump and the case became live. Equipment is often knocked or dropped by both staff and patients, but is it always checked by competent technicians afterwards? The nursing adviser at the MDA advocates a 'drop policy', whereby any device which is dropped is immediately taken out of service to be checked and repaired (Glenister, 1996; Wilkinson, 1992).

Defective items should always be investigated and modified or removed from service, and the MDA believes that all adverse incidents should be reported, even if they might seem trivial at the time.

Once reports are registered they are investigated by an expert, cooperating with the person who reported the problem and the manufacturer of the device. Other users are warned of potentially dangerous problems, either immediately, by a hazard notice or, in less urgent situations, by a safety notice which is reported in the Safety Action Bulletins circulated bimonthly. Safety reps should have access to these.

Preventive measures

The MDA emphasises the importance of reporting defects so that action can be taken. But it also stresses the need for equipment to be thoroughly checked by technicians before it comes into use, so that faults can be picked up before anyone is put at risk.

Equally, regular inspection and maintenance are vital once the apparatus is in service; the RCN tells its safety reps to bear the following five points in mind when completing their inspection checklists:

- The equipment's suitability for the purpose for which it is provided.
- Proper maintenance.
- Information, instruction and training in the safe use and maintenance of the equipment and in what to do if things go wrong.
- Full compliance with the Provision and Use of Work Equipment Regulations (1992).
- How work equipment provided since 1 January, 1993 is checked to ensure it complies with the regulations, including the following:

    - suitable guarding for mechanical hazards;
    - protection against burns and scalds from hot or cold equipment or its products;

- control devices which are visible, identifiable, marked and located outside danger zones, and control systems which are safe;
- work equipment which is stabilised by clamping or other means and sufficient lighting provided when equipment is used;
- where there are health and safety hazards, work equipment is marked clearly and incorporates warnings.

MDA studies show that operational difficulties arise from design errors, breakdowns in quality, lack of maintenance, operator misuse and the age of the apparatus. Resources clearly play a part, as money is needed for inspection and maintenance as well as replacing outmoded or worn-out stock. Helen Glenister, principal nursing adviser for the MDA, suggests that, 'Health care professionals have a particular role in ensuring that [medical devices] are used properly and in the manner intended by the manufacturer' (Glenister, 1996).

References, contact organisations and resources on equipment safety

Glenister, H. (1996) 'Safety first', *Nursing Management*, vol. 3, no. 6 (October), pp. 14–5.

MDA (1995) *Corporate Plan 1995–2000*. London: Medical Devices Agency, Department of Health.

MDA (1997) *MDA Annual Report and Accounts. 1996–1997*. London: Medical Devices Agency, Department of Health.

NHSME (1993) *Reporting adverse incidents and reactions, and defective products relating to medical and non-medical equipment and supplies, food, buildings, and plant and medicinal products*, HSG93.13. Leeds: National Health Service Management Executive.

RCN (1994) *Safety Representatives' Manual*. London: Royal College of Nursing Labour Relations Department.

TUC (1997) *Hazards at Work: TUC Guide to Health and Safety*. London: Trades Union Congress. See especially Chapter 18, 'Work Equipment. . .'; Chapter 22, 'Maintenance Hazards'; Chapter 23, 'Electrical Safety'; Chapter 24, 'Office Hazards'; Chapter 25, 'Display Screen Equipment'.

Wilkinson, R. (1992) 'Machine age killers', *Nursing Standard*, vol. 6, no. 43 (15 July), pp. 44–5.

Contact organisations

Medical Devices Agency (Head Office), Hannibal House, Elephant and Castle, London SE1 6TQ. Tel.: 0171 972 8000.

Medical Devices Agency – European and Regulatory Affairs (ERA) Responsible for the MDA's regulatory role as the UK's Competent Authority for the European Union Medical Devices Directives. ERA assesses manufacturers' protocols for clinical investigations, issues regular bulletins and gives directives affecting medical devices. Tel.: 0171 972 8300. Fax: 0171 972 8112.

Medical Devices Agency – Device Technology and Safety (DTS). Responsible for investigation of adverse incidents associated with medical devices; issues device bulletins, hazard and safety notices to UK health services. DTS also provides technical advice on devices, including support and development of standards underpinning EU directives.

Medical Devices Agency – Adverse Incident Centre (AIC) receives reports from users and manufacturers and coordinates investigations. To report Adverse Incidents:

In England: Tel.: 0171 972 8080. Fax: 0171 972 8109.

In Scotland: Scottish Healthcare Supplies, Trinity Park House, South Trinity Road, Edinburgh EH5 3SH. Helpline: 0131 551 8333. Emergency: 0131 552 6380. Fax: 0131 552 6535

In Wales: Welsh Office, Cathays Park, Cardiff CF1 3NQ. Tel.: 01222 825479.

In Northern Ireland: Northern Ireland Department of Health and Social Security, Defect Investigation Centre, Eastern Services Directorate, Stoney Road, Dundonald, Belfast BT16 0US. Tel.: 01232 523714. Fax: 01232 483299.

Medical Devices Agency – Device Evaluation and Publications. Manages independent medical device evaluations and publishes reports about safety, performance and user experience. Reports include pathology equipment, infusion pumps, neonatal incubators, patient monitors, defibrillators, anaesthetic workstations and diagnostic imaging equipment. A catalogue is available. Tel.: 0171 972 8181. Fax: 0171 972 8105.

Medical Devices Agency – Clinical Team (CLIN). Gives specialist expertise, as support and to raise awareness of the MDA in the NHS and with professional bodies. For medical issues: tel. 0171 972 8123, fax. 0171 972 8111, or write to The Medical Director. For nursing issues: tel. 0171 972 8128, fax. 0171 972 8103, or write to the Nursing Director. E-mail: mda__mail@mda.win-uk.net World Wide Web: http://www.open.gov.uk/mda/mdahome.htm

Nurses working in specialised settings, especially where complex and sophisticated equipment is used, need to be aware of the particular hazards they face. General safety guidance may not cover all these complexities and it is advisable for each specialist area to appoint a safety representative who can familiarise herself with the specific information needed, for example in the operating theatre.

The range of equipment used by nurses is so great that it would be impossible to list all the possible hazards here. Instead we will look in more detail at four specific areas: sharps, electrical equipment, lasers and computers.

Sharps

Every nurse knows about the dangers of 'sharps' – hypodermic needles, broken ampoules, scalpels and so on – yet accidents arising from the improper use or disposal of these objects are still very common. Failure to dispose of them safely can also harm other health workers: porters and other ancillary staff involved in waste disposal report many such injuries.

Surveillance studies show that around two thirds of reported sharps injuries happen to nurses (McCormick *et al.*, 1991), although researchers suggest that doctors may have a higher rate of sharps injury (de Vries and Cossart, 1994). An injury of this sort is painful and unpleasant, but it can have more serious consequences for health care workers. An injury which pierces the protective layer of the skin increases the risk of infection from the following:

- Serum hepatitis B, C or D (one in 1000 people carries the Australian antigen).
- Herpes simplex – a highly infectious virus which can cause painful and septic sores (whitlows) around the nails.
- Syphilis.
- Staphylococcal and streptococcal infections.
- Local or systemic sepsis from *Clostridium tetani.*
- HIV.

These infections are very dangerous, and employers should make staff aware of the procedures to follow if they receive a sharps injury from equipment used with a patient, such as a needle or scalpel. A suggested response is as follows:

- Encourage bleeding at the site of the injury.
- Wash the wound with soap and hot water.
- Dry hands.
- Apply povidone iodine to wound.
- Cover with an occlusive dressing (preferably waterproof).
- Report the incident immediately to your line manager and occupational health department
- Complete an accident form.
- Identify the source of needle contamination if possible (Russell, 1997).

A blood sample should be taken from both patient and nurse. If contamination is suspected and immunisation is considered necessary, it must be given within 48 hours. Testing for HIV and hepatitis B or C in the source of contamination is recommended but consent must be given. If it is positive for any infection, the employee should be tested over a period of at least six months for sero-conversion (Hanrahan and Reutter, 1997). Non-immunised or susceptible staff exposed to hepatitis B may receive two immediate doses of hepatitis B immune globulin, which is repeated a month later. This is reported to be up to 75 per cent successful in preventing the development of hepatitis B (Centers for Disease Control, 1990).

Box 8.1   *British Standard specification for sharps containers*

- British Standards Institution (BSI) kitemark on the container.
- Clear instructions for assembly.
- Clear markings on the sharps container, indicating when it is three quarters full.
- Secure closing and locking mechanisms.
- The presence of a handle to enable the user to carry a full sharps container away from the body.
- The use of sturdy material to prevent penetration by hypodermic needles or leakage of blood or blood fluids.
- The presence of biological hazard warning signs on the outside of the container.
- Sharps containers that are indestructible by incineration.

Source: Russell, 1997.

Thoughtlessness is often at the root of sharps-related injuries; needles carelessly left among linen or swabs used on patients, for example, and discovered by the nurse clearing the trolley afterwards. A significant proportion of injuries are associated with the collection or disposal of waste – using inadequate or overfilled containers, through laziness, lack of time or lack of supplies. Accidents can also occur when nurses take catheter specimens of urine from ports in the plastic tubing leading to the drainage bag, an illustration of the need to report and rectify badly designed equipment.

Preventive measures, therefore, depend on staff education as well as the provision of proper facilities: education of all staff in the careful handling of sharps, clear and well monitored infection control procedures, and provision by managers of adequate facilities for safe disposal (Box 8.1).

Staff education

Safety reps, occupational health departments and infection control nurses have organised local education campaigns based on input to induction courses for new staff and nursing students, in-service training and posters. Guidelines on the safe disposal of clinical waste have been issued by the Health and Safety Commission. The DoH and the BMA (1990) also make recommendations on sharps. Hospitals have been very innovative in staff education on the handling and disposal of sharps, with campaigns linking bad practice with the risk of self-inflicted injury and infection and public praise of staff for good practice. One hospital in Nottingham used a football-style 'yellow card' and 'red card' system to get the message across (*Health Service Journal*, 1997).

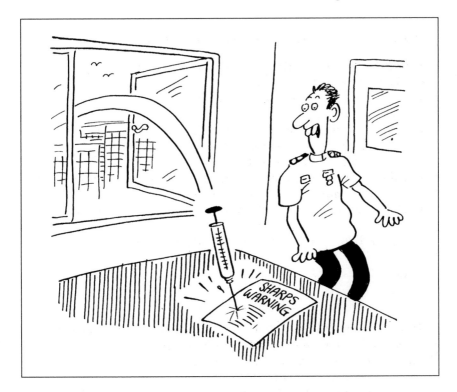

The key to safety with sharps is continually to promote safe practice, with all the rationales behind it, and to minimise risk by such policies as:

- No resheathing of needles.
- Ready access to sharps disposal boxes in all clinical areas.
- Evaluation of new, potentially safer products.
- Monitoring of workplace policies.
- Monitoring and publicising the incidence of sharps-related injuries.
- Examination of other factors, such as poor lighting, cramped work areas, improvised equipment.

References and further reading on sharps

British Medical Association (1990) 'A code for the safe use and disposal of sharps', London: BMA.

Centers for Disease Control (1990) 'Protection against viral hepatitis: recommendations of the Immunisations Practices Advisory Committee'. Atlanta, Georgia. (ACIP), Morbidity and Mortality Weekly Report no 39 (supplement), pp. 1–25.

Hanrahan, A. and Reutter, L. (1997) 'A critical review of the literature on sharps injuries: epidemiology, management of exposures and prevention', *Journal of Advanced Nursing*, vol. 25, no.1 (January), pp. 144–54.

Health and Safety Commission (1992) *The Safe Disposal of Clinical Waste*, ISBN 0717604470. London: HMSO.

HSJ (1997) 'Special Report: Infection Control: 4', *Health Service Journal*, vol. 107, no. 5577 (30 October), pp. 1–16.

McCormick, R., Meisch, M., Ircink, F. and Maki, D. (1991) 'Epidemiology of hospital sharps injuries: a 14 year prospective study in the pre-AIDS and AIDS eras', *American Journal of Medicine*, vol. 70, no. 91 (supplement), pp. 301–7.

Mercier, C. (1994) 'Reducing the incidence of sharps injuries', *British Journal of Nursing*, vol. 3, no. 17 (22 September), pp. 897–8, 900–1.

Murdoch, S. and Cowell, F. (1993) 'Sharp shocks', *Nursing Times*, vol. 89, no. 2 (13 January), pp. 64–8.

Russell, P. (1997) 'Reducing the incidence of needlestick injuries', *Professional Nurse*, vol. 12, no. 4 (January), pp. 275–8.

TUC (1997) *Hazards at Work, TUC Guide to Health and Safety*. London: Trades Union Congress. See especially pp. 126–7.

Vries, B. and Cossart, Y. (1994) 'Needlestick injury in medical students', *Medical Journal of Australia*, vol. 160, pp. 390–400.

Electrical hazards

Electrical hazards are a good example of safety risks which are so common that we barely notice them. Moreover, apart from the obvious dangers of old wiring, overloaded circuits and trailing flexes, the growth in complex technology means more electrical apparatus is being used in treatment and care, particularly in specialised departments such as theatres and intensive care.

The subject is not exactly a turn-on, and as Bishop (1979) points out, 'the existing education for nurses on their handling of electrical apparatus is slightly less than a housewife receives when buying a new vacuum cleaner'. Electric shocks and burns to nurses could also result from insufficient safety checks.

EU regulations attempt to enforce the isolation of all electrical apparatus used on patients. The RCN says that all equipment should be correctly and regularly maintained, appropriate for the task in hand and used in accordance with the manufacturer's instructions. Defects should be reported immediately and the equipment should normally be withdrawn until the fault has been corrected. All equipment should have the right plugs, and on no account should systems be overloaded.

Employers' duties

Employers must ensure that live parts of electrical equipment are inaccessible in normal operation and that suitably trained and competent people maintain it.

Electrical safety is covered under the Health and Safety at Work Act (1974), and several other sets of regulations:

- Electricity at Work Regulations 1989: general health and safety principles, regarding actual and foreseeable risks.
- Low Voltage Electrical Equipment (Safety) Regulations 1989: implementing EU regulations harmonising the laws of member states.

References and further reading on electrical hazards

Bishop, V. (1979) 'It can be lethal in the care unit', *Nursing Mirror*, vol. 149 (11 October), pp. 20–1.

HSE (1994) *Maintaining portable and transportable electrical equipment*, HS(G) 107. Sudbury: Health and Safety Executive.

McConnell, E. (1996) 'Clinical dos and don'ts. Ensuring electrical safety', *Nursing 96*, vol. 26, no. 10 (October), p. 20.

Wilkinson, R. (1992) 'Machine age killers', *Nursing Standard*, vol. 6, no. 43 (15 July), pp. 44–5.

Lasers

The need to be aware of the hazards not only of familiar equipment but also of new apparatus is well illustrated by the increased use of lasers. Many doctors are eager to rush into using new technology, an enthusiasm fostered by manufacturers who stand to make good profits, and there is a risk of insufficient research and testing before the equipment is put to use. Too often, staff using such equipment are inadequately trained and lack knowledge of the risks involved.

Referring to the increasing use of lasers in health services, the RCN says that all staff should be warned of the risks, the correct safe working procedure and any protective clothing or equipment required. Some clinical studies have been published, for example Gibbs (1990), Hall (1991) and Frost (1993), but the detailed MDA guidlines (MDA, 1995) may not be readily available to nurses.

Lasers are contributing to significant advances in medical practice in many specialities, including ophthalmology, gynaecology, neurosurgery, dermatology, respiratory medicine and dentistry, but the way they are generated and used can be dangerous. The main hazard is permanent eye damage, which can result from accidental exposure, either from the direct beam or from reflection off surfaces such as walls. The hands and face may also be damaged and/or sensitised and the use of lasers on particular materials releases poisonous dust, fumes and smoke (laser plumes). Some lasers use gases such as chlorine, bromine and fluorine, and gas leakage may cause a chemical hazard. Electric shocks, explosions and fires are possible, particularly in the presence of oxygen or anaesthetic gases (MDA, 1995, p. 10). Risk assessment under the COSHH regulations must therefore be carried out in areas of laser use.

The British Standards Institution sets out guidelines which classify types of laser according to their strength, which directly relates to their potential hazard. Class 4, the most hazardous, is also used most often in medicine. The DoH follows much of the BSI's advice (although in a weaker form) and states that a laser protection advisor should be appointed when Class 3A lasers and above are in use. Guidance on the maximum permissible exposure levels is given in the British Standard document BS EN 60825-1, based on exposures causing the minimum injury that can be caused clinically (MDA, 1995). The MDA offers advice on subjects which should be covered in the training of laser users (ibid.) There is also a recommended symbol, which should be displayed on all lasers.

Safety policies

As with ionising radiation safety, laser use requires the drawing up of local rules, and the MDA (1995) offers the following suggestions on the issues which should be covered:

- Nature of the hazard to persons.
- Controlled and safe access.
- A register of authorised users.
- Nominated keyholders and keyholders' responsibilities.
- Need for training.
- Methods of safe working.
- Definition of simple, pre-use safety checks.
- Personal protective equipment, especially eye protection.
- Prevention of use by unauthorised people.
- Normal operating procedures.
- Adverse incident procedures.
- Contact point for laser protection adviser.
- Limits of the laser controlled area.

To follow RIDDOR requirements and Department of Health and EU directives for medical devices, any adverse incidents should be reported to the Department of Health and the MDA.

Specific safety measures

- Eye protection – all who are at risk should have eye protection appropriate to the laser type being used, and ensure its safety and suitability before use.
- Fire risks – since laser beams could light anaesthetic gases, these should be protected from the laser beam. The MDA notes the particular

importance of fire precautions during ENT surgery. The MDA also suggests that tissues surrounding the treatment site should be protected by applying moist dressings and avoiding alcohol-based skin preparations. Laser plume should be removed by suction.

- Reflective surfaces – the MDA warns against the use of instruments with reflective surfaces (such as dental mirrors) near the laser beam, and suggests that matt-finished instruments be acquired.

References and further reading on lasers

BSI (1994) *Radiation safety of laser products, equipment classification, requirements, and user's guide*, BS EN 60825-1:1994. London: British Standards Institution.

Frost, J. (1993) 'Clinical application of lasers', *Professional Nurse*, vol. 8, no. 5 (February), pp. 298, 300, 302–3.

Gibbs, J. (1990) 'Action on the environment: a closer look at lasers', *Nursing Times*, vol. 86, no. 46 (14 November), pp. 33–4.

Hall, F. (1991) 'Our experience of laser work', *Natnews: British Journal of Theatre Nursing*, vol. 28, no. 3 (March), pp. 9–10.

Medical Devices Agency (1995) *Guidance on the Safe Use of Lasers in Medical Practice*. London: Department of Health.

Computers

Over the past 20 years, nurses have become increasingly accustomed to using computers in the course of their work – clinical, education and research. Studies, however, have highlighted the health risks from spending protracted periods at work on the computer. These include repetitive strain injury (RSI), which according to the TUC, is a major problem in one in three work places (Hazards, 1996); furniture design-related muscle spasm and strains; postural fatigue; computer vision syndrome (CVS), which involves headaches, sore eyes, blurred vision and eye strain (Hazards, 1997a); and electrosensitivity to display screen equipment (DSE), manifested as hypersensivity to both screen flicker and radiation emissions and recognised in Sweden as an industrial disease (Hazards, 1997b).

The relevant legislation on this issue is the Health and Safety (Display Screen Equipment) Regulations 1992. Following EU directives, these regulations require employers to:

- Identify 'users', 'operators' and DSE workstations.
- Assess workstations to determine risks.
- Reduce any risks identified in assessments.
- Ensure new workstations meet the minimum requirements.
- Plan daily work to provide breaks and changes of activity.
- Provide training and information so that staff can work safely and without risk to their health.

Concern has also been expressed about the possible risk, particularly to reproductive health, from radiation emissions from display screen equipment. Reports from Canada and the USA have linked miscarriages, premature births and birth defects with DSE use, although the Health and Safety Executive (HSE, 1996a) maintains that there is no conclusive evidence that DSE usage poses any increased risk during pregnancy. The TUC (1997) notes concern about 'abnormal pregnancy outcomes' linked to DSE use but acknowledges there is no consensus about the causes.

The only measurable levels of radiation from display screen equipment have been in the very low frequency (VLF) and extra low frequency (ELF) bands, which have not been shown to affect human biological systems and processes. The TUC suggests that until more comprehensive research is available, unions should negotiate agreeements that give pregnant women the right to move to other work or to take leave during pregnancy without loss of employment rights. Agreements on the right to transfer from DSE work should be seen as relating to all potential causes of reproductive hazards, not just radiation, and should also cover those planning to become pregnant.

References, contact organisations and further reading on computers

Doyal, L. (1995) *What Makes Women Sick: Gender and the Political Economy of Health*. Basingstoke: Macmillan.

Hazards (1996) 'Design RSI Out', *Hazards*, vol. 56 (Autumn), p. 12.

Hazards (1997a) 'Computer Vision syndrome', *Hazards*, vol. 58 (April/June), pp. 8–9.

Hazards (1997b) 'Screen sensitive', *Hazards*, vol. 59 (July/September), p. 5.

HSE (1993) 'Health and Safety (Display Screen Equipment) Regulations 1992', Health Services Sheet no. 5. Sudbury: Health and Safety Executive.

HSE (1996) *Working with VDUs*, IND(G)36(L). Sudbury: Health and Safety Executive.

RCN (1995) 'Hazards for Pregnant Nurses: An A-Z Guide', Health and Safety at Work leaflet no. 4, re-order no. 000 496. London: Labour Relations Department, Royal College of Nursing.

TUC (1997) *Hazards at Work: TUC Guide to Health and Safety*. London: Trades Union Congress. See especially Chapter 25, 'Display Screen Equipment', pp. 225–40.

Contact organisations

City Centre, Sophia House, 32–35 Featherstone Street, London EC1Y 8QX. Provides information and advice on hazards, and subjects such as sexual harassment, racial discrimination for office workers. Publishes the *Safer Office Bulletin*. Tel.: 0171 608 1338. The VDU Workers Rights Campaign is based at City Centre too.

Hazards Magazine, PO Box 199, Sheffield S1 1FQ. Information magazine aimed at safety reps. Frequently publishes articles and news items about work-related equipment and hazards. Tel.: 0114 276 5695.

Labour Research Department, 78 Blackfriars Road, London SE1 8HF. Tel. 0171 928 3649. Produces leaflets for trade unionists (prices higher for non-labour movement bodies). Includes 'VDUs & Health and Safety – a user's guide' (1991).

Other sources of information: the **TUC**, the **GMB**, the **Transport and General Workers' Union UNISON**, and **Hazard Centres** in many UK cities. Full details are provided in Appendix 2 at the end of this book.

9 Reproductive hazards

Hazards at work can cause a range of adverse reproductive effects, including infertility, stillbirth, miscarriage, congenital abnormalities and childhood cancer (Box 9.1). The risks come from harmful agents such as chemicals or radiation; or from work conditions such as stress or heavy manual work (Box 9.2) (Williams, 1996).

A comprehensive analysis of the risk is difficult. It is impossible to assess the proportion of reproductive problems caused by occupational hazards or to produce a definitive list of dangerous substances and circumstances. Little research has been done and much of the available evidence is derived from animal data, which can be highly unreliable. For example human reproduction can be harmed by doses of chemicals that produce no effect in animals. Thalidomide, the drug that tragically did more than anything to alert the public to reproductive risks, had no effect on pregnant rats when tested prior to marketing.

Recognising reproductive effects can also be difficult. Early miscarriages, for example, can be mistaken for heavy periods and there are no reliable statistics for miscarriage rates. Some reproductive problems such as miscarriage and subfertility are relatively common anyway, and can too easily be attributed to factors unconnected with work. So any evidence tends to be controversial and can be easily dismissed.

This may be reinforced by the male bias of research in occupational health (Doyal, 1995). Karen Messing of the University of Quebec, speaking at the 1996 inaugural International Congress on 'Women, Work and Health', stated that 'Past exclusion of women from scientific studies has produced evidence of health problems only among men, resulting in reluctance to study women . . . because of the prejudice that women's work is safe, there are few prevention programmes in areas where women work' (Paul, 1996).

Nevertheless there is evidence that health workers are at risk, and the fact that the majority of health workers are women should in any case alert employers to the need for special precautions and care. It is also important to remember that men as well as women face risks, both to themselves and to their families. Lowered sperm count, damaged sperm, loss of libido and impotence have all been connected with work conditions. There is evidence of an increased miscarriage rate in the partners of men in certain occupational groups, while other research has suggested an increased incidence of cancer in the children of male workers exposed to lead.

Box 9.1   *Adverse reproductive effects*

Pre-conception:
Menstrual disorders	Reduced libido
Hormone imbalance	Male impotence
Reduced fertility (male or female)	Sperm disorders
Infertility	Lower age at menopause

During pregnancy:
Spontaneous abortion (up to 28 weeks)	Chromosomal damage
	Altered sex ratio
Late fetal death, stillbirth	Maternal illness during pregnancy:
Retarded fetal development (physical or mental)	toxaemia, haemorrhage

After delivery:
Premature births	Mental retardation
Congenital abnormalities	Low birth weights
Behavioural disorders	Child morbidity
Child cancer	

Box 9.2   *Sources of risk*

Chemicals:
Anaesthetic gases	Toluene
Mercury	Ethylene oxide
Formaldehyde	Ethylene dichloride
Lead	Arsenic and compounds

Drugs:
Cytotoxic drugs	Warfarin

Physical agents:
Radiation	Excessive noise levels

Work conditions:
Heavy manual work	Stress
Shift work	

Biological agents:
Varicella zoster (chicken pox)	Hepatitis
Rubella (German measles)	Cytomegalovirus
Herpes	

Anaesthetic gases

The main risk to reproductive health in operating theatres lies in the exposure of staff to anaesthetic gases, in particular nitrous oxide.

Evidence of a link between anaesthetic gases and miscarriage first emerged in the 1970s. More recently, several reports have indicated that there are significantly more congenital abnormalities in the children of women exposed to anaesthetic gases and a significantly increased frequency of spontaneous abortion (Guirguis *et al.*, 1990; Eger, 1991; Foley, 1993; Donaldson and Meechan, 1995). Partners of male operating theatre staff have been found to face a slightly increased risk of miscarriage and there is also some evidence of a link between waste anaesthetic gases and congenital abnormalities in the offspring of operating room staff (Guirguis *et al.*, 1990).

Nitrous oxide, halothane, penthane, triluene, ethane and cyclopropane have all been identified as potentially harmful, particularly to anaesthetists, theatre nurses and theatre technicians who face continuous low-level exposure. The HSE only introduced occupational exposure standards for anaesthetic gases in 1993, and updated them in 1996 (Johnston, 1993; Cooper, 1994; JNM, 1996). However while in the USA the National Institute of Occupational Safety and Health (NIOSH) in 1977 set a threshold limit of 25 parts per million for an eight-hour exposure, in the UK the exposure limit introduced in 1994 was 100 parts per million (Johnston, 1993).

Green's excellent British study on nitrous oxide and other anaesthetic hazards in the peri-operative environment is a valuable summary of research into hazards in operating theatres, and suggests a disturbingly low level of health and safety awareness amongst operating theatre staff (Green, 1996). Green concludes that 'contamination of the operating environment with trace concentrations of waste anaesthetic gases is . . . inevitable'. She emphasises the continued lack of staff awareness of exposure hazards, some mistakenly believing that scavenging eliminates gas pollution and that nitrous oxide is innocuous when clearly it is not.

Under the Management Regulations 1992 and COSHH 1988 statutory actions, risk assessments should be made in operating departments. Employers are required to establish the true extent of waste anaesthetic gas hazards, to monitor exposure levels and to eliminate or minimise risks. All staff should be given adequate information about the problem and be aware of their responsibility to maintain a safe environment.

Contamination can come from three sources:

- Leakages from faulty equipment.
- As the anaesthetist administers the gas.
- From the patient's breath in the immediate post-operative period.

The most effective preventive measure is adequate theatre ventilation and scavenging systems: all operating theatres have been required by the HSE to use active scavenging systems since 1996, when revised occupational exposure standards became effective for anaesthetic gases (HSE, 1996b; 1997c). However further research into the potential reproductive hazards of anaesthetic gases has been undertaken in the USA, and it has been shown that high concentrations of waste gases exist even when scavenger systems are used (AAOHN, 1995).

Action checklist

- Ask your managers for staff education and information on the health and safety regulations affecting theatres, especially related to maximum exposure limits and occupational exposure standards.
- Use your safety rep to press for regular monitoring of contamination in theatres and recovery rooms. Checks should be carried out at least every three months.
- Find out if the theatres you work in are properly ventilated or scavenged. If not, press for equipment to be installed, used and maintained.
- Find out if low-flow anaesthesia methods and laryngeal mask airways are used to reduce exposure levels (Green, 1996).
- If you are pregnant, avoid working in anaesthetic rooms or recovery rooms and press for transfer elsewhere without loss of pay or seniority. If possible, avoid theatre work altogether.
- Try not to expose yourself to the patient's breath post-operatively. Some anaesthetic gases have been detected in the end-expired air of patients for 10–18 days post-anaesthesia.
- Urge management to ensure that all staff who may become pregnant are aware of the risks – damage to the fetus is most likely before pregnancy is discovered or confirmed.

Biological risks

Some infectious agents can cause birth defects when they cross the placenta and infect and damage the fetus at a particularly vulnerable time, usually during the first eight weeks of pregnancy. Rubella (German measles) is probably the best known and can cause miscarriage or deafness, cataracts, mental retardation or abnormalities in bone or heart formation. The risk is avoidable if the mother is already immune through immunisation or having had the disease, probably in childhood. Public awareness of the risk is now such that all schoolgirls in the UK are tested for immunity and vaccinated at the age of 16, while the combined measles, mumps and rubella (MMR) vaccination during infancy is reducing the incidence of the disease in childhood. All nurses, however – particularly those working with children as they are more likely to be exposed to the rubella virus – should be screened for immunity on employment.

Rubella may be the best known risk, but it is not the only one. A US study estimated that about 2 per cent of all congenital malformations were due to maternal infections during pregnancy (Kalter and Warkany, 1983). Other potentially harmful viruses and diseases are:

- *Varicella zoster* (chicken pox): may cause development defects, stillbirths or infant mortality.
- Coxsackie: development defects, stillbirths, infant mortality.
- Cytomegalovirus: development defects.
- Herpes simplex: development defects, infant mortality.
- Hepatitis: stillbirths, infant mortality.
- Influenza: developmental defects.
- Syphilis: developmental defects, stillbirths.
- Toxoplasmosis: developmental defects.

However, the evidence is strongest for rubella, cytomegalovirus (CMV) and toxoplasmosis (Pillay, 1996). Most patients with HIV excrete CMV in their urine and faeces, and the Royal College of Nursing recommends that pregnant nurses do not nurse patients who are HIV positive or have AIDS.

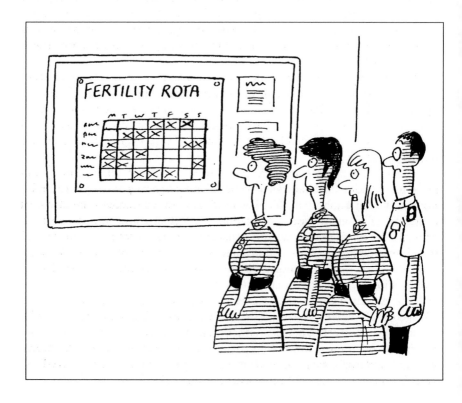

With some of the viruses mentioned, those responsible for influenza for example, the risk may come from the increased body temperature that accompanies the infection – at certain times during pregnancy this may present a risk of fetal malformation, and it can also reduce fertility in men.

Certain organisms are directly implicated in male infertility, notably those causing mumps and syphilis.

Radiation

Radiation is discussed at length elsewhere in this book, but is mentioned here to highlight its specific effects on human reproduction. There are two types of radiation, ionising and non-ionising. Non-ionising radiation is electromagnetic and comes from microwave frequencies and radio frequencies. It is emitted in varying degrees from all types of electrical equipment, including computer display screen equipment (DSE). There has been much recent controversy about the effects of DSEs on pregnant women. 'Clusters' of miscarriages have been reported among computer operators. The Health and Safety Executive has declared DSEs safe. Its conclusions are based on recorded levels of radiation emitted from the equipment (HSE, 1996a), but other experts argue that low-frequency radiation coming from the machines is not fully detected by normal measuring equipment. The posture of computer operators may also have some bearing on reproductive health (TUC, 1997).

While there remains considerable doubt about the risks, it would seem sensible to take precautions, such as restricting the amount of time all operators, but especially pregnant women, spend at the machines. Nurses' work with computers is limited, although increasing rapidly, and there is no reason why such work could not be avoided during pregnancy, if the nurse herself wishes to avoid it.

Ionising radiation includes X-rays, alpha, beta and gamma rays, and neutron radiation. Obviously the type of most concern to the nurse is X-ray radiation. Ionising radiation is harmful because it changes the electrical charge of some atoms and molecules in our cells by removing an electron from the atom. These changes can alter enzymes, structural proteins, cell membranes and genetic material. Pregnant women are most at risk because the developing fetus, with rapidly dividing cells, is more susceptible to radiation than any other part of the body.

The reproductive risks of high doses of radiation, such as that experienced after atom bomb explosions, include developmental defects, especially central nervous system defects, and childhood cancers. There is very little research into reproductive outcomes in radiation workers, especially health workers, although there is evidence to suggest that chronic, low-dose radiation might be harmful to pregnant women (McAbee *et al.*, 1993).

Extra precautions must be taken with radiation if you are pregnant or planning to be (see Box 9.3). Do not work in a unit where there are frequent X-rays, such as coronary care units, and do not look after a patient with a radioactive implant. Keep as far away as possible when an X-ray is being taken. If possible do not hold a patient who is being X-rayed. In New York State, all women of childbearing age are forbidden to hold any patient, adult or child during X-ray procedures.

Workload and stress

Does working through pregnancy generally have any adverse effects? Some studies into the effect of employment on pregnancy have found a link between low birth weight and working late into pregnancy. Other research has not borne this out, however, and one study found that perinatal mortality rates, prematurity and low birth weights were higher among non-working mothers (Murphy *et al.*, 1984). There is some new evidence of a direct link between stress and miscarriage in a US study of 600 women lawyers, which showed a clear link between long office hours in the first three months of pregnancy and a threefold increase in miscarriages (Hazards, 1997).

The long hours, shift work, heavy lifting and physical and mental tiredness involved in nursing may therefore affect pregnancy, and possibly contribute to preterm labour and low birth weight. It can also have indirect effects by encouraging smoking and under- or overeating.

Employees' rights

Given the risk to reproductive health inherent in the work of many nurses, what rights and protection do you have if you are pregnant or hoping to become so, or if you are a new mother?

Alternative employment

The EU Pregnant Workers directive, implemented through the Management of Health and Safety at Work (Amendment) Regulations 1994 and 1997, obliges employers to consider workplace and workplace hazards which could affect women of child-bearing age, the new or expectant mother (defined in the regulations as a worker who is pregnant, has given birth in the previous six months or is breastfeeding), or her baby. They must either remove the hazards or offer alternative working arrangements such as reduced or flexible hours of work, or if this is not possible, suspend the person for as long as necessary to avoid the risks.

Nurses in clinical areas, for example, can expect their managers to advise them to move from higher-risk areas, such as operating theatres and radiotherapy, chemotherapy and radiology units. The regulations are detailed if rather jargon-laden, and require consideration of 'processes or working conditions, or physical, biological or chemical agents' and 'any infectious or contagious disease', for their potential risk or effects on breastfeeding.

If night working is considered a risk, the employee is obliged to provide a certificate from a doctor or registered midwife, stating that she should not work in that area for a specified period. It is important to note that if you don't provide the certificate, your employer doesn't have to carry out the risk assessment, nor to move you or suspend you from night duty on full pay.

Women may take legal action against their employer if they do not fulfil their duties under these regulations (HSE, 1997), for example if suitable alternative work is available but not offered, and the employee is dismissed rather than suspended for health and safety reasons. The Royal College of Midwives advises its safety reps to be alert to employers dismissing pregnant workers instead of redeploying or temporarily suspending them (RCM, 1997).

Maternity rights

All of these hazards could be greatly reduced by improved conditions of employment for pregnant women, such as a shorter working week and extended maternity leave. Maternity rights for NHS employees are laid down in the Whitley Council Handbook, but are viewed by some as less generous than the basic minimum contained in the Employment Protection (Consolidation) Act of 1978 (Bennett, 1994; Howard, 1994). All employees have the right to return to work after the baby is born and the right to maternity pay, as long as four conditions are met:

1. You must carry on working until immediately before the beginning of the eleventh week before the expected date of delivery.
2. You must have completed at least 26 weeks with the same employer at the start of the fifteenth week before the expected week of childbirth, and normally earn at least £57 a week.
3. You must inform your employer (in writing) at least 21 days before taking maternity leave, or in the event of premature birth as soon as reasonably possible, that you will be absent because of pregnancy and that you wish to return to work for a minimum of three months, if that is the case.
4. You must provide, not less than 21 days before taking maternity leave, a statement from a doctor or practising midwife of the expected date of delivery.

Return to work

Your employer must keep your job for you as long as you return to work before the end of the 29th week after delivery. The employee is entitled to 'the job in which she was employed under the original contract of employment and on terms and conditions not less favourable than those which would have applied to her if she had not been so absent'. The wording of this is somewhat ambiguous, however, and does not necessarily mean a job on the same ward or department, as long as your pay and conditions of service are not disadvantaged.

Under NHS (Whitley) regulations, if you do intend to go back to work after the baby is born your employer is entitled to write to ask you for confirmation, no earlier than 49 days from the date or week of the expected confinement, and you must notify him or her at least three weeks before the day you wish to return. The first condition can cause problems as many women have no idea whether they will be able to go back to work so soon. Alternatively if you say in advance that you are not coming back you may change your mind or you may even lose the baby, and you have said goodbye to your job. Statutory provision allows a return to work after 14 weeks, without the requirement for notification, so those on Whitley contracts may want to query the consistency of this with their employers.

There is certainly room for employers to be flexible and most health trusts have an 'undecided option', allowing employees to postpone the final decision until after the birth. It is probably safest to say you want to return anyway.

Maternity pay

You are entitled to six weeks' statutory pay – nine tenths of a normal week's pay less the flat-rate maternity allowance – providing you have been continuously employed by the same employer for at least 26 weeks up to the fourteenth week before the expected week of birth (EWB), working full-time for two years or 16 hours a week for five years. You are entitled to six weeks' pay at 90 per cent of earnings (calculated on normal weekly earnings for the eight weeks preceeding the 14th week before the EWB), and £52.50 for up to twelve weeks – that is eighteen weeks statutory maternity pay in total.

Time off during pregnancy

You are entitled to time off work with pay for antenatal care, as long your appointment was made on the advice of a registered doctor, midwife or health visitor.

Breastfeeding

The RCM advocates that trusts should make a commitment to the promotion and facilitation of breastfeeding, and suggests practical measures such as staff being enabled to leave the workplace temporarily for this purpose, with provision of appropriate accommodation, rest areas and refrigerators for expressed milk to be stored near the workplace.

Childcare

There is a continued dearth of affordable, flexible childcare for health care staff, especially that tailored to nurses' shift patterns. There are huge opportunities for employers to do more in this area, both through the direct provision of affordable child care and through flexible working arrangements which make it easier for those with children to work. These include job shares, part-time contracts and flexible holiday arrangements, for example to allow staff to take extra, unpaid leave during school holidays. Many such arrangements have been introduced in commercial companies in other sectors as employers see the value of retaining skilled, qualified staff after childbirth.

The statutory requirements of maternity leave and other parental leave should be seen as a baseline, linked to post-natal provision that is responsive to the individual needs of staff. Beyond acknowledging parental rights and responsibilities, employers should see the health and well-being of all staff as a priority, and we return to this topic in Chapter 12, 'The healthy nurse'.

Box 9.3   *Pregnancy risk assessment*

Frenchay NHS Trust decided that an Institute of Personnel Development (IPD) student would be seconded to work with the occupational health manager to develop an advice leaflet for employer and employees. This collaboration resulted in the production of two leaflets – one for line managers and one for pregnant employees. The launch of these leaflets was supported by training sessions for managers on undertaking pregnant worker risk assessments. The original print run of 500 copies of each leaflet in 1994 has been repeated twice. Managers confirm that they feel more confident about their risk management process, whilst employees understand both their responsibilities and their rights, and only exceptional cases are now referred for advice.

During 1996 the leaflets were shown to the Department of Health midwifery team by a trust employee working on a special project. The leaflet excited considerable interest and permission was sought from and given by the occupational health service and the trust for the leaflets to be distributed as examples of good practice, with the trust's copyright acknowledged. Contact Frenchay Healthcare NHS Trust, Frenchay Hospital, Frenchay Park Road, Bristol BS16 1LE. Tel.: 0117 975 3810. Fax: 0117 975 3826

Source: DoH, 1998, p. 21.

References and further reading on reproductive hazards

AAOHN (1995) 'Reproductive hazards: an overview of exposure to health care workers', *AAOHN Journal*, vol. 43, no. 12 (December), pp. 614–21

Badgwell, J. (1996) 'An evaluation of air safety source-control technology for the post anaesthesia care unit', *Journal of Perianaesthesia Nursing*, vol. 11, no. 4 (August), pp. 207–22.

Bennett, K. (1994) 'Your rights at work. Watered down. . .', *Health Visitor*, vol. 67, no. 12 (December), p. 440.

Cooper, N. (1994) 'The measurement of anaesthetic gases – legal requirement', *British Journal of Theatre Nursing*, vol. 3, no. 10 (January), pp. 29–30.

DoH (1998) 'Occupational Health Nursing: contributing to healthier workplaces'. London: Department of Health, with the ENB, Association of Occupational Health Nurse Practitioners (UK) and the RCN Society for Occupational Health Nursing.

Donaldson, D. and Meecham, J. (1995) 'The hazards of chronic exposure to nitrous oxide: an update', *British Dental Journal*, no. 178, pp. 95–100

Doyal, L. (1995) *What Makes Women Sick: Gender and the Political Economy of Health*. London: Macmillan.

Eger, E. (1991) 'Fetal injury and abortion associated with occupational exposure to inhaled anaesthetics', *AANA Journal*, vol. 59, no. 4 (August), pp. 309–12

Foley, K. (1993) 'Update for nurse anaesthetics – occupational exposure to trace anaesthetics: Quantifying the risk', *AANA Journal*, vol. 61, no. 4 (August), pp. 405–12

Green, S. (1996) 'Nitrous oxide – a potential hazard', *British Journal of Theatre Nursing*, vol. 6, no. 6 (September), pp. 27–33.

Guirguis, S. *et al.* (1990) 'Health effects associated with exposure to anaesthetic gases in Ontario hospital personnel', *British Journal of Industrial Medicine*, no. 46 (July), pp. 490–7

Hazards (1997) 'Miscarriages rise with stress', *Hazards*, vol. 59 (July–September), p. 5.

Howard, G. (1994) 'The new maternity rights', *Occupational Health*, vol. 46, no. 4 (April), pp. 133–4.

HSE (1996a) 'Working with VDUs', leaflet IND(G)36(L). Sudbury: Health and Safety Executive.

HSE (1996b) *Anaesthetic Agents: Controlling Exposure under COSHH*. ISBN 0-7176-1-43-8, Sudbury: Health Services Advisory Commitee/Health and Safety Executive.

HSE (1997) 'New and Expectant mothers at work: A Guide for employers', leaflet HS(G)122. Sudbury: Health and Safety Executive.

HSE (1997) *Occupational Exposure Limits*. EH 40. Sudbury: Health and Safety Executive.

Johnston, J. (1993) 'Nitrous oxide: your health, not theirs', *British Journal of Theatre Nursing*, vol. 3, no. 6 (September), pp. 29–30.

Journal of Nursing Management (1996) 'New guidance on controlling exposure of health services staff to anaesthetic agents', *Journal of Nursing Management*, vol. 4, no. 3 (May), p. 181.

Kalter, H. and Warkany, J. (1983) 'Congenital malformations', *New England Journal of Medicine*, no. 308, pp. 424–31

Labour Research Department (1991) *VDUs & Health and Safety*. London: Labour Research Department.

Labour Research Department (1997) *Maternity rights – an LRD guide to the law and best practice*. London: Labour Research Department.

McAbee, R., Gallucci., B. and Checkoway, H. (1993) 'Adverse reproductive outcomes and occupational exposures among nurses: an investigation of multiple hazardous exposures', *AAOHN Journal*, vol. 41, no. 3 (March), pp. 158–60.

Murphy, J., Dauncey, M. and Newcombe, R. (1984) 'Employment in pregnancy: prevalance maternal characteristics, perinatal outcomes, *Lancet*, vol. 1, no. 8387 (26 May), pp. 1163–6.

National Institute of Occupational Safety and Health (1977) *Waste Anaesthetic Gases and Vapours*. Cincinatti, Ohio: NIOSH.

Paul, J. (1996) 'Women, Work & Health', TUTB Newsletter no. 3 (June). Brussels: Trade Union Technical Bureau for Health and Safety (ITUH House, 155 Bd Emile Jacqmain, B-1210, Brussels, Belgium. Tel.: 00 322 224 0560).

Pillay, D. (1996) 'Maternal infections 2: cytomegalovirus', *Modern Midwife*, vol. 6. no. 1 (January), pp. 20–4.

RCM (1997) 'The European Pregnant Workers Directive', *RCM Health & Safety Representatives Bulletin*, issue 1 (January), pp. 8–10.

RCN (1995) *Hazards for pregnant nurses*, re-order No 000. London: Royal College of Nursing, Labour Relations Department.

RCN (1994) *A Beginner's Guide to New Maternity Rights*. London: Royal College of Nursing, Labour Relations Department.

TUC (1997) *Hazards at Work. TUC Guide to Health and Safety*. London: Trades Union Congress. See especially pp. 21–2, 'New and Expectant Mothers'.

Williams, N. (1996) 'Hazards to pregnant women at work', *Modern Midwife*, vol. 6, no. 3 (March), pp. 28–30

10 *Manual handling: time to stop?*

'No one working in a hospital, nursing home or community setting should need to lift patients manually any more' (RCN, 1996a). Such a statement would have been thought fanciful by most nurses as little as a decade ago. Since the introduction of the Manual Handling Operations Regulations in 1992, however, it is a realistic goal for most safety and cost-conscious health care employers.

This chapter will look first at the cost to nurses which manual handling has levied, second at the nature and significance of the manual handling regulations, and third at the available guidelines and practice for manual handling and safer patient handling policies. As stated in the chapter title, underlying all of these issues is the question: is it time to stop?

The costs of manual handling

Back injury is easily the most widespread working hazard faced by the nursing profession. One in every three nurses has time off with back injury every year, and it is estimated by Pheasant and Stubbs (1992) that nurses have almost 30 per cent more days off per year due to back pain than the general population, a median time off (seven days) that is over twice the median for all other occupations (two days), and a higher incidence of back-injury-related work absence than any other working group, including miners and construction workers.

The NHS loses over £50 million a year through nurses' absence with back injuries, a staggering 1.5 million working days. The impact can be measured in several other ways:

- The loss of trained, experienced nurses, either temporarily or permanently through early retirement or redeployment.
- Increase in staff turnover.
- Cost of extra, temporary staff.
- Lost productivity.
- Effects on quality and continuity of care.
- Cost of injury benefit payments.
- Litigation and personal injury claims by nurses against their employers.

For the people concerned, the loss of earnings and the consequent strain on personal budgets are significant and enduring, but the costs are more than financial. Many are unable to resume their chosen career and have chronic conditions such as reduced mobility, persistent pain, neurological symptoms, loss of concentration, insomnia, social isolation, depression and low self-esteem, as well as a disrupted family, domestic and social life.

Nearly 40 per cent of a sample of injured working nurses surveyed by the RCN (1996d) had experienced a previous injury, with two thirds of that group having been injured during the previous five years, one third within the previous 12 months.

Although three quarters of the sample had told their employers of their continuing symptoms, a significant minority had chosen not to. There is a tradition that nurses must cope and carry on regardless. Time off for back pain continues to be regarded with suspicion and the feeling persists that it should somehow be accepted as an occupational hazard, despite the Manual Handling Regulations. Nurses with back injury are frequently regarded as malingerers and as work-shy. One nurse, less than a fortnight after being injured, was visited at home by the line manager and told that 'some of the staff don't believe you have a back injury'. The nurse was told by a work colleague that the manager had already removed the nurse's photograph from the public staff identity board.

The nurse with back pain or injury

A recent survey (Smith and Seccombe, 1996) revealed no gender differences in the percentage of nurses taking sick leave for back injury – 5 per cent for both sexes, with a similar figure within age groups, except for the 40–44 year-old group, which had a 7 per cent reported absence. Slightly more community nurses than nurses in hospital settings reported back pain and, significantly, community nurses reported less access to handling equipment. Nearly 40 per cent of the nurses surveyed worked in general medical or surgical areas and nearly 20 per cent in elderly care units. A smaller but significant number with time off for a back injury worked in critical care and theatres, and a much smaller number worked in mental health, paediatrics or GP practices.

The fact remains, however, that it takes just a single incident, lasting only a matter of seconds, to affect a nurse's health, career and life, often permanently. Smith and Seccombe (ibid.) state that twice as many of the respondents with regular back pain said they would leave nursing if they could, compared with those not experiencing regular back pain. In an earlier study, Seccombe and Ball (1992) noted that nurses with back injury were three times more likely to leave nursing and /or paid employment than were people in other occupations.

These are the bare facts about the costs of manual handling to nurses. Why is the problem so widespread and persistent, and why are nurses so much at risk?

Nurses at risk

Looking at the legislation, regulations and guidance on manual handling, one might expect that health services would be exemplary in fulfilling their obligations to their employees, but the reality is not so rosy.

Traditionally, the lifting tasks involved in nursing have been as heavy as those in the hardest manual labour and the circumstances frequently worse. Patients do not conform to neat size or weight limits. They may be unpredictable, frequently uncooperative, and need to be handled with much more care and attention than an inanimate object. If the load suddenly becomes unbearable, you cannot just drop it.

Even allowing for the fact that the load is often shared between two nurses, nurses often lift excessively heavy patients or those who are difficult to lift. Nurses are subject to prolonged wear and tear injuries; slips and trips; poor building and equipment design such as narrow doorways, small toilets and bathroom areas; lack of space around bed areas where nurses have to manoeuvre patients, fixed bed heights; and unsuitable uniforms.

These factors are compounded by staff shortages, greater proportions of high-dependency, acutely ill patients, earlier discharge into the community and faster throughput of patients.

Yet before the 1992 regulations (detailed below) very few hospitals had specified safe procedures for lifting. Even now, there are not enough mechanical lifting aids and many are not used enough, due to lack of training, lack of space and a general mistrust on the part of both nurses and patients. Patients' dislike of lifting equipment is often cited by nurses as a reason for not using it (White, 1997). Although nurses are now legally obliged to use the available equipment, the RCN's occupational health adviser, Carol Bannister, believes that back injuries have become more common since the new legislation. Since employers are required by law to provide manual handling training to employees, this points back to the original question – is it time to stop? If manual handling training does not result in reduced incidence of back injury and back pain among nurses, it seems likely that manual handling is unsafe.

Nurses represented by the RCN won over £8 million in damages for back injury from the NHS in 1996, an illustration of the huge cost to trusts and the continued flouting of regulations by trust managers. The HSE has fined some employers for failures in this area – Southern Derbyshire Health Authority was fined £12,000 in 1993, for example – but it doesn't yet appear to be a sufficient deterrent. It seems employers would rather pay large litigation claims and fines than spend more on handling equipment and safe systems of work. Will it take more litigation, larger fines and higher insurance costs to force health service managers to implement policies which are so obviously in their best interests?

The regulations

Even before 1992, manual handling training was obligatory under the Health and Safety at Work Act. If a nurse injured her back at work and could prove employer negligence, she could sue for damages; but it was a difficult task, and rarely successful.

The Management of Health and Safety Work Regulations (1992) and the Manual Handling Operations Regulations (1992) are part of the 'Six Pack' bundle of EU regulations aimed at setting out employer duties and encouraging a more systematic and better organised approach to health and safety.

The Management Regulations require employers to:

- Assess the risks to employees and others affected by work activity.
- Make arrangements to implement measures which follow risk assessment.
- Provide health surveillance where necessary.
- Appoint competent people to devise and apply these measures.
- Set up emergency procedures.
- Provide employees with clear information about health and safety.
- Cooperate with other employers on the same site.
- Ensure that employees have adequate health and safety training and can avoid risks in their work.
- Provide temporary workers with appropriate health and safety information.

The Manual Handling Operations Regulations require employers first to *avoid the need for hazardous manual handling*, so far as is reasonably practicable. The HSE guidelines on the regulations include such questions as 'Can you take the treatment to the patient, not vice versa?' Clearly, many episodes of patient handling could be avoided, but this option must be appraised alongside the patient's wishes and the nursing plan to encourage independence and mobility. The phrase 'so far as is reasonably practicable' may be applied narrowly or stretched broadly; one NHS solicitor, however, remarks that 'What is novel about the regulation is that it places a positive duty on employers to consider whether the lift can be avoided, in other words, to consider the safety of the employee alongside the needs of the patient' (Bevan Ashford, 1992).

Second, *assess the risk of injury from any hazardous manual handling that can't be avoided*. Assessment involves consideration of the following four factors (see also Table 10.1, p. 211).

(a) The task. This relates to the mechanics of an activity, for example clinical procedures carried out on a patient in the bed, turning the patient in bed, moving the patient up and down the bed, assisting the patient from a

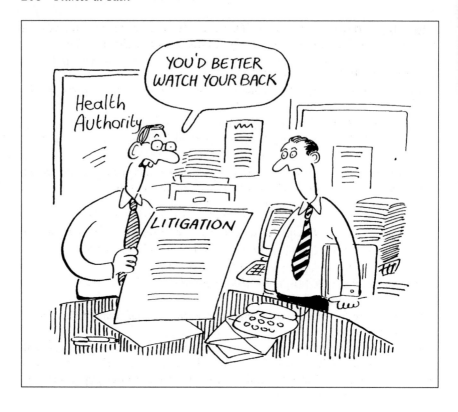

lying to a sitting position and *vice versa*, bed-bathing the patient, getting the patient in and out of bed. Questions to ask might include the following:

> Does the task involve holding the patient away from the body?
> Would you be twisting, stooping or reaching upwards?
> Are large, vertical movements involved (for example floor to overhead)?
> Are there long carrying, pushing or pulling distances?
> Would you be taking up an awkward posture, or hand/limb position or grip?
> Is there sufficient rest or recovery time during the task?

(b) The load. Questions to ask might include:

> Is the patient heavy, bulky or unwieldy, because of other equipment such as infusion pumps, dressings, drains?
> Is the patient unstable or unpredictable, for example recovering from a cerebro-vascular accident or anaesthesia, agitated or confused?
> Is the patient *potentially* harmful, for example has sharp fingernails or a known history of aggression?
> Is the patient difficult to grasp, for example has a hemiplegia, exposed wounds or painful limbs?

(c) The working environment. This includes the space constraints of a ward, clinic or community setting. Questions to ask might include:

Are there restrictions of posture?
What is the state of the floor, for example slippery, uneven, cluttered?
What are the lighting conditions?
Are there extremes of temperature?
Does the nurse's clothing restrict or inhibit movement?

(d) Individual capacity. This refers to the knowledge, training, ability and competence of the worker. Questions to ask might include:

Does the task need unusual capability (or height or strength)?
Is there any danger to individuals with existing health problems, for example to someone with asthma or a previous back injury?
Is it hazardous for a pregnant woman to perform?
Is special information or training required?

Third, *reduce the risk of injury from hazardous manual handling,* as far as reasonably practicable.

Reducing the risk should involve actions taken in response to assessment of the four factors described above: task, load, working environment and individual capacity. Manual handling assessments are pointless unless the necessary changes are made as a result.

The task:

Could the twisting, stooping or reaching be eliminated?
Could lifting from floor level or above shoulder height be avoided?
Could repetitive manual handling be avoided?
Could staff be rested after manual handling activity?

The load:

Can mechanical equipment take the strain (for example hoists, adjustable beds, examination couches)?
Is the existing equipment fit for the purpose and available in all areas when and where required? Equipment should be modern and appropriate for the patients. It is not satisfactory for wards to share hoists or to have fixed-height beds.
Can equipment such as infusion pumps be temporarily disconnected during manual handling, or at least attended to by designated staff?
Is the manoeuvre essential – can it wait until a patient is more comfortable, calm or lucid? For example drug administration such as analgesia or sedation could be planned to precede manual handling.

The working environment:

> Can obstructions to free movement and suitable posture be removed?
> Can the floor be made firm, even and uncluttered?
> Can the lighting and room temperature be improved?
> Could more appropriate staff clothing be designed and issued?

Individual capacity:

> Are the strongest people undertaking the tasks?
> Is consideration taken of individual nurses' health needs?
> Are appropriate adjustments made for pregnant staff?
> Do staff have adequate information about the handling tasks?
> Have all staff had recent and sufficient manual handling training?

Employees' responsibility

The Manual Handling Operations Regulations place a responsibility on the employee to make full and proper use of any system of work, equipment or training provided by the employer.

Guidance on manual handling

The implementation of the Manual Handling Operations Regulations has been cascaded from the European Union through the member states, in the UK through the HSE and from the NHS Executive to NHS trusts. The NHS employer has a statutory obligation to provide guidance on manual handling, within the framework outlined here.

Training programmes

The Health Services Advisory Committee suggests that manual handling training programmes should include:

- Information about back care.
- An ergonomic approach to risk assessment.
- The practical use and care of manual handling equipment.
- Guidance on manual handling techniques.
- Factors affecting an individual's capabilities.

According to Smith and Seccombe (1996) four fifths of nurses reported receiving manual handling training since qualifying, and more than half had received training in the previous 12 months.

Back care advice

Access to back care advisers varies markedly across the UK, according to Smith and Seccombe, from nearly 30 per cent of respondents in Northern

Table 10.1 *Risk assessment for lifting and handling*

SUGGESTED RISK-ASSESSMENT CHART FOR LIFTING AND HANDLING PATIENTS

Each person should initially be assessed using the following scoring system. The factors listed below will influence the potential risk of injury to the attendant during the moving and handling of this person. A score of above 12 indicates high risk, and therefore a full assessment is needed. The patient should be re-assessed if any of the factors change. Circle the appropriate score, estimating if you do not have the information

Height

1.5m or less	1
1.6m	2
1.7m	3
1.8m	4

Weight

50kg or less	1
51–60 kg	2
61–70kg	3
71kg–80kg	4
81kg or above	5

Age

30 years or below	1
40 years	2
50 years	3
60 years	4
70 years or over	5

Mobility

Able to bear weight and balance	1
Able to bear weight and balance	2
ICU equipment	3
Bears weight but unstable	5
Unable to bear weight	7

Level of consciousness

Conscious and cooperative	1
Conscious and confused/forgetful	5
Conscious and uncooperative	6
Unconscious/semiconscious	6

Special risks

Pain and stiffness	5
Peripheral vascular disease	5
Hypo-/hypertension	5
Diabetes	5
Paraplegia	6
Hemiplegia	7
Quadriplegia	8
Muscular spasms	5
Amputation	5
Rigidity	5
Vertigo	8
Major surgery/trauma first 24 hours	3
Orthopaedics/spinal	3

Hydration

Well hydrated	1
Dehydrated	3
Peripheral line	2
Central line	2

Medication

Hypotensive	2
Chlorpromazine sedatives	5

Total Score

[ ]

* A total score below 12 indicates a low risk
* A score above 12 indicates need for a full assessment
* A score above 5 in any individual category may indicate need for full assessment

Patient's name [ ]

Source: Fay Reid, chairwoman, National Back Exchange

Ireland to 20 per cent of respondents in Scotland, and with wide variation between regions. One third of respondents in England, Scotland and Wales didn't know if they had access to back care advice or not.

Trades unions and professional groups

Although the structures of manual handling are laid down in legislation, much of the best guidance and practice on the subject has been produced by organisations such the TUC, Unison, the RCN, the Chartered Society of Physiotherapy and voluntary groups (see 'Contact Organisations and Resources' at the end of this chapter, and Appendix 2). It is to such groups that nurses and other health care workers should turn in seeking information and advice which they might usefully pass on to their managers. If you feel underinformed or think that your place of work does not conform to safe working practices, you could discuss the situation with your union steward or safety rep, and together approach your line manager. The provision of information may be an employer obligation, but employees are also responsible for their own safety and that of their colleagues.

Safer patient handling policies

Manual lifting must be regarded as a last resort if the incidence of back pain and injury is to be reduced. For many nurses, this will require a fundamental change of thinking; even now, the use of lifting devices is often the last resort.

One of the most radical recent suggestions concerning manual handling in the UK has been the RCN's proposal that manual lifting of patients should be eliminated in all but exceptional circumstances and that a 'safer patient handling policy' (see below) should be introduced. Several hospitals have introduced a 'no lifting policy', a rare few as long ago as the 1980s.

In this final section of the chapter we discuss these proposals and their practicability in clinical situations.

Lifting devices

Lifting devices are unpopular with nurses. Frequently, there are not enough of them, and one hoist may be shared between several wards. Community nurses are unable to access appropriate equipment for their patients. Lifting devices are assumed to be large and unwieldy, time-consuming and complicated to use, and patients may express dislike of them, feeling uncomfortable, insecure and undignified.

However, manufacturers are constantly improving the design of their products, making them simpler to use, more easily manoeuvred and more comfortable for patients. A range of equipment is available, from electrical or mechanical hoists and transfer devices to simple slings and sliding boards.

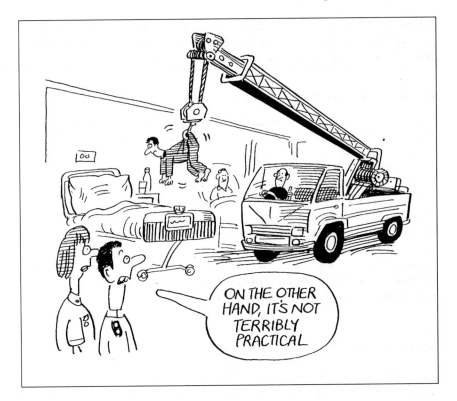

The Disabled Living Foundation, which has branches throughout the UK, can provide comprehensive catalogues and give advice on equipment. Companies are generally keen to demonstrate their products, often provide training sessions and may loan equipment for a trial period.

- Budget holders should give one member of staff overall responsibility for advice, maintenance and use of lifting devices, in liaison with appropriate groups such as trust safety committees.
- Each unit should have an accurate inventory of lifting aids in that workplace and monitor their use.
- All potential users of equipment should know where it is stored and be confident in assessing the appropriateness of the equipment for particular situations.
- Suppliers and manufacturers should be approached with suggestions for modifications and improvements.

A safer patient handling policy

The RCN contends that any organisation which has not adopted a safer handling policy is breaking the law and that the simple decision to introduce such a policy would accelerate change, committing employers to reduce risk and forcing staff to review their habitual working practices. Such a policy might state:

> 'the manual lifting of patients is to be eliminated in all but exceptional or life threatening situations.'
> 'patients are encouraged to assist in their own transfers.'
> 'handling aids must be used wherever they can help to reduce risk, if this is not contrary to a patient's needs.' (RCN, 1996a)

The RCN also suggests that manual handling should only involve giving a patient light assistance, such as support or horizontal movement using a sliding aid.

Of course simply making a statement or proclaiming a policy doesn't make it happen. That requires three principal prerequisites:

- Sufficient equipment.
- A suitable working environment.
- Adequately trained and informed staff.

As described in Box 10.1, there is a small but growing body of evidence to demonstrate the success of the safer patient handling policies and similar initiatives. Other measures of success might be found in the number of incident or accident reports filed, audits of occupational health referrals, and the amount of litigation. Less tangibly, staff morale might be raised, both through the improved working practices and through being actively involved in setting up the policy.

Box 10.1   *The first 'no-lifting' policy*

Nurses at Broomhill Hospital, Glasgow, set up a 'no-manual lifting zone' in their hospital over ten years ago. Within a year the incidence of back injuries had reduced by 50 per cent and subsequently was almost eliminated.

In 1994 the Wigan and Leigh NHS Trust introduced a safer patient handling policy and reduced sickness absence by 84 per cent.

Source: RCN, 1996a.

Risk assessments and monitoring

Once a policy is in place, it must be maintained and monitored. All working environments and the normal range of tasks should be assessed, and a step-by-step plan devised for modifying the environment and the tasks, starting with the minimum acceptable, aiming towards the optimum, with a target date schedule.

Nurses are used to planning individual care for their patients, relating to their personal, physical, psychological, social and spiritual needs; so planning for their handling needs and capabilities should not be difficult.

Simplicity and clarity, accessibility and universality should be key words in any handling assessment. Those who devise patient-handling assessment tools and forms should take account of the busy and stressful workload of nurses in most settings and ensure that the minimum of detail is required, and that the intention of the assessment is expressed in clear language.

Assessment should be made at the first appropriate moment – obviously, in life-threatening situations in a casualty department this is not a priority.

For assessments to be used, they should be accessible, for example kept in a prominent part of a care plan folder, either the front or back; the specific location isn't important, provided it is agreed and known by all who work with a patient. There is also a greater chance of assessments being used consistently if their form and content is universally agreed across trusts or work-places.

Just as each patient should be individually assessed, it should also be remembered that all nurses' capabilities are different. Assessment of an individual's knowledge, suitability and capacity for patient handling might form part of that person's development programme. The assessment could be devised by the designated manual handling operations trainer in a work-place, perhaps with a self-administered questionnaire. Individual confidentiality should be maintained, but the outcome could be a mandatory consideration of each person's permitted role in patient handling.

'Manual handling certificates' would seem unnecessary, but the UKCC 'Scope of Professional Practice' and PREP requirements support the idea that staff should work to the capacity at which they are confident and competent.

The myth of acceptable weight limits

Some of the assessment documents in use, including the HSE guidance, include numerical charts showing the apparently safe or acceptable weights which can be lifted or lowered by an 'average' person, close to and at arm's length from the body. The 1993 RCN *Code of Practice for the Handling of Patients*, for example, suggests that no single nurse should take the full weight of any patient weighing more than 30 kilos, and no two nurses should take the full weight of any patient weighing more than 50 kilos.

Such figures are deceptive and generalised and do not take sufficient account of the individual variations in ability to lift. Since relatively few adult patients come within these limits, the logical outcome of using such a code would be the ending of manual handling in nursing practice. Given that around 80,000 nurses a year hurt their back and at least 3600 of these have to retire early, isn't it time to stop?

References, contact organisations and further reading

Alderman, C. (1996) 'Back in control', *Nursing Standard,* vol. 10, no. 44 (24 July), pp. 22–4.

Bevan Ashford (1992) 'Legal Implications of the EC Directive on "Handling of Loads"', Bevan Ashford (Solicitors), Oxfordshire.

Brewer, S. (1993) 'The back injury battle', *Nursing Standard,* vol. 7, no. 40 (23 June), pp. 20–1.

Carrington, A. (1993) 'New law – old habits', *British Journal of Theatre Nursing,* vol. 2, no 11 (February), pp. 16–7.

Croner's Health and Safety at Work: Manual Handling (1995) Kingston Upon Thames: Croner Publications Ltd.

Dixon, R., Lloyd, B. and Coleman, S. (1996) 'Defining and implementing a "no lifting" standard', *Nursing Standard,* vol. 10, no. 44 (24 July), pp. 33–6.

Duffy, M. (1993) 'Implementing the Manual Handling regulations', *Occupational Health,* vol. 45, no. 5 (May), pp. 161–5.

Hollingdale, R. (1997) 'Back pain in nursing and associated factors: a study', *Nursing Standard,* vol. 11, no. 39 (18 June), pp. 35–8.

HSE (1992a) *Manual Handling Operations Regulations,* ACoP. L21. Sudbury: Health and Safety Executive.

HSE (1992b) *New Health and Safety At Work Regulations,* IND(G)143L. C5000. Sudbury: Health and Safety Executive.

HSE (1992c) *Manual Handling: Guidance on the Regulations,* L22. Sudbury: Health and Safety Executive.

HSE (1995) *Lighten the load. Guidance for employers on musculo-skeletal disorders,* IND(G)109L(rev) C500. Sudbury: Health and Safety Executive.

HSE (1996) *Getting to grips with manual handling,* IND(G)143L C1300. Sudbury: Health and Safety Executive.

Love, C. (1997) 'A Delphi study examining standards for patient handling', *Nursing Standard,* vol. 11, no. 45 (30 July), pp. 34–8.

McGuire, T. and Dewar, B. (1995) 'An assessment of moving and handling practices among Scottish nurses', *Nursing Standard,* vol. 9, no. 40 (28 June), pp. 35–9.

McGuire, T., Hanson, M. and Tigar, F. (1996) 'A study into clients' attitudes towards mechanical devices'. *Nursing Standard,* vol. 11, no. 5 (23 October), pp. 35–8.

MDD (1993) *Disability Equipment Assessment: Mobile Domestic Hoists,* no. A3, Medical Devices Directorate. London: HMSO.

MDD (1994) *Disability Equipment Assessment: Moving and Transferring Equipment,* no. A19, Medical Devices Directorate. London: HMSO.

Naish, J. (1996) 'Campaign aims to change the culture on manual lifting', *Nursing Times,* vol. 92, no. 15 (10 April), pp. 27–9.

Pheasant, S. and Stubbs, D. (1992) 'Back pain in nurses: epidemiology and risk assessment', *Applied Ergonomics,* vol. 23, no. 4, pp. 226–32.

RCN (1993) *Royal College of Nursing Code of Practice for the Handling of Patients,* re-order no. 000 126. London: Royal College of Nursing.

RCN (1996a) *Introducing a Safer Patient Handling Policy,* re-order no. 000 603. London: Royal College of Nursing.

RCN (1996b) *RCN Code of Practice for Patient Handling,* re-order no. 000 604. London: Royal College of Nursing.

RCN (1996c) *Manual Handling Assessments in Hospitals and the Community: An RCN Guide,* re-order no. 000 605. London: Royal College of Nursing.

RCN (1996d) *Hazards of Nursing. Personal Injuries at Work,* re-order no. 000 692; *Summary of key findings,* re-order no. 000 693. London: Royal College of Nursing.

RCN (1997) 'Annual Report for the RCN Employment Policy Committee from the RCN Advisory Committee for Back Pain in Nurses. April 1996 to March 1997. London: Royal College of Nursing.

Seccombe, I. and Ball, J. (1992) *Back Injured Nurses: A Profile*. London: Institute of Manpower Studies/Royal College of Nursing.

Seymour, J. (1996) 'Patient Handling: Safe practice', Special Report, *Nursing Times*, vol. 92, no. 32 (7 August), pp. 46–8.

Smith, G and Seccombe, I. (1996) *Manual Handling: Issues for Nurses*. London: Institute for Employment Studies, Brighton/Royal College of Nursing.

White, C. (1997) 'Benefits of new legislation for moving and handling', *Nursing Times*, vol. 93, no. 27 (2 July), pp. 60–4.

Williams, K. and Cowell, R. (1996) 'Handle with Care', *Nursing Standard*, vol. 10, no. 28 (3 April), pp. 26–7.

Willis, J. (1996) 'Moving and Handling. Guidelines for back care', *Nursing Times*, vol. 92, no. 49 (4 December), pp. 48-50.

Wright, C. (1996) 'A safe place to work?', *Nursing Times*, vol. 92, no. 42 (16 October), pp. 20–1.

Contact organisations and resources

Disabled Living Foundation, 380–84 Harrow Road, London W9 2HU. Tel.: 0171 289 6111.

National Back Exchange, 82 Muswell Hill Road, Highgate, London N10 3JR. Tel.: 0181 444 5386.

National Back Pain Association (NBPA), 16 Elmtree Road, Teddington, Middlesex, TW11 8ST. Tel.: 0181 977 5474. The NBPA, with the RCN, produced the authoritative *Guide to the Handling of Patients*. In 1995 the NBPA produced a very useful and comprehensive directory, then priced £6.95. It provides lists of member professionals throughout the UK and abroad who may be consulted for assessment, treatment and advice. It also lists different therapies, hospitals, clinics and trusts who offer back pain treatments, and lists of professional associations.

Royal College of Midwives, *Handle with care – A Midwife's Guide to Preventing Back Injury* (May 1997, £7.50) is a clear and comprehensive guide which covers employers' duty of care, health and safety issues, a healthy working environment and principles of good manual handling practice in midwifery. Available from the Royal College of Midwives, 15 Mansfield Street, London, W1M 0BE. Tel.: 0171 872 5100.

Trades Union Congress, *Hazards at Work* (1997) has an excellent section on manual handling and the Operations Regulations. See Chapter 13, 'Physical Hazards'.

Unison has produced a number of good, clear and detailed guides, including one for each of the 1992 'Six-Pack' Regulations, and one on risk assessment. These are all listed in Appendix 1 and may be obtained from Unison, 1 Mabledon Place, London WC1H 9AJ (free to Unison members).

Disability Information Trust, Mary Marlborough Centre, Nuffield Orthopaedic Centre, Headington Oxford OX3 7LD. Tel.: 01865 227 592. Fax: 01865 227 596. Publications include *Hoists, Lifts and Transfers* (1996) (a 'research based tool for all who need access to lifting equipment'), and *Walking and Standing Audit* (1997).

Equipment and design: *The Arjo Handbook for Architects and Planners of Hospitals, Elderly Care Units and Nursing Homes*, Malmo, Sweden (1996).

11 *Work injury and work-related illness*

'The NHS chews you up, sucks you dry, and spits you out.' Many nurses feel like this about working in the health service, but it is surely unacceptable. In an ideal world no nurse would have an accident or develop an illness as a result of her work; although these things do happen, it is not enough simply to try to pick up the pieces *ad hoc*. Health service employers should actively develop good employment and human resources policies and practice to respond to individual and corporate needs in a humane, balanced and sympathetic manner. The reality is less than ideal, however, and often it is the unfortunate nurse who is blamed, discriminated against, left to muddle through or even summarily dismissed.

Marginalisation is the common experience of injured or ill nurses, who are often isolated and depressed. They receive little or no support from their managers, their colleagues have to fill the gap left by their absence, and their family and friends may not understand what is happening. This chapter looks at what causes accidents, what a nurse can do if she has a work-related injury or illness, and what a good employer can do to support and assist her, whether through rehabilitation to a return to the same work, redeployment or early retirement.

Accidents

The focus on accidents is often on individual mistakes, and even illness may be attributed to carelessness or inattention. Thorough investigation leads to different conclusions. The HSE has analysed accidents closely, and suggests that carelessness causes very few – most result from unsafe systems of work. It is the employer's legal responsibility to maintain a safe working environment, although employees also have a responsibility to follow safe systems of work.

Reduction of accident rates is a key goal of the Health Education Authority/NHS Executive 'Health at Work in the NHS' initiative, but there is little research on the causes of accidents. The inadequacy of accident reporting has been noted already, but two recent studies highlight useful findings and make recommendations.

The Institute for Employment Studies (1994) described the general defects of accident reporting: that emphasis is on reporting procedures, hazard identification and risk assessment, not on safety; there is a lack of standard definitions in accident reports; and only a third of ward managers receive accident injury information. The cost of accidents is hard to quantify, but the current trends in work accidents are reported in an RCN study (1996b):

- Age: younger nurses incur more lifting and handling injuries, while older nurses have more slips, trips and falls.
- Experience: the incidence of accidents is significantly higher among nurses who have been qualified for 11 years or more.
- Grade: most accidents occur to D and E grade nurses.
- Work environment: over 80 per cent of accidents occur in the NHS, 76 per cent in hospitals; two thirds of accidents in the community occur in private homes and nursing/residential homes.
- Time of day: 40 per cent of accidents occur during early shifts, and especially during the first quarter of any shift (which corresponds with increased activity).

Stress, caused by staff shortages, poor equipment, poor working conditions and poor management, was seen as significant by over three-quarters of those who have had accidents. Similar findings emerge from a National Audit Office report, *The Cost of Accidents in the NHS*, in which the HSE estimates that 5 per cent of NHS trust revenue is lost through poor safety management.

Action on monitoring and prevention

- Look at the accident forms and reporting procedures in your workplace to see if they focus on safe environments and safe practices and learning. If not, ask your safety rep to suggest a review of accident monitoring.
- Ask your line manager to provide monthly information and statistics on accident injuries in your workplace.
- Discuss ways of calculating the real costs of accident injury with the budget holder, and publicise it.
- Ask for an audit of manual handling, with a view to introducing or reviewing your patient handling policy, and regular refresher courses for all staff at least once a year.
- Look at shift patterns and systems of work to find ways of incorporating safety improvements, such as spreading work activity away from the end of night shifts and from the first quarter of shifts, and pass on your suggestions to the safety rep and/or safety committee.
- Contact your union and the Health and Safety Executive for up-to-date leaflets on health and safety, and ask how well your employer is promoting your health and safety.
- Consider becoming a steward, safety rep or link member for your workplace.

Stress is discussed in detail in Chapter 4, including its interaction with other hazards and employment issues. It is important to emphasise here that stress, along with musculo-skeletal disorders, has been identified as one of the two main causes of work absence (see, for example, Bird, 1995). Instead of looking for punitive measures to combat absence or linking pay rises to attendance records, managers should be looking at the organisation as a whole to identify and reduce the causes of stress. So-called 'sickness absence counselling' for nurses, sometimes even after one day off sick, has become a tool to intimidate staff into returning to work, even if they are not well enough, thus putting themselves, colleagues and patients at risk. To quote Bird, 'unless or until morale within the NHS is improved no managers on earth will be able to deal with sick leave', and nurses will continue to behave rationally and sensibly by taking time off to escape the stressful environment.

Reporting accidents: first actions

Your employer is legally required to report accidents to the HSE under the Reporting of Injuries, Diseases and Dangerous Occurrences Regulations (1995), and you should make sure this happens. If you are involved in an accident at work, or on the way to or from work, you should report it as soon as possible to:

- Your immediate superior, and fill out the official accident book.
- The DSS (on form B195), if it could be classed as an industrial accident, so that you can claim Industrial Injuries Benefit.
- Your union steward or safety rep, so that you can receive continuous and expert support. Discuss the incident with your union rep before writing an accident report, and focus on what happened, not on your feelings. Make sure you keep a copy of the completed accident form, make an early appointment with your general practitioner so that the accident is in your health record, and discuss the events with your occupational health nurse. Begin to keep your own file of all forms, correspondence, appointments, treatment, medications and investigations – this is valuable in terms of keeping control of your situation, and also vital if you pursue a legal claim for damages or compensation. If you are ill or injured for more than a few weeks, your file will become very thick.

Supporting the work-injured nurse

The first line of support may be the work-injured nurse's union representative. This person may be sympathetic, but a little detached from the situation. Family and friends are important, too, but may find it difficult, especially if you are ill or in pain. Your doctor may be a great help, but specific advice and support is best sought from those experienced in occupational health issues. Practical advice and legal support is far harder to come by if you do not belong to a union, and you are less likely to receive consistent and continued attention. For example, if you are in the RCN, the

Work Injured Nurses Group (WING) will provide practical advice, support and information, through a direct line to the adviser and local link members. WING has produced a comprehensive guide and leaflets about benefits, pain control and rehabilitation. The sooner you contact it, the more support it can offer. If you are still ill or injured after a year, WING gives generous grants to cover household bills, equipment such as TENS machines and courses for returning to work or retraining.

WING is a world leader in supporting work-injured and ill nurses, but some similar advice and support is given by other unions such as the Royal College of Midwives and Unison. Most unions offer personal accident insurance, which gives some financial support, and access to physiotherapy and osteopathy. Other good sources of support are Citizen's Advice Bureaux, claimants' advice groups, the RCN's Nurseline and the Samaritans. It's easy to become isolated, and until you take the first step you may feel very low. Contacting these groups may not resolve all your difficulties, but it reduces the feeling of isolation and powerlessness, which can inhibit you from action.

Nurses' experience of ill-health is varied, and their treatment by their employers no less so. Some nurses find they are sidelined, suspended, disciplined or dismissed at an early stage, and the situation is retrieved only by skilful and assertive union support. Things should never get to that stage,

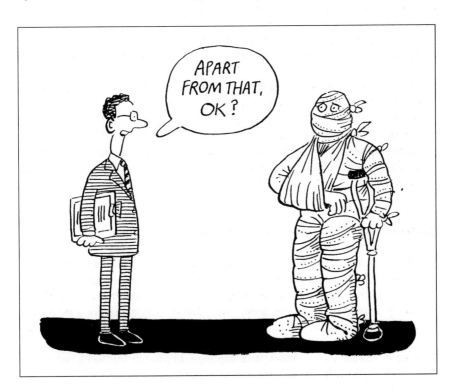

yet they can and do because there are no clear and systematic national guidelines for responding to long-term sickness and injury absence. Three words sum up the ideal employer–employee relationship: communication, consultation and cooperation. All these can be applied to maintain good practice. There are practical reasons for both employee and employer to maintain good communications. The following points give guidance on what should be considered.

Financial issues

NHS injury benefits

Employees on sick leave must submit regular medical certificates to their employer, for the employer to pass on to the DSS. Copies are required by the personnel/human resources and salaries departments, especially after the nurses begin to receive NHS Temporary Injury Benefit, when their income falls below 85 per cent of pre-injury/illness levels. Conditions such as hepatitis, if attributable to work, can entitle nurses to NHS injury benefit, Temporary Injury Allowance during employment and Permanent Injury Allowance after early retirement. The amount is calculated to take account of other income such as social security benefits.

Pay entitlements

For nurses employed on NHS trust contracts, the terms and conditions of service vary from place to place, but for those on a Whitley or pre-trust contract, sick pay entitlement is six months on full pay and six months on half pay. Beyond 12 months, levels of pay are discretionary. As soon as it is clear you will be off sick for a prolonged period, this should be explained to you by your line manager and/or human resources manager. You should be informed by your manager when the six-month and twelve-month periods of sick leave are approaching.

Management issues

Financial and/or sick leave communications are sometimes the only ones that injured or sick nurses receive from their employer. This seems harsh and uncaring. While managers are not entitled to receive confidential health information on employees, it is in everybody's interests to show a tactful interest in an absent nurse, and for the nurse to keep the manager informed in general terms of health progress, and possibly investigations – by phone, by letter with medical certificates, or in personal meetings. The balance lies between showing so much interest as to pressurise the nurse into returning to work prematurely, or make other decisions prematurely, and showing so little interest that she or he feels abandoned.

It has been common in the NHS to call a 'disciplinary hearing' to discuss an employee's long-term sickness absence. This is inappropriate, and compounds the stress of an already anxious situation. The rationale for the treatment of sickness as a disciplinary offence is that although you cannot be disciplined or dismissed for being sick, you can be disciplined for being absent because you are sick. If you feel you are under this sort of pressure, you should consult your union rep – the intervention of a union representative can be constructive and transforming.

There are no requirements for managers to meet sick or injured employees until the approach of six or 12 months' continuous absence. This seems a pity – if nurses were to meet informally every so often with their manager, together with a human resources manager and the union rep or other supporter, there would be a clearer picture of the likely outcome of the absence, and alternatives could be discussed without pressure.

For each case before the '12 months' meeting, if not earlier, the manager should discuss the situation with the human resources department in order to become familiar with the alternatives available, the requirements of employment law, the terms of the nurse's contract, and the possible application of disability discrimination legislation (for example the Disability Discrimination Act). The meeting with the nurse should be informal, and could be a home visit. If early recovery is likely, the manager should agree to continue the nurse's sick pay, subject to regular review. If the prospect of an early return to work is unclear, the manager might request a medical report from the nurse's GP, hospital consultant or the occupational health department. The nurse has a right to see this report before it is sent to the manager.

On receiving the medical report, another meeting with the manager, nurse and human resources officer should be arranged, making sure that there is plenty of time to allow all parties to attend. The nurse is entitled to attend

---

Box 11.1   *On the scrapheap?*

After examination and interview by an occupational health physician, a work-injured nurse employed in a small community NHS trust saw the letter to his line manager. It read:

> After examining X again, and noting that the symptoms and level of pain have not lessened, in fact may have deteriorated, I consider that he is not fit to return to his previous post. We discussed options for redeployment, and agreed that limited hours in a clerical or research post, of perhaps two to three hours a day, with hourly breaks of ten or fifteen minutes, would be a suitable option. I don't suppose there is anything suitable, is there?

Unsurprisingly, given the cue, the manager's response was No.

with her or his union rep or supporter if desired. When this more structured meeting is arranged, a number of options should be available for discussion, and these should be outlined in advance. For example:

1. Return to the same job, before or after sick pay entitlement ends.
2. Redeployment to alternative employment.
3. Dismissal on grounds of incapacity to work due to ill-health.
4. Retirement on grounds of ill-health.

Returning to the same job

Returning to the same job after a full recovery poses the fewest problems, but is not without pitfalls. Prolonged absence may mean that nurses have to adjust rapidly to changes of personnel and working practices, and their colleagues have to allow time for these adjustments. In some ways it is more difficult than starting a new job, because you expect things to be the same, and superficially they may seem to be. Managers should offer nurses returning to work a period of adjustment, perhaps reduced hours, to assist the process.

Redeployment

Before the Disability Discrimination Act 1996 there was little pressure on employers and managers seriously to consider redeployment options for returning ill or injured nurses. The DDA is an unsatisfactory law, defining disability by a medical rather than a social model (labelling people as 'disabled' by their medical conditions, rather than acknowledging that it is social structures and attitudes which are the disability), but at least it does require employers not to 'treat any employee less favourably because of their disability', and to consider making a 'reasonable adjustment' to the workplace in order to employ a person with a disability.

Its impact is not yet clear, but unions such as Unison and the RCN are determined to test its value in representing their members. As Carol Bannister, RCN occupational health adviser, says: 'Hundreds of nurses are retired each year due to injury. That could be transformed into hundreds of claims of discrimination.' Perhaps the employment of nurses with disabilities can be encouraged by suggesting that it is the workplace which is disabled, not the person. With flexibility and imagination, employers, their human resources and occupational health staff, and union reps could devise employment policies which fit jobs to people, not *vice versa* (see Boxes 11.1 and 11.2). It should be possible to recruit and retain qualified people, not discard them because of reduced mobility, chronic pain or visual or hearing impairments; these are hidden disabilities that may alter the manner and extent to which people can work, but should not be used as a bar to employment.

Jobs cannot be created out of nothing, but there are examples of employers finding posts for injured nurses which take account of their knowledge

Box 11.2   *Innovative practice*

The occupational health service at St James' Hospital, Leeds, looked at how back injury cases were handled. Cases were not always followed through, scant attention was paid to actual work activities and more attention was paid to the physical examination of an individual than in combining the examination with a work-based assessment. It was decided that the actual activities of a job should be observed, rather than relying on a job description. Multi-disciplinary advisors – occupational health nurses and physicians, physiotherapists, occupational therapists – would provide reports. The 'circle of carers' became standard practice: now all staff with problems affecting their ability to work or to return to work receive a full assessment and get help from various support networks, to stay in work if at all possible, instead of wasting their knowledge and experience, which had been gained at great expense and could only be replaced after similar expenditure.

Source: ENB/DoH, 1998.

and experience, focusing not on what they can't do, but what they can. Nurses have health knowledge, management, teaching, research and multi-task skills, for example, which can be deployed outside clinical practice.

NHS staff spend their lives caring for others, which in the long term may be detrimental to their own health. Loss of a worker to ill-health retirement or dismissal on the ground of medical incapacity is not always the answer for the individual and rarely for the NHS. Many millions of pounds are spent on the training and development of health care professionals, their skills are honed to perfection and their expertise is difficult to replace. It makes good financial sense to provide them with the best occupational health care available. Take heart: in one hospital, a senior ward sister was off sick for five months with a slipped disc. She had a great deal of experience, knowledge and skills which the unit could not afford to lose. The manager fully supported all action and recommendations made by the OHS, which resulted in some mechanical adaptations and equipment purchases which enabled the sister to remain there.

Dismissal on the grounds of incapacity to work due to ill-health

This option should be opposed in most cases as inappropriate, and may be cause for an industrial tribunal for unfair dismissal. In one case, a nurse was told on a Friday of a disciplinary hearing to be held the following Tuesday, at which a decision would be made on her options (including a medical report). The nurse was warned that non-attendance might result in decisions being made regardless. She was unable to get the regional union officer to attend at short notice, but the officer contacted the human resources department to query the appropriateness of disciplinary proceedings (the nurse had been off sick for 15 months with a chronic non-specific back injury), and mentioned the possibility of an industrial tribunal if the disciplinary hearing went ahead. The human resources officer offered an alternative date and agreed to arrange a consultative rather than a disciplinary meeting. Why was this not considered in the first place?

Retirement on the grounds of ill-health

At first, this option might shock an ill or injured nurse, but it can be creative and liberating, not a depressing end to her or his career. Consideration of ill-health retirement, at whatever stage, need not lead to retirement – return to normal duties or redeployment may turn out to be the best alternative. If retirement on the ground of ill-health seems a possibility, members of the NHS Pension Scheme (contributors to superannuation) must make an application for a pension through their human resources department. This should be confidential: there is no reason or excuse for human resources or occupational health staff to inform your manager that you are considering or have applied for early retirement. Breach of confidentiality is a good reason for invoking the grievance procedure, but it shouldn't happen.

Pensions

Nurses in the NHS Pension Scheme considering early retirement can obtain an estimate of their entitlement from the Pensions Agency (in Fleetwood, Edinburgh and Londonderry), usually through their employer's wages and salaries department. It is based on the number of contributory years, at a proportion of final pay for each year's employment, with a lump sum and enhancement in ill health retirement. The lump sum is three times the yearly pension payment, and the enhancement means that employment between five and ten years is counted double, and over ten years but under 20 it is counted as 20 years, or increased by six and two thirds years, up to the maximum possible entitlement at age 60. Therefore if you have, say, been in the pension scheme for nine years you may be entitled to 18 years. Note that a pension estimate is not the same as acceptance of a pension claim.

Pension claims are made by submitting a form and having a medical examination by your GP or occupational health doctor, and/or your consultant, for their opinion on whether you are unable permanently to do your job. Making a successful claim is not always easy. Probably the most important factor affecting the outcome is the wording of the medical reports – make sure that they include the word 'permanent' or its equivalent in relation to your medical condition or the grounds for ill-health retirement, and in relation to your inability to return to nursing. If this wording is absent, your claim is likely to be rejected. Nurses with gross and obvious disc damage, such as a prolapse, will probably be successful. Those with a non-specific back injury (no definite cause of the symptoms – at least 80 per cent of cases) will have a harder task, and may have to go through several appeals, with additional medical reports from sympathetic consultants, before being awarded a pension. The advice and support of your union rep is essential, and the intervention of your MP can be helpful.

Other nurses who may experience difficulty with the Pensions Agency include those with mental health problems, chronic fatigue syndrome (myalgic encephalomyelitis or ME) or work-related stress. As with non-specific back injury, the burden of proof is on the applicants to convince the agency that their condition is permanent.

Until recently, almost all ill-health retirement applications were approved on the nod by the Pensions Agency. Some past claims were undoubtedly made as a way of dismissing staff without risking unfair or constructive dismissal claims. Since the pension scheme became an 'executive agency' it has had far tighter budgetary constraints, and it appears to have been pressurised to be more rigorous in vetting applications. The extensive and open misuse of early retirement in the teachers' pension scheme, as a means of leaving an increasingly pressured and unhappy profession, probably had a significant effect on the unannounced NHS Pensions Agency policy changes, making it a more arbitrary, less accountable body.

Many nurses were duped into opting out of the NHS Pension Scheme into private schemes in the 1980s, and are still trying to gain compensation and return to the NHS scheme. But all staff with at least five years' NHS service, including those outside the pension scheme, may be eligible for the NHS Permanent Injury Allowance, which is calculated as a percentage of potential earnings lost, following a medical examination and report from a Pensions Agency-nominated doctor. Nurses dismissed from the NHS on ill health grounds who have a lower income, and nurses who remain in the NHS but on permanently reduced hours, may apply for this allowance. Ensure that any dismissal letter states the grounds of ill-health, and that the Permanent Injury Allowance claim is made at that time.

Union reps and pensions advisers in salaries departments may be able to advise on NHS benefits and social security benefits such as Industrial Injuries Benefit, Incapacity Benefit and the Disability Living and Disability Working Allowances. Once awarded, Permanent Injury Allowance is payable for life.

Support and rehabilitation

Nurses in UK health services are generally treated badly – they are not valued, respected, or their health and safety well protected (see Box 11.3). Ill or injured nurses quickly learn that the pecking order prevails against them, too. Crudely put, a flock of hens will attack an ill or injured bird, rather than support or care for it. Nursing is a 'blame' culture where praise is uncommon, and managers are far more likely to accentuate errors or shortcomings than achievements and abilities. The 'low status, high stress' nature of nursing work, the damage to self-esteem from 'giving' to others and receiving little back, and the lack of control over one's own work is emotionally damaging, and perhaps overloads nurses, increasing the potential for accidents.

Doyal (1995) discusses this issue for women's work in general, and Smith (1992) examines the emotional labour of nursing, which like many aspects of 'caring' work remains underresearched. Individuals are held responsible for their stress, injuries or illness, when more often poor organisation and systems of work are major factors. Additionally, the workload pressures resulting from sickness absence are rarely alleviated by extra staff, so adding to the work and stress of the nurse's remaining colleagues.

The neglect of nurses with injury is astonishing, given the high incidence and costs involved. Following musculo-skeletal injury, for example, current rehabilitation thinking is that early intervention is crucial to the outcome. A swift diagnosis, combined with a planned rehabilitation programme of physiotherapy, exercises and pain management will lead to a full or optimum recovery for most, and enable injured nurses to return to some clinical posts. Unfortunately the reality is very different. Many managers do not inform the occupational health department of staff injuries, and few trusts have any policy to promote swift rehabilitation of their staff. One trust OH doctor, questioned on this, said that such a policy would be impossible, because the health services were not permitted to give preferential treatment to staff. Meanwhile thousands of nurses every year join the lengthy waiting lists for consultant appointments, diagnostic tests, physiotherapy and specialist pain and symptom control.

According to the Clinical Standards Advisory Group (1994), 'once someone is off work for six months with backache, they only have a 50% chance of returning to their previous job. Once they are off work for two years, or have lost their job because of back pain (which may happen very much earlier than two years), they will have great difficulty returning to any form of work.' The best alternative is the virtual elimination of manual handling (see Chapter 10), which would drastically reduce the incidence of musculo-skeletal injuries to nurses. Once an injury has occurred, however, rehabilitation and symptom management courses offer the best prospect for changing the experience of people who feel as if they have been written off.

There are few good rehabilitation courses. Either they are in the NHS and have long waiting lists, such as St Thomas' Hospital Pain Management Centre in London, or they are private and costly, such as the Spring Medical Active Rehabilitation Centre. These both offer intensive assessment and exercises, a mixture of physical treatment and group exercise, and individually tailored exercises. The group ethos of such courses is very stimulating to participants, who can discuss their problems and draw strength from losing their feeling of isolation and powerlessness. As many participants say, such programmes should be an early alternative, not a last resort.

There are a number of centres for the management of chronic pain which offer individual treatment and some counselling, but waiting lists are long, resources are in short supply, and beyond physical treatments, few can offer much in the way of rehabilitation. It is difficult to assess what proportion of injured nurses try complementary therapies, and most must be obtained privately. Osteopathy, chiropractic, homoeopathy, aromatherapy and acupuncture are the principal treatments of choice for people with musculoskeletal injuries. More information is needed to help nurses choose the best options, with monitoring of the results.

Disability discrimination in health care

The Disability Discrimination Act, which offers a similar legal framework to race and gender legislation, arose from prolonged political pressure and campaigning by disability rights groups, and replaces previous legislation such as the Disabled Persons (Employment) Act 1994. It defines disability as 'a physical or mental impairment which has a substantial and long-term adverse effect on a person's ability to carry out day-to-day activities'. Physical impairment is taken to mean 'affecting the senses, such as sight and hearing'. Mental impairment includes 'learning disabilities and mental illness (if it is recognised by a respected body of medical opinion)'. 'Substantial' means 'must be more than minor'; 'long-term' means lasting more than 12 months, or likely to, or likely to last for the rest of a person's life. The Act also covers people with severe disfigurements, progressive conditions such as cancers, HIV or multiple sclerosis, and 'people who have had a disability' and have 'recovered'. This a medically based definition – people are seen as being disabled by their conditions, rather than by the barriers that society puts in front of them.

Box 11.3 *Worse treatment than in industry*

'Too little is being done to get nurses who have been on sick leave back to work. . . . Senior nurses were worried about litigation and were reluctant to allow nurses to return to work on "light duties". . . . The nursing hierarchy was concerned that staff who had been off work with back problems or a leg injury would be unable to cope in an emergency. . . . It is worth noting that one third of all job applicants at the Bethlem and Maudsley Hospitals had a previous mental health problem. NHS staff are treated worse and supported less than those in industry.' (Dr Pamela Rogers, Bethlem and Maudsley Hospitals occupational health physician, quoted in Friend, 1994.)

Case studies on injury and neglect: the double whammy

Diane Bosley was a nurse tutor at a London teaching hospital, with five years' teaching and 25 years' clinical experience, when she contracted what she felt was a bad case of flu. After six months she was diagnosed as having myalgic encephalitis and diabetes and lost her job and almost her home.

When her employers requested a consultant's report, he said she was likely to make a full recovery within a year and she felt quite optimistic about her return to work. However, soon after, on the day she was expecting a visit from her line manager, the personnel manager and a union representative at home, she was woken by an early morning telephone call to say her job had gone.

'I then had a letter saying "We are very sorry but because of your ill health we have to dispense with your services." I felt as if the whole thing had been done behind my back. 1 didn't know they could do that – I thought it only happened in cases of gross misconduct. I thought if you were unwell you would be supported until you could return to work, take on a part-time post or retire on health grounds,' she says.

Although she received a lump sum of money from the hospital, it took Ms Bosley one extremely stressful year to achieve retirement on health grounds, and in the meantime she came perilously close to having to sell her home. She had no telephone call from her employers to find out how how she was getting on or offering her counselling. She overcame her sense of isolation by making contact with other nurses who had undergone similar experiences.

'My feeling was that, although what my employers did was perfectly legitimate, it was abysmal. After 30 years in nursing it felt like a slap in the face. Their lack of sensitivity was unbelievable. And they call it the caring profession,' she said.

Valerie Munro had been a nurse for four years and saw her career stretching ahead when, at the age of 26, she injured her back at work. Now, at 33, there are days when she cannot get out of bed. She was off work for two years, was redeployed in a clerical post after hard lobbying by an RCN representative, and successfully sued her health authority for negligence over the accident. She has since been forced to retire on health grounds.

Ms Munro is bitter about the way she was treated after her injury, both by management and her former colleagues. 'I had no back-up at all. I was just left. The problem is that once you go off sick and have no idea when you are going to return, you lose contact and find yourself completely alone. Colleagues fall away very quickly because they can't cope with long-term sickness.

'My occupational health department was not involved until they retired me from my nursing post. It was diabolical. Now I'm on the scrap heap. I was devastated by the injury. Giving up my nursing career has been very difficult. You go through a grieving process. Everything revolves around my back now, it impinges on every avenue of my life.'

Kate Howard-Jones has just completed her training at the Middlesex Hospital in central London and is now applying for jobs. This achievement is significant. She has a hearing impairment. Now aged 24, and hearing-impaired since the age of four, she has learnt to cope with the help of two hearing aids and finely honed lip-reading skills. She had no trouble getting a place at college after being asked to submit a copy of her audiogram to the hospital's occupational health department.

During her training Ms Howard-Jones found her college, Bloomsbury and Islington College of Nursing and Midwifery, extremely supportive - it bought her a £225 stethoscope with an amplifier attachment - but overall she has had little contact with management. 'My personal tutors and the college have been wonderful. But I don't think the hospital management even know I am here.'

She received some initial guidance from the OH department in her bid for a special amplified telephone, something she is still trying to acquire, but nothing since. 'They pointed me in the direction of the job centre but didn't bother to chase it up to see if I had been successful. Nobody has come and said to me: "Are you alright?".'

Ms Howard-Jones always makes a point of informing fellow nursing staff of her hearing problem but sees no reason to tell patients unless they ask. In general colleagues have been extremely supportive. Once or twice her confidence has taken a bashing when other nurses have raised the question of how she could cope but, she says, 'I decided it was their problem, not mine.'

She freely admits that things have not always been easy. 'The telephone is always going to be a problem for me but it is not the most important thing about nursing. The most important thing is delivering patient care and being responsible and accountable.'

Source: Taylor, 1995b.

The Act makes it illegal for employers with 20 or more employees to discriminate against a person for a reason relating to their disability in a way that is not applied to others, and if this treatment is unjustifiable. Thus 'discrimination ' is only justifiable if a person cannot do a job, and there is no practicable or 'reasonable' adjustment. Unlawful discrimination in employment covers recruitment and retention, promotion and transfers, training and development and dismissal procedures.

Reasonable adjustments could be to physical features such as access, furniture and equipment, or to employment arrangements such as application forms and selection and interview procedures. The Act gives examples such as allocating some duties to another person, transferring a person to fill a vacancy, altering working hours, assigning a person to a different workplace, permitting a person to have assessment, treatment or rehabilitation during working hours, modifying equipment, providing a reader or interpreter and providing supervision.

Complaints of unlawful discrimination must be made through an industrial tribunal, so if you want to complain you should contact your union rep or Citizen's Advice Bureau. There have been few test cases to date, and pressure groups such as the Disability Income Group, Unison and WING are looking to establish how effectively the Act can be applied.

Even now, several years after the Act became law, employers have shown no marked willingness to recruit or retain nurses who have been ill or injured, and they continue to focus on their disabilities, not their abilities. This is surprising, considering the experience and skills which are being lost and the rising average age of the nursing workforce. It shows that health care employers do not recognise that employing people with disabilities might boost their reputation as good employers.

Conclusion

It's difficult to be optimistic about the way health services treat their injured or ill staff – the record to date has been poor. Action on four particular points would bring about improvement. First, the adoption by line managers and human resources managers of systematic protocols. Second, a more sympathetic and humane approach to injured or ill nurses, giving them the support and information described as good practice in this chapter. Third, an effort to record work accidents more accurately and learn from them by studying their causes. Fourth, the planning of safe working environments and safe systems of work, so that healthy staff will work in a healthy workplace. This last point is included in the proposals in this book's closing chapter on 'The Healthy Nurse'.

References, contact organisations and further reading

Bird, J. (1995) 'Sick nurses or a sick NHS?', *Nursing Standard*, vol. 9, no. 49 (30 August), pp. 18–9.

CSAG (1994) *Report on Back Pain*. London: Clinical Standards Advisory Group.

Cole, A. (1994) 'Staff hide back pain for fear of dismissal, survey shows', *Nursing Times*, vol. 90, no. 16 (20 April), p. 9.

Cowell, R. (1994) 'Backs to the wall', *Nursing Standard*, vol. 9, no. 7 (9 November) p. 46.

Cowell, R. (1995) 'Isolated, abandoned and blamed' *Nursing Standard*, vol. 9, no. 48 (23 August), p. 53.

Doyal, L. (1995) *What Makes Women Sick: Gender and the Political Economy of Health*. London: Macmillan.

ENB and DoH (1998) *Occupational Health Nursing: Contributing to healthier workplaces*. London: English National Board for Nursing, Midwifery and Health Visiting and Department of Health.

Friend, B. (1994) 'Injured nurses fail to get back to work', *Nursing Times*, vol. 90, no. 27 (6 July), p. 9.

Institute for Employment Studies (1994) *Health at Work in the NHS: Key indicators*, report for the Health Education Authority. London: IES.

RCM (1997) *Handle with Care: A Midwife's Guide to Preventing Back Injury*. London: Royal College of Midwives.

RCN (1994) *An RCN Guide for Work Injured Nurses*. London: Royal College of Nursing.

RCN (1995a) *Reporting Accidents*, Health and Safety at Work no. 2, re-order no. 000 344. London: Royal College of Nursing.

RCN (1995b) *Accidents at Work: Your Financial Rights*, Health and Safety at Work no. 3, re-order no. 000 344. London: Royal College of Nursing.

RCN (1996a) *Guide to the Disability Discrimination Act 1995*. London: Labour Relations Department (RCN Work Injured Nurses' Group) Royal College of Nursing, London.

RCN (1996b) *Hazards of Nursing. Personal Injuries at Work*, re-order no. 000 692. London: Royal College of Nursing.

Sarfas, H. (1993) 'Ill health retirement in health workers', *Occupational Health* vol. 45, no. 3 (March), pp. 101–3.

Seccombe, I. and Ball, J. (1992) *Back Injured Nurses: A Profile*. London: Institute of Manpower Studies (with the RCN).

Smith, G. and Seccombe, I. (1996) *Manual Handling: Issues for Nurses*. Brighton: Institute for Employment Studies (with the RCN).

Smith, P. (1992) *The Emotional Labour of Nursing: how nurses care*. London: Macmillan.

Taylor, A. (1995b) 'Shattered Dreams' (Nurses talk about their experience of disability), *Nursing Times*, vol. 91, no. 40 (4 October), pp. 26–9.

Taylor, A. (1995a) 'Absence record', *Nursing Times*, vol. 91, no. 23 (7 June), pp. 20–1.

Unison (1996) *Women's health and safety*, stock no. 818. London: Unison/ Labour Research Department.

Unison (1997) *Work – it's a risky business. Guide to risk assessment for Unison health and safety representatives*, stock no. 1351. London: Unison.

Contact organisations and resources

On the Disability Discrimination Act: 'Disability – on the agenda' is a series of free booklets produced for the Minister for Disabled People:
(1995) A Brief guide to the Disability Discrimination Act (DL 40).
(1996) Definition of Disability (DL 60).
(1996) Employment (DL 70).
(1996) Access to Goods, Facilities and Services (DL 80).
(1996) Letting or Selling Land or Property (DL 90).
(1996) Education (DL 100).
(1996) Public Transport Vehicles (DL 110).
(1996) National Disability Council and the Northern Ireland
Disability Council (DL 120).
All are obtainable from Disability on the Agenda, FREEPOST, Bristol BS38 7DE. tel: 0345 622 633.

RADAR (The Royal Association for Disability and Rehabilitation) has produced *The Employer's Guide to the DDA*, available from RADAR, 12 City Forum, 250 City Road, London EC1V 8AF. Tel.: 0171 250 3222.

The Trades Union Congress has produced *Trades Unions and Disability Law* (and many other useful documents). Available from TUC Publications, Congress House, Great Russell Street, London WC1B 3LS.

Detailed guidance booklets on the Act are also available from non-governmental groups listed in Appendix 1 and Appendix 2.

The NHS Executive has issued official guidance, *Employing Disabled People in the NHS: A Guide to Good Practice.* Stewards, safety reps and union officials might wish to refer to this and check whether employers are aware of it.

Union reps who are supporting an injured or ill nurse might suggest that employers make contact with external support such services as the Employment Service, which has disability employment advisers; placement, assessment and counselling teams (PACT); and the Access to Work scheme. These agencies can provide advice and assistance in helping employers to make 'reasonable adjustments' in recruiting or retaining injured or disabled nurses.

Work Injured Nurses Group, RCN – see Appendix 2 for full details

12 *The healthy nurse*

Working in an environment so fraught with hazards and risks, it may seem there is very little your work could actually do to promote health; most employers still have a long way to go in properly tackling hazards. Yet a great deal can be done to create a healthy working environment, one that encourages health and healthy living instead of threatening it. As organisations that are supposedly concerned with health promotion, health services are appallingly bad at this, and many private companies do far better in all areas, from recreational facilities to health screening. This final chapter looks at the positive dimensions of health and safety and provides a charter for the healthy nurse.

Personal commitment

Nurses are constantly urged to set a good example in health promotion, which is now regarded as an integral part of their role. Individual lifestyle plays a vital part in enhancing personal health, and an unfit nurse who smells of cigarettes is hardly an advertisement for good health. But it is notoriously difficult to apply the principles preached to patients to our own lives. The stresses and demands of the job, inconvenient shift work, hastily taken meal breaks and unpalatable institutional food make it all too easy to reach for a cigarette, skip a proper meal in favour of a bar of chocolate, or collapse in front of the TV instead of going for a swim, a run, aerobics or a work-out at the fitness centre.

While each one of us is responsible for trying to live a healthy life and act as a positive role model, employers can help and encourage this in many ways. There is a vast difference between health education, which simply informs people of the effects and benefits of a healthy lifestyle, and health promotion, which seeks to create an environment that makes it possible to choose a healthy lifestyle.

Physical fitness and exercise

To maintain physical fitness, the Health Education Authority's Good Health Guide recommends the following:

- Thirty minutes of vigorous activity a day (that is, enough to increase the heart rate); twist and turn all the major joints through a full range of movements to keep supple.

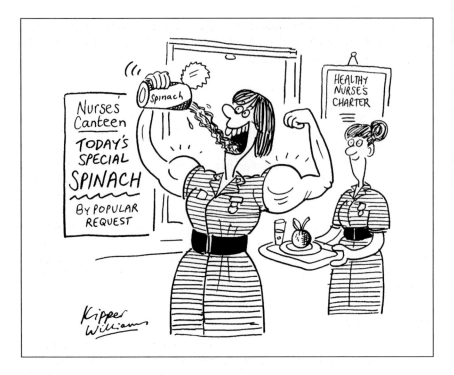

- Be on your feet for at least two hours a day to help the circulation and maintain bone density (no problem for most nurses there!).
- Lift a heavy load (with correct lifting techniques) for at least five seconds a day to maintain muscle tone (ditto!)

Most general nurses would reckon they easily maintain and far surpass that level of activity simply through the physical demands of their job. But the problem with nursing is that it requires intense physical activity in concentrated bursts, which often leave nurses so exhausted at the end of the day that they cannot face doing anything else. And although much of nursing is undoubtedly physical, it does not necessarily provide the appropriate sorts of activity to promote good health. Excessive or poor lifting, for example, inflicts cumulative damage to the back. Prolonged stooping when carrying out nursing procedures strains muscles and affects posture. Furthermore, to obtain the maximum benefit from physical activity it should be enjoyable. A competitive game of squash, a robust swim or a vigorous dance class leaves you feeling tired but invigorated, instead of exhausted and drained.

Physical exercise outside work is very important, but requires a great effort of will. Shift patterns make it difficult to attend exercise classes regularly or commit yourself to a team sport. Sports facilities may be some distance away and they are often expensive. The work environment should therefore be structured to encourage exercise, through providing sports and exercise facilities or opportunities, and encouraging exercise in other ways, such as providing bicycle racks and adequate shower facilities to make it easier for people to cycle to work.

Action points on fitness and exercise

- The provision of sports facilities at work, including swimming pools, tennis and squash courts and even playing fields may sound prohibitively expensive, but many medical schools and universities already have these facilities; they should be made universally accessible. One of the benefits of nursing education's move into higher education has been the widening of recreation facilities for nursing students, and these could also be made available to qualified staff.
- Local sports and fitness centres may be prepared to offer staff discounts at off-peak times, or in return for cooperation on sports medicine provision.
- Aerobics and exercise classes could be organised within the workplace, coinciding with shift patterns. These facilities should be attractively publicised.

Healthy eating

A healthy diet is one of the most important requirements for a healthy body. Nurses are well aware of this and are often closely involved in monitoring and advising their patients on diet and nutrition. Yet many nurses eat badly, and few would truly claim to apply to their own diet the principles they adopt with their patients.

Nurses face huge pressures which discourage healthy eating. Meal breaks are short or often non-existent, so food is eaten quickly and not properly digested before the nurse rushes back to work. Institutional food is often unpalatable and high in fat and carbohydrate. The 'healthy' alternatives may lack variety, and may not be attractively presented or encouraged, though they have improved greatly in recent years. Nurses under financial pressure may choose hospital canteen food as an easy option to catering more healthily for themselves.

Meanwhile nurses are subject to the same media pressure as the rest of the population to eat unhealthy foods – compare the millions spent on advertising high-sugar, high-fat foods with the minuscule promotion of the wholefood industry. Much of the food available in shops and supermarkets is highly processed, with added chemical preservatives, flavourings and colourings. Even though more wholefoods are now available, they are usually more expensive: wholemeal bread, for example, can cost at least 25 per cent more than white.

Healthy eating cannot be achieved simply by providing information about a healthy diet. It means increasing the food choices available in line with nutritional goals; providing healthy food that tastes good and looks attractive.

Two major reports in the 1980s provided the basis of nutritional guidance in the UK. The COMA report, published in 1984 by the DHSS, specified the links between diet and health, recommending less salt, less saturated fat, no more sugar than at present and an increase in dietary fibre. These recommendations echoed the advice of the Health Education Council, although the latter also stressed manufacturers' responsibilities in cutting the fat, carbohydrate and salt levels in food and in limiting the use of chemical additives.

Although the emphasis was different, the central message of the two reports was the same and provided the first national guidelines to health authorities on the fat, sugar, salt and fibre content of diets. A few took up the challenge, drawing up district food and health policies and actively seeking to incorporate the guidelines into their catering, but most hospital canteen food remained high in fat, sugar and carbohydrates and low in fibre. In 1992 the NHS Executive advised health authorities to include specific nutritional standards in their purchasing contracts with hospitals, and a nutrition task force was included in the Health at Work in the NHS initiatives (House of Commons Committee of Public Accounts, 1994). However, as Alan Langlands, chief executive of the NHS, stated, 'One can send out clear guidelines, one can send out orders. It is not possible sitting in an office in Whitehall to ensure that 90 million meals served every year in the NHS reach a proper level of perfection'.

Action points on healthy eating

- Health authorities and trusts should draw up food and health policies stating their nutritional aims and how these are going to be achieved.
- Catering managers should survey staff and patients for their views on hospital food.
- Information on healthy eating should be circulated in leaflets and posters, emphasising key points. Added fibre can be provided through wholemeal bread, wholemeal flour, high-fibre breakfast cereals, wholewheat pasta, brown rice, fresh fruit and vegetables and jacket potatoes. To cut down on fat intake, food should be grilled rather than fried, leaner cuts of meat used, more chicken and fish dishes eaten and polyunsaturated fat spreads used instead of butter or margarine. Less sugar should be added to food (artificial sweeteners do nothing to educate the taste buds towards a less sweet taste).
- This advice should be reflected in meals for staff and patients. Healthy food should taste good and be attractively presented.

Smoking, alcohol and drugs

Nurses smoke as much as corresponding groups in the general population despite directly witnessing the effects of smoking on health. Undoubtedly the stresses of the job are a major contributory factor, yet other health professionals such as doctors have drastically cut their smoking. Simple education about the effects of smoking is clearly not enough to encourage nurses to stop. It requires a more sensitive understanding of the reasons why nurses smoke and the provision of all possible support to help them to quit.

Action points on smoking, alcohol and drugs

- Set up stop-smoking groups, convened in work time, to provide practical advice and support.
- Limit smoking on staff premises to well-defined areas, with separate sections in eating and recreational facilities, making it less easy to smoke and providing a smoke-free environment for non-smokers (this has been a positive recent development throughout UK health services).
- Post clear no-smoking signs in non-smoking areas.
- Launch information campaigns on the health hazards of smoking, urging the positive rather than the negative, and including tips on how to give up. These campaigns should be a continuous process, rather than a one-week burst of activity.
- Alcohol and drugs problems among staff should be readily recognised and dealt with sympathetically. Independent counselling should be provided and the strictest confidentiality maintained. Alcoholics Anonymous groups can be formed in the workplace in the same way as stop-smoking groups, although individual help must be made available to any nurse who requires it.

Working conditions and the working environment

It is impossible to maintain a healthy lifestyle in an unhealthy workplace; working conditions are crucial in promoting health at work. Too many nurses work in shabby surroundings with dilapidated buildings, outdated and inadequate facilities, dingy paintwork and poor standards of hygiene – conditions that are at best depressing, at worst positively dangerous. Inconvenient and inflexible shift patterns, lack of child care facilities and problems in finding accommodation add to the pressures of the job, and do not promote a healthy workforce. And it's hard enough for safety representatives to deal with trying to contain the overt hazards of the workplace, let alone making it a pleasant environment in which to work.

Health at Work in the NHS

The Health at Work in the NHS campaign, set up with the Health Education Authority, is a particularly interesting initiative – a health promotion programme aimed at encouraging a healthier lifestyle and safer conditions for staff. It centres on health and safety policy and risk management (HEA, 1994).

Health-promoting Hospitals

Linked with the Health at Work programme is the Health Promoting Hospitals initiative, a Europe-wide partnership programme launched in 1988 by the World Health Organization. This is a logical but novel idea, because hospitals focus on sickness rather than health. The HPH has set up pilot hospital projects, national and regional networks, models of good practice and information exchange. By the end of 1997, there were 288 participating hospitals (NHSE 1994; see also 'Contact Organisations and resources' below). The goals of the movement include:

• The hospital as a healthy workplace.
• Clinical centres of excellence with patients as partners.
• Hospitals as partners in comprehensive care with primary care, community services, home care and informal helpers.
• The hospital as an ally for public health, providing a database for community-based health promotion, linked with improving clinical practice and the maintenance of healthy staff.

Money is management's perennial excuse for the dismal conditions in which many health services staff work. Yet saving money on building maintenance is a false economy. Neglected paintwork can lead to wet and dry rot, which is far more costly to repair in the end; pest infestation causes outbreaks of infection, which puts an extra burden on resources. Buildings should be kept in good repair, decorated regularly in bright, attractive colours, and kept clean. Pest infestation must be abolished, rubbish collected regularly and grounds kept neat. Carpeted floors muffle noise and are more pleasant than vinyl flooring. Pictures and plants make the institutional setting more homely. Morale will be higher in a bright, clean and pleasant working environment, with a knock-on effect on recruitment, staff retention rates and sickness levels.

Staff facilities

Staff canteens can be made more attractive, providing a more relaxing environment for a quick break. Meals should be provided with nurses' shifts in mind, with hot meals available in the evening and at night – too many hospitals cater properly only for their daytime workforce. There should be areas other than the canteen where staff can relax during breaks. In many hospitals, on-site shops, banks, laundrettes and even hairdressers help to save staff time. There should be secure staff car parks and adequate, safe public transport late at night. If staff residences are situated away from the workplace, transport should be provided to and from work. Staff changing rooms and cloakrooms should be roomy, with a personal locker for each nurse, showers and a sufficient number of toilets. Hospital wards should have a private staff area.

Many of nursing's current recruitment problems would be solved if health services provided child care facilities. For an organisation predominantly staffed by women, it is incredible that so little is done to help women with children return to work. Many mothers take night work so that they can look after their children during the day, snatching a few hours' sleep before returning to work – a regime that is hardly conducive to good health. Health employers should provide (or ensure easy access to) creches and nurseries, preschool play groups and facilities for caring for children after school hours if their parents are still working.

Nurses' homes

While they are mostly consigned to history, those nurses' homes that remain seem to be a department of the hospital rather than a place for people to live in. Many are grim institutions in a poor state of repair, with up to 100 staff sharing one kitchen and inadequate bathroom and toilet facilities. Dangerous wiring, faulty cookers and inadequate fire precautions make some positively lethal. The ideal layout for nurses' homes is in flats with a bath, toilet and kitchen for every four to six people or fewer. They should be in a quiet area so that staff on night duty can sleep properly, with bike and car parking and laundrette facilities. They should be properly maintained, with regular safety inspections, fire escapes and fire extinguisher equipment, and regular refuse collection.

Following a cost-cutting review in 1984, health authorities sold off much of their residential property, providing accommodation only for student nurses and staff on call. While it may be difficult today to provide residential accommodation for as many nurses as require it, rooms could be available for those with long journeys home who are required to work a late shift followed by an early one, or at other unsocial times. Shift patterns make it difficult to get to work on public transport, and accommodation provided on site, or with transport arrangements, makes getting to work easier and safer.

Shift work

Providing 24-hour care is an inescapable reality for most nurses, especially hospital nurses, so shift work is inevitable. It can impose an enormous strain on nurses' physical and mental health, and play havoc with social life and relationships, as well as with eating and sleeping routines (Healy, 1997). Yet, planned properly, the risks of shift work can be minimised and it can even become preferable to the grind of a nine to five, Monday to Friday week. It can be useful and enjoyable having time off during the week when shops, transport, cinemas, theatres and restaurants are less crowded.

Shift work must be well planned, which means avoiding gruelling 10-day stretches that leave nurses in no state to enjoy their days off. It should be organised to a regular pattern wherever possible, so nurses know well in advance when their time off will be. Last-minute changes should be avoided except as a final resort, as should split shifts (Barton *et al.*, 1995).

Shifts can also be made more flexible to accommodate family commitments – fitting in with school hours, for example. Nurse banks can be established to employ nurses who wish to work more flexible hours, and more part-time nurses could be employed on permanent contracts, including in more senior posts. All these arrangements would make it easier for women with children to nurse (RCN, 1997; Totterdell *et al.*, 1995; Unison, 1996).

European directives

Few nurses are happy (or healthy) under the current shift patterns, but the EU Working Time Directive (Council Directive 93/104/EC, 23 November 1993), which covers important health and safety issues, offers the hope that something will be done about it. Its main provisions are:

- A maximum 48-hour working week, including overtime, averaged over four months.
- A minimum 11 consecutive hours' rest per day.
- Thirty-five consecutive hours' rest per week.
- A rest break in any working day after six hours – its length to be set by collective agreement or national law and practice; each member state may decide if Sunday should be included in the rest period.
- Four weeks' paid annual leave per year (three weeks is acceptable until 1999), the qualifying conditions to follow national law and practice.
- Work organisation should take account of health and safety needs.

Night work is defined in the directive as 'not less than seven hours and must include at least three hours between midnight and 5 am'. This includes anyone who is likely to work a certain proportion of their working time during the night. The directive prescribes a maximum night shift of eight hours for hazardous or stressful work, and requires workers to have the right to transfer to appropriate day work on medical grounds, whenever possible, and that free health assessments are available for this purpose.

On health and safety, the directive states that 'every worker must enjoy satisfactory health and safety conditions in his working environment', and that the employer should take account of the general principle of adapting work to the worker.

Due to become law in 1996, the directive was delayed by the Conservative government, which believed that working hours was not a health and safety issue and secured a seven-year opt-out, so that workers may 'voluntarily' work more than 48 hours a week. The employer must ensure that these workers' agreement has been obtained, and keep records of those who work over 48 hours. No worker should be penalised for being unwilling to work more than 48 hours. The HSE, trades unions and environmental health officials should have access to these records.

Other 'derogations', or departures from the directive, are optional, and relate to workers who can be excluded from the rest period and night shift provisions, but they must be agreed collectively and exchanged for equivalent rest periods. Note that employers may not impose shift changes under the pretext that they are complying with the EU directive. If this is suggested, contact your union steward or officer.

The Labour government has not yet clarified its views on implementation, so the directive does not directly affect nurses at present, and explicitly excludes 'areas of continuous production or service, such as hospitals, emergency services and utilities' and 'doctors in training' from the mandatory provisions, although the European Commission may alter that soon. Yet even if the government does not apply the directive to nurses or health services, it contains some important statements about the inherent hazards and risks of work, and the good employer would be well advised to take account of it when planning working policies. Joint union/staff and management groups should discuss its implications alongside the recommendations with which this section concludes (see below).

Recommendations for action on the working environment and working conditions

- Provision of a clean, attractive and safe working environment.
- Good staff facilities, including canteens, shops, recreational facilities, car parks and changing rooms.
- Child care facilities on site or nearby for all staff who require them.
- Good residential accommodation for those who request it, well designed and maintained, available at reasonable rents.
- Shifts should be well planned and as flexible as possible to fit in with family commitments.
- Public transport should be adequate, with cooperation between employers and the providers of public transport services to ensure that timetables fit with the beginning and end of shifts.

Occupational health services

Decisive government and management action are desperately needed to improve nurses' working conditions. But the fight for better health and safety also needs an institutional focus in the NHS in the form of an occupational health service (OHS). In Chapter 1 we looked at the political and historical background to find out why progress on developing such a service has been so slow; here we sketch out what such a service might look like.

The Royal College of Nursing and the Health and Safety Commission's health services advisory committee agree on most of the key principles. Many of their views have now been endorsed by the government and the issue has been given a welcome boost in the new policy focus on public health, of which workplace health and safety is an important subset (see below for further discussion). The World Health Organization says that OH programmes should aim to promote and maintain the health of employees. This involves identifying and controlling all chemical, physical, psychosocial and other agents that may be hazardous to health, matching people's capabilities to their work, and protecting those who are specially vulnerable to adverse working conditions.

Other authors, unions and pressure groups put greater emphasis on the dynamic, preventive role of an OH service. Lunn and Waldron (1991), for example, advocate a nationally coherent service run by specially trained nurses who have expertise in epidemiology and other relevant disciplines, and actively seek out hazards rather than wait for the problems to come to them. Carol Bannister, the RCN's occupational health adviser, says that the lack of regulation and the variations in the work of occupational health services in the NHS are major causes for concern, but sees positive signs in policy and practice development for OH nurses.

There are various descriptions of the aims and functions of an OH service; the RCN's 1991 document gives a comprehensive account, and provides a useful framework for discussion. All health authorities and trusts should, in conjunction with staff representatives, draw up a similar plan for their own service as a basis for development; the planning group should include at least one health authority or board member, who can act as a direct link with the employer. The OHS should be independent of management, accountable to the trust board or equivalent, and have its own designated staff and budget.

Health supervision

Assessment and supervision of the nurse's health before and during employment is a key function. Medical screening of applicants for nursing training is controversial and there have been complaints of unjustified discrimination on health grounds, for example against people with epilepsy or diabetes. Other areas where difficulties arise include physique, back problems, chronic skin disease and mental health problems. While it is to no one's advantage that a student nurse should prove unable to do the job, any assessment – if it is thought necessary on completion of a health questionnaire – should be conducted on the basis of clear health criteria. These should be drawn up by the OHS, the school of nursing and management, using guidance from the appropriate government health department and nursing statutory body. Employers should use the Disability Discrimination Act's criteria on employment as a model of good practice, with risk assessment and advice on appropriate 'reasonable adjustments'. Carol Bannister advocates adjusting health assessment criteria to the needs of a job: 'The occupational health service isn't there to decide who should or shouldn't be employed. That's a management decision.'

Staff health can be monitored during employment in various ways, but above all it must not be seen to be part of a disciplinary procedure. If managers think a health assessment is needed for a member of staff, that person must agree, and both parties must be given the results. Use of the OHS must be voluntary, so the uptake of its facilities will depend very much on how it presents itself, its reputation and its relations with staff of all grades. It is useful to do a needs assessment of the organisation and individual nurses as a basis for prioritising interventions; health assessment interviews could be held after long sickness absences or a change of job in order to determine the need for 'reasonable adjustments' to support staff back to work. Collecting sickness and absence records is a management responsibility, but personal health records stay with the OHS and must be strictly confidential (DoH, 1993a).

Any necessary immunisation programmes should follow agreed guidelines – for TB, polio, tetanus, typhoid, rubella and hepatitis B. Nurses working in clinical areas may be at high risk and the benefits of immunisation are obvious. The government's expert advisory committee on hepatitis (DoH, 1993b) recommends that people who can't seroconvert (show immunity to hepatitis B) should not be required to participate in exposure-prone procedures such as in renal units, theatres and intensive care, but this doesn't exclude them from most other areas of nursing.

There is disagreement about whether an OHS should provide general screening programmes for diseases which are not thought to be related to work hazards. Best OH practice should be to prioritise access to health needs assessment and risk assessment. An OHS can play an active part in organising services or access to them, avoiding duplication of NHS services. A good example is provided by Leicester General Hospital, which offers physiotherapy referral for staff for rapid rehabilitation of musculo-skeletal injuries, with an evaluation of its effectiveness. It cannot safely be assumed that nurses' proximity to health services means they make full use of them.

Health promotion

Programmes should be developed in response to perceived needs, and also by finding out what staff want; a user group is another way of finding out whether the service is meeting people's needs. They may deal with specific work hazards, or tackle problems such as smoking and drinking. The OHS should participate in training and refresher courses for new and qualified staff where there are opportunities for health promotion on work hazards such as moving and handling. Individual consultations may also provide an opportunity for advice and investigation, for example for a nurse who complains of back pain. Does her or his ward lack hoists, is it short-staffed, are staff using the correct techniques? The OHS staff should regularly visit all premises in their patch to see for themselves the kind of education needed, and should regard the workplace rather than the clinic as their real base.

Occupational safety

The OHS should be notified by management of all incidents and accidents, so the trends and causes can be investigated and tackled. The staff should be seen as experts on safety, working closely with trust safety officers, managers, safety committees and union reps, and being involved in drawing up codes of practice for safe working procedures.

Environmental monitoring

Closely linked with its occupational safety functions is the OHS's responsibility for environmental monitoring – identifying hazards in the workplace. It should investigate, evaluate and review all activities which could present health risks to staff. Sometimes it may be necessary to call in expert advice from within or outside the NHS; effective liaison with specialists in fields such as radiation and infection control should be a matter of course. Data collected for environmental monitoring should be used in epidemiological analysis, on a small or large scale, to assess the health effects of particular hazards or working in particular wards or specialties. Research and epidemiological skills should form part of OH training but staff may also seek help from academic institutions, the TUC, trade unions and others (see, for example, the risk assessment and reporting work of unions such as the TGWU, GMB and Unison, and reports by the Labour Research Department and *Hazards* magazine).

Counselling

The workers' confidence in the skills and integrity of the OHS will lead some to seek counselling on personal problems which may or may not be related to work. OHS staff should all have adequate training in counselling to enable them to deal empathetically with such approaches and identify when referral elsewhere is desirable. Nursing students may be especially vulnerable to work stress and should have access to a full range of services in university health centres. 'Interested, available, no local axes to grind' was the counsellor's job description suggested by one student. Qualified nurses also need plenty of emotional support. Again strict confidentiality, adhering to British Counselling Association codes of practice, is crucial, with an outside telephone line and a secluded waiting area.

First aid and treatment

The main role of the OHS should be preventive, and it should avoid duplicating NHS treatment services. However it may, on request, continue treatments prescribed by a GP or outpatient department, such as a course of injections. It should monitor accidents for which staff are treated at work through the notification system. The OHS also provides advice on the facilities and training required under the First Aid Regulations 1981 (and 1997 Approved Code of Practice).

Rehabilitation and redeployment

Trusts should have an agreed policy that adheres to the national require-ments for the recruitment of disabled people and for dealing with those who are disabled during employment. These policies should meet at least the minimum requirements of the Disability Discrimination Act, and preferably exceed them. Nurses returning to work after a long illness should be able to choose work which will not overtax them. The NHS has a poor record on redeployment and the OHS can help improve this with advice on changes in working methods, alternative work and rehabilitation. The Act should be seen as an opportunity to make the most of all nurses' skills and experience.

Records

The OHS has an important role in interpreting statistics on sickness and absence, accidents and work-related ill-health, but must take account of Data Protection Act requirements. Individual health records are confidential and must not leave the OH department or be shown to or discussed with non-OHS staff without the person's prior written consent, unless directed by court order or a professional judgement of 'public interest'. Reports on health to management should refer not to confidential health information, but to a nurse's ability to do the job, linked to the job description. A standardised computer system with closed access is most convenient for record-keeping and research, but personnel and other trust staff should not be able to access the system.

These are the principal areas of activity which should be developed in a trust-wide OHS. Detailed advice on premises, security arrangements, accommodation and other issues is available in DoH, Unison, TUC, RCN and HSAC guidelines.

The staffing of the service is the key to its success. Every nurse and doctor it employs should be specially trained in occupational health, or offered the training as a condition of employment. Even those who have the required qualifications, however, may not regard themselves primarily as preventive health workers. Davies' thesis on the problems encountered by injured and ill nurses seeking to return to work shows that many OH nurses see themselves as management gatekeepers rather than advocates for their clients (Davies, 1994). Unless OH nurses take their preventive role more seriously, including its health promotion component, they will see the initiative for such work pass to others.

The OH nurse has traditionally been regarded as the doctor's assistant, which is inappropriate in any health care, and no less so in OH, where the emphasis should not be on medical treatment but on active prevention. Far more nurses than doctors possess appropriate OH qualifications but they must be prepared to take up the challenge and show the true worth of their expertise. They could form the foundation of a humane and caring advocacy for their own nurse colleagues in the NHS. It is to be hoped that the current review of occupational health by the Health Services Advisory Committee of the Health and Safety Commission will reflect these ideals.

Government health strategy and occupational health nursing

The 1998 report *Occupational Health Nursing: contributing to healthier workplaces*, published by the Department of Health and the English National Board in association with the Association of Occupational Health Nurse Practitioners and the RCN Society for Occupational Nursing, is an important aspect of the government's public health strategy 'Our Healthier Nation'. It brings welcome and long overdue recognition of the value of OH nursing. Highlighting many examples of good practice, it should help OH nurses to develop current practice, prevent ill-health and promote health in the workplace, and it addresses many of the issues highlighted in this book.

The report aims to share good practice and be illustrative rather than prescriptive. It asks seven key questions:

1. How can employers work with qualified OH professionals to manage workplace risks and improve the health of the workforce?
2. How can OH nurses use their expertise to maximise new opportunities and contribute to meeting business needs?
3. How can OH nurses increase their influence and impact in the workplace?
4. How can the workplace be used best to promote healthy practices among the workforce?
5. How can OH nurses work with colleagues in multiprofessional OH teams to improve the health of the workforce?
6. How can the needs of small and medium-sized businesses be met by OH nurses?
7. How can educational programmes meet the needs of OH nurses?

Innovative practices along these lines already exist. For example a Healthy Workplace Initiative (for Health at Work in the NHS) has been developed in

---

Box 12.1 *Occupational health nursing: approaching the millennium with optimism?*

New occupational health and safety guidance for the NHS in Scotland and for OH nursing in England give good grounds for approaching the millennium with optimism.

The Scottish Office/NHS Executive guidelines (Scottish Office, 1995) suggest that OH services in the NHS exist to:

- Promote and maintain the physical, mental and social well-being of all staff.
- Help management to protect staff from physical and environmental health hazards arising from their work or conditions of work, and to provide advice on the working environment.
- Contribute to increasing the effectiveness of the organisation, by enhancing staff performance and morale through reducing risks at work which lead to ill-health, staff absence and accidents.
- Assess applicants for employment, to ensure they are fit and to recommend placement in appropriate work.
- Help management to protect patients, visitors and others from physical, environmental and health hazards in NHS settings.
- Advise on environmental issues in the NHS.

---

a project involving the Wessex Institute for Health Research and Development, together with purchasers and OH staff from the South and West Regions. The outcomes include a 15-point NHS OH Service Standards document and a 12-point Healthy Workplace Indicators plan, which may be used in purchasing contracts and in trusts to assess progress in OH and workplace health promotion.

A similar philosophy has been advocated in Scotland (see Box 12.1).

Conclusion

Every trust or its equivalent and every private institution in the UK should establish without delay a fully funded, independent, confidential and comprehensive OH service for all its employees. Its main function should be to prevent ill-health and promote staff health through rigorous monitoring and control or abolition of hazards in the workplace. Its principal activities should include health needs assessment for employment, health supervision during employment, health promotion and education, advice on occupational safety, environmental monitoring, counselling, rehabilitation and resettlement.

OH services established on these lines would do a great deal to improve nurses' health and safety. Success in setting them up, and their subsequent record, will depend heavily on the extent to which staff are involved in planning and participation. The OHS should be viewed not as a paternalistic institution bestowed by a kind employer, but as an aspect of every nurse's right to work in safe and healthy conditions, in the fullest sense.

The need for a vigilant monitoring service would in any case diminish if the health services became more responsive to the needs of staff – and the best way of ensuring this sensitivity is to involve staff fully in decision-making at all levels, as advocated in the 1997 English government white paper *The New NHS*. The UK lags behind many other countries in this respect, and policy discussions of worker participation have rarely made progress despite the known benefits. We might expect that democracy would be welcomed rather than feared, even after years of undermining of the public service ethos of the NHS. Unlike private industry, where the demands of workers for better pay and conditions and the desire of owners for bigger profits often come into conflict, all NHS staff appear to have common goals.

The reality, though, is that the NHS is a constant battleground. The needs of patients and different groups of staff are not always compatible, and some groups have much more say than others. Nurses became acutely aware of this after the introduction of general management and the replacement of multidisciplinary management teams by a single powerful chief executive, which led to the exclusion of many senior nurses from decision making and the muffling of the nursing voice. The nurse's place at the top table is no longer guaranteed, but depends largely on the attitudes of the chief executive and the skills of the senior nurse.

As well as management shortcomings, it is tempting to blame every problem on a lack of resources. The key point, however, is how the billions poured into health services are actually spent. Even when (or perhaps especially when) money is tight, some groups of staff and some specialties fare better than others. There is evidence throughout this book to suggest that the workers at the sharp end, those in the wards, clinics, kitchens and sluices, are low on the list of priorities, and suffer even more during recessions or when a government wants to appear to be financially strict.

An individualistic, victim-blaming approach to the wide-ranging problems associated with health and safety can do little more than apply sticking plasters. Nor is it enough to rely on the goodwill of the employers, as experience has shown. The reforms recommended in this book should be seen as part of a broader plan to put more power in the hands of the staff who keep the service going 24 hours a day, but have the least status and fewest rewards. Talk of democracy in the NHS now focuses on restoring accountability and openness within the regional and trust structures, while there is some likelihood of restoring some of the powers which were gradually stripped away from the trade unions. There is scope for proper representation of staff interests, not just through a token professional or trade union presence on a board, but through more substantial worker involvement in many decision-making arenas.

Grass-roots staff should be better represented in the management and policy-making structure, but the traditional hierarchy makes this difficult. There are many ways in which staff could be involved and consulted, and nurses must be more assertive in putting their views forward. The professional advisory machinery is one neglected channel of communication; it has an officially sanctioned role and a nurses' committee should be part of every trust and HA.

We have frequently alluded to the vital part played by staff organisations in defending and promoting their members' interests, and their major contribution in pushing for better health and safety standards and the enforcement of legislation. Without them, measures such as the Health and Safety at Work Act would be little more than a dead letter. The previous government attempted to curb their powers but the unions continue to act as a major force, pressing for improvements through their stewards, safety reps, branches and national officials. On health and safety issues rival unions have muted their traditional antagonisms and TUC unions work closely with non-TUC organisations, notably the RCN and the Royal College of Midwives. The RCN now has 1600 safety reps who are adopting a more proactive approach, while its labour relations officials and Forum for Occupational Health Nurses continue to do valuable work. The role of the unions as independent organisations through which workers can promote their interests should be strengthened rather than weakened, and nurses should be encouraged to play a more active part in them.

Our research for the updated edition of this book showed us, regrettably, how little has changed ten years on in the continuing exploitation of nurses. The lack of attention paid to their health, safety and welfare, with constant lip service paid to their angelic qualities of compassion and selflessness, is a graphic indication of the wide gap between myth and reality. One important remedy is for nurses to secure more autonomy, both as individuals and as an occupational group. This does not mean working in isolation or ignoring others, but giving nurses their due as full members of the health care team. Their physical and mental health and their job satisfaction will be vastly improved if an occupational structure is established which enables them to earn good salaries by remaining as practitioners, with ample opportunity for continuing education. The lack of full opportunities for personal and professional growth underlies many of the less tangible but equally dangerous threats to health and safety. Wide-ranging reforms, incorporating the many practical recommendations we have outlined, are vital to ensure that the shoemaker's children are not barefoot but properly shod.

Recommendations for empowering and caring for NHS workers

- Health care staff at all levels should have more say in planning and decision-making.
- Resources should be allocated in a more equitable manner.
- More attention should be paid to the welfare of employees.
- Health service employers should be more democratic and more sensitive to the needs and views of staff.
- Health service structures should be more democratic and less hierarchical.
- Nurses should make better use of their professional advisory machinery.
- The role of the trade unions should be strengthened.
- Nurses should be more active in union affairs.
- The autonomy of nurses, individually and collectively, should be secured.
- Clinical grading and career paths should be thoroughly reexamined, better to achieve their original intentions.
- The personal and professional needs of every nurse should be met as far as possible – starting with action to ensure their safety at work and the maintenance of good health.

A charter for the healthy nurse

- A healthy individual lifestyle, promoted by the employer through healthy diet, sports facilities and support to help nurses avoid health hazards such as smoking, drugs and alcohol.
- A safe and healthy working environment in which health hazards are rigorously monitored, controlled and abolished wherever possible.
- Good working conditions, including extensive staff facilities, canteens, changing rooms, shops and banking facilities, recreational activities, child care facilities, residential accommodation for those who need it, and well planned and flexible shift arrangements.
- An occupational health service that is independent of management and totally confidential, providing a comprehensive and fully funded resource for preventive health care, counselling, health education and screening, monitoring work conditions, controlling and abolishing work hazards, and record-keeping.
- The inclusion and involvement of nurses in all decisions affecting the conditions, environment and hazards of the workplace, through individual and trade union representation.

References, contact organisations and further reading

Association of National Health Service Occupational Physicians (1996) *The Role of Occupational Health in the Process of Managing Sickness Absence.* ANHOPS Executive, West Midland Occupational Health Audit Group, Birmingham.

Bannister, C. and Coakley, L. (1995)'The best laid schemes', *Occupational Health*, vol. 47, no. 9 (September), pp. 428–9.

Barton, J., Spelton, E., Totterdell, P., Smith, L. and Folkard S. (1995) 'Is there an optimum number of night shifts?', *Work & Stress*, vol. 9, no. 2/3 (April–September), pp. 109–23.

British Medical Association (1994) *Environmental and Occupational Risks of Health Care.* London: BMA.

Bunt, K. (1993) *Occupational health provision at work,* HSE Contract Research Report no. 57. Sudbury: Health and Safety Executive.

Davies, G. (1994) *Factors helping or hindering nurses returning to work following illness or injury.* London: MSc thesis, City University.

DHSS (1984) *Report of the Committee on Medical Aspects of Food Policy, Diet and Cardiovascular Disease* (COMA Report). London: HMSO.

DoH (1991) *Report of the Panel on Dietary Reference Values of the Committee on Medical Aspects of Food Policy.* London: HMSO.

DoH (1993a) *The management of occupational health services for healthcare staff,* NHS MEL. London: HMSO.

DoH (1993b) *Protecting health care workers and patients from Hepatitis B.* Expert Advisory Group on Hepatitis B. London: DoH.

DoH and ENB (1998) *Occupational Health Nursing: contributing to healthier workplaces.* London: Department of Health with the English National Board for Nursing, Midwifery and Health Visiting, in collaboration with the Association of Occupational Health Nurse Practitioners (UK) and the RCN Society for Occupational Health Nursing.

Glover, W. (1997a) 'The Working Time Directive – what it means for you', RCN *Newsline* vol. 22, no. 9 (September), p. 3.

Glover, W. (1997b) 'Nurse sagas: working time directive still not implemented in UK', RCN *Euroforum*, no. 3 (Autumn), p. 4.

Gulland, A. (1997) 'Nurses triumph with Euro shifts', *Nursing Times*, vol. 93, no. 27 (2 July), p. 10.

Health Education Authority (1994) *Health at Work in the NHS: working well – a guide to success.* London: HEA.

Healy, D. (1997) 'Blues in the night', *Nursing Times*, vol. 93, no. 15 (9 April), pp. 26-28.

House of Commons Committee of Public Accounts (1994) *National Health Service: Hospital Catering in England,* 49th Report. London: HMSO.

Lunn, J. and Waldron, H. (1991) *Concerning the Carers. Occupational health for health care workers.* London: Butterworth Heinemann.

NHS Executive (1994) *Health Promoting Hospitals.* Leeds: NHSE.

RCN (1991) *A Guide to an Occupational Health Nursing Service,* 2nd ed. London: RCN Society of Occupational Health Nursing.

RCN (1993) *The Occupational Health Nurse: Opportunities for Developing Professional Practice,* re-order no. 000 336. London: Royal College of Nursing.

RCN (1995) *Health Assessment: Advice to Managers,* re-order no. 000 555; *Advice for Occupational Health Nurses,* re-order no. 000 556. London: Royal College of Nursing.

RCN (1996) 'Occupational Health Nursing Guidelines', 15 fact sheets. London: Royal College of Nursing.

RCN (1997) 'Shifting the balance: Towards best practice in shift working and patient care', Health and Safety at Work leaflet no. 6, re-order no. 000 733. London: Royal College of Nursing.

Reid, T. (1995) 'Improving working conditions: occupational health'. *Nursing Times*, vol. 91, no. 24 (14 June), pp. 26–7.

Scottish Office: National Health Service in Scotland Management Executive (1995) 'Occupational Health and Safety Services for the NHS in Scotland', SOHHD/NHSE NHS Circular GEN.

Totterdell, P., Spelton, E. and Pokorski, J. (1995) 'The effects of nightwork on psychological changes during the menstrual cycle', *Journal of Advanced Nursing*, vol. 21, no. 5 (May), pp. 996–1005.

Unison (1996) *Women's health and safety: a trade union guide*, Unison stock no. 818. London: LRD Publications.

Contact organisations and resources

Action on Smoking and Health (ASH), 109 Gloucester Place, London W1H 3PH. Tel.: 0171 935 3519. Fax 0171 935 3463.

Alcoholics Anonymous, 11 Redcliffe Gardens, London SW10 9BG. General Service Centre: tel: 01904 644026. London Regional Telephone Service (10am–10pm): Tel.: 0171 352 3001.

Association of Occupational Health Nurse Practitioners (UK), 33 Beechdale, Winchmore Hill, London N21 3QG. Tel.: 0181 882 5695.

British Nutrition Foundation 52–54 High Holborn, London WC1. Tel.: 0171 404 6504.

Health Education Authority, Hamilton House, Mabledon Place, London WC1. Tel.: 0171 383 3833.

London Food Commission, 94 White Lion Street, London N1 9PF. Tel.: 0171 8372250.

RCN Society of Occupational Health Nursing, also has Forums for Occupational Health Nurses in the NHS and for Occupational Health Nursing Managers. 20 Cavendish Square, London W1M 0AB. Tel.: 0171 409 3333.

Scottish Health Education Group, Woodburn House, Cannen Lane, Edinburgh, EH10 4SG. Tel.: 0131 536 5500.

Sports Council, P.O. Box 480, Crystal Palace National Sports Centre, Leadrington Road, London SE19. Tel.: 0181 778 8600.

Unison, *The European Working Time Directive: a Unison negotiator's guide* (1996) is an excellent, comprehensive booklet, giving a summary of the political context, legal position and numerous checkpoints of advice for negotiators. *Women's health and safety: a trade union guide* (1997) was produced for Unison by the Labour Research Department. Unison Stock no. 818.

WHO Health Promoting Hospitals Project. Information is available from the Hospital Programme Health Care Delivery Unit, World Health Organization Regional Office for Europe, Scherfigsvej 8, DK-2100 Copenhagen, Denmark. Tel.: 00 45 39 17 15 77. Fax: 00 45 39 17 18 65, or e-mail: mgb@who.dk or kja@who.dk. Publications on HPH include Pelikan, J., Lobnig, H. and Krajic, K. 'Health Promoting Hospitals', *World Health*, 3 (May–June 1997), pp. 24–5; 'The Vienna Recommendations on Health Promoting Hospitals' (1997) and 'The WHO Health-Promoting Hospitals European Project' (1997), Copenhagen: WHO European Regional Office.

Appendix 1   Information

This appendix summarises the relevant official guidelines and circulars, inquiry reports, trade unions and pressure group publications and journals.

Official guidelines and circulars

UK government departments and the NHS Executive

AIDS/HIV infected health care workers – guidance on the management of infected health care workers, NHS Management Executive letter (NHS MEL) 31 (1994).

Advisory Committee on Dangerous Pathogens, *HIV, Hepatitis*, Department of Health (1995).

Car Parking, Health Facilities Note 21, Department of Health (1996).

Committee on Medical Aspects of Food Policy, Diet and Cardiovascular Disease, COMA report, HMSO (1984).

Disability Equipment Assessment Publications & Device Evaluation and Publications Catalogue, Medical Devices Agency (1997).

Estate Management. An exemplar estate strategy, NHS Estates (1996).

Food Hygiene. Assured Safe Catering, Department of Health, HMSO (1993).

Food Hygiene. Guidelines for the Safe Production of Heat Preserved Foods, Department of Health (1994).

Guidance notes for the protection of persons against ionising radiations arising from medical and dental use, National Radiological Protection Board, HMSO (1988).

Health and safety in the NHS: reporting on injuries, diseases and dangerous occurrences regulations 1985 (RIDDOR), NHS MEL 97, NHS Executive (1993)

Health of the Nation – A Strategy for Health in England, HMSO (1992).

Health Notices on Legionnaires' Disease, Department of Health. (May 1987).

Health Services – Guidelines: Infection Control, Department of Health (1996).

Health Services – Guidelines on Post-Exposure Prophylaxis for Health Care Workers Occupationally Exposed to HIV, Department of Health (1997).

Health Services – Health awareness for NHS staff, NHS circular PCS(GC)93/2 (1993).

Health Services – Health Promoting Hospitals, NHSE (1994).

Health Services – The Prevention and Control of Tuberculosis in the United Kingdom. Recommendations for the Prevention and Control at local level, Department of Health (1996).

Health Services – The Prevention and Control of Tuberculosis in the United Kingdom: Tuberculosis and Homeless People, Department of Health (1996).

Health Services – Management. Fire Precautions in New Hospitals, HC(87)2, (1987) DHSS.

Health Services – Management. Health and Safety at Work: Crown Immunity, HC(87)3, DHSS (1987).

Health Services – Management. Health and Safety Management in the NHS, HSG(97)6, Department of Health (1997).

Health Services – Management. Disability Discrimination Act: a Guide for presenters, EL(97)5, Department of Health (1997).

Health Services – Management. Disability Discrimination Act: implications for NHS trusts and health authorities, EL(96)70, Department of Health (1996).

Health Services – Management. Ionizing Radiations Regulations 1985, HC(85)31, DHSS (1985).

Health Services – Management. Occupational Health Services for healthcare staff, NHS MEL, DoH (1993).

Health Services – Management. Risk Management in the NHS, Department of Health (1994).

Health Services – Security in the NHS, EL(96) 13, and Security in A & E, EL (97)34, Department of Health (1997).

Health Services – Health Service use of ionising and non-ionising radiation, NHS MEL 79, Department of Health (1993).

Immunisation against infectious disease, HMSO (1992).

Guidance on the Safe Use of Lasers in Medical and Dental Practice, Medical Devices Agency (MDA). (1995)

Medical Devices Agency. *Annual Report and Accounts 1996–1997*, London: The Stationery Office. (1997).

Medical Devices Agency Corporate Plan 1995–2000, MDA (1995).

NHS Estate Management and Property Maintenance, Audit Commission (1991).

Occupational Health Nursing: contributing to healthier workplaces, Department of Health and the English National Board for Nursing, Midwifery and Health Visiting, in collaboration with the Association of Occupational Health Nurse Practitioners (UK) and the RCN Society for Occupational Health Nursing (1998).

Protecting health care workers and patients from Hepatitis B, Expert Advisory Group on Hepatitis, DoH (1993).

Reporting of hazards and potential hazards, NHS Circular GEN 24 (1991).

Reporting defects in medicinal products, NHS Circular GEN 25 (1991).

Residential Accommodation for Staff, Hospital Building Note 24, DHSS (1986).

Revised Guidance on Asbestos in NHS Premises, Safety Information Bulletin, SIB (84)16, DHSS (1984).

Risk Management in the NHS, DoH (1993).

Safety Action Bulletins, regularly issued to managers.

The management of occupational health services for healthcare staff. NHS MEL 119. HMSO (1993)

The Safe Use of Ionizing Radiations: A Handbook for Nurses, HMSO, Edinburgh (1973).

Safe working and the prevention of infection in the mortuary and post-mortem room, HMSO (1991).

Safe working and the prevention of infection in clinical laboratories, HMSO (1991).

Scotland's Health: a challenge to us all, HMSO (1992).

Scottish Office Home and Health Department:

   Decontamination of equipment prior to inspection, service or repair, SHHD/DGM 66 (1987).

   Framework for Action: impact on NHS staff 1991–92 (1992).

   Health education in Scotland – A national policy statement (1991).

   Scotland's Health: a challenge to us all, HMSO (1992).

Health and Safety Commission

Health and Safety at Work etc. Act 1974; Advice to Employees (HSC 3), *Advice to Employers* (HSC 5), *Writing a safety policy statement. Advice to Employers* (HSC 6), *Safety committees; guidance to employers whose employees are not members of recognised independent trade unions* (HSC8).

Industrial Advisory Committee Report, *Safety in Health Service Laboratories: the Labelling, Transport and Reception of Specimens*, HMSO (1986).

Respiratory protective equipment: A practical guide for users, HSG53 (1990).
A short guide to the Personal Protective Equipment at Work Regulations, IND(G)174 (1992).

Health Services Advisory Committee

AIDS, Prevention of Infection in the Health Services, HSC Factsheet (December 1986).
Management of Occupational Health Services for Healthcare staff, HMSO (1993).
Guidance on manual lifting of loads in the health services, HMSO (1992).
Management of Health and Safety in the Health Services (1994).
The Safe Disposal of Clinical Waste, HMSO (1992).
Violence to Staff in the Health Services, HMSO (1987).
Waste Anaesthetic Gases, Health Services Information Sheet no. 7, HSAC (1994).

Health and Safety Executive

Anaesthetic agents: Controlling exposure under COSHH, ISBN 0 7176 1043 8 (1996).
Asbestos Medical Series MS12, (1998).
Carriage of Dangerous Goods by Road Regulations 1996, L89 (1996).
Control of Asbestos at Work Regulations 1987, ACoP, L27 and L28 (1993).
First Aid at Work, The Health and Safety First Aid at Work Regulations 1981 Approved Code of Practice (ACoP) and Guidance, L74 (1997).
First Aid at work -- your questions answered, IND(G)214. HSE (1997)
Basic advice on first aid at work, IND(G)215. HSE (1997)
Health and safety in kitchens and food preparation areas, HSG55 HSE (1990).
Health and safety in residential care homes, HSG104, (1993).
Health surveillance of occupational skin disease, MS24 (1991).
Introducing the Noise at Work Regulations, INDG75.
Information approved for the classification and labelling of substances and preparations dangerous for supply, CHIP 96 and 97, L76 (1996/97); CHIP 97 L100 (1997).
How to deal with sick building syndrome, HSG132 (1995).
Legionnaires' Disease, Guidance Note EH48, HMSO (1987).
Control of legionellosis including Legionnaires' disease, HSG70 (1993); IACL27 Legionnaires' Disease.
Mercury and its inorganic divalent compounds, EH17 (1996).
Mercury and its inorganic divalent compounds: Criteria document for an Occupational Limit, EH65/19 (1995).
Mercury: Medical guidance notes, MS12 (1996).
Management of health and safety at work, Management of Health and Safety at Work Regulations 1992, ACoP, L21 (1992).
Noise at Work: Noise assessment, information and control, HSG56 (1990).
Sound solutions. Techniques to reduce noise at work, HSG138 (1995).
Slips and trips: Guidance for employers on identifying hazards and controlling risks, HSG156 (1996).
Preventing trips, slips and falls at work, IND(G)225 HSE (1996).
Guide to the Reporting of Injuries, Diseases and Dangerous Occurrences Regulations (RIDDOR) 1995, L73, (1996).
Everyone's Guide to RIDDOR 95, HSE31 (1996).
Passive smoking at work, IND(G)63 (1995).
Preventing asthma at work, L55 (1994).
Taking action on stress at work: A guide for employers, HSG116 (1995).
Respiratory sensitisers and COSHH, IND(G)95 (1995).
The Ventilation of Buildings – Fresh Air Requirements, Guidance Note EH22, HMSO (1988).

Step by step guide to COSHH, HSG97; *COSHH: the new brief guide for employers*, revised, IND(G)136; *General COSHH ACoP: a brief guide to the changes*, L99F (1996).
The costs of accidents at work, HSG96 (1997).
The costs to the British economy of work accidents and work related ill health, HSG101 (1995).
VDUs: An easy guide to the regulations, HSG90 (1994). *Working with VDUs*, IND(G)36 HSE.
Wear your dosimeter (poster pack), IND(G)206P (1995).
Violence at Work, IND(G)69 (1997).

Major legislation, guidance and approved codes of practice (ACoP)

Health and Safety at Work Act (1974) *A Guide to the Health and Safety at Work etc Act 1974*, L1 (1992). *Management of health and safety at work.*
Management of Health and Safety at Work Regulations 1992, ACoP, L21 (1992); *Information for Managers* (1997); *Safety representatives and safety committees (The Brown Book)* ACoP and guidance, L87 (1996).
Work equipment: *Provision and Use of Work Equipment Regulations 1992*, guidance, L22 (1992).
Manual handling: *Manual Handling Operations Regulations 1992*, guidance, L23 (1992).
Workplace health, safety and welfare: *Workplace (Health, Safety and Welfare) Regulations 1992*, ACoP and guidance, L24 (1992).
Personal protective equipment at work: *Personal Protective Equipment at Work Regulations 1992*, guidance, L25 (1992).
Display screen equipment: *Health and Safety (Display Screen Equipment) Regulations. 1992*, guidance, L26, (1992).
First aid: *The Health and Safety (First Aid) At Work Regulations 1981*, ACoP and Guidance, L74 (1997).
Fire safety: Home Office (1997) *Fire Safety Legislation for the Future. A Consultation Document.*

Inquiry reports and strategy documents

A Vision for the Future. The Nursing, Midwifery and Health Visiting Contribution to Health and Health Care, NHS Executive (1993).
Testing the Vision: A report on progress in the first year of A Vision for the Future, NHS Executive (1995)
First Report of the Committee of Inquiry into the Outbreak of Legionnaires' Disease in Stafford in April 1985, Badenoch report (1986), London: HMSO.
The Allitt Inquiry: Independent inquiry relating to deaths and injuries on the children's ward at Grantham and Kesteven General Hospital during the period February to April 1991, Clothier report (1994), London: HMSO.
Health Education Council, *Proposals for Nutritional Guidance for Health Education in Britain* (NACNE report), London: HEC (1983).
Improving the Health of the NHS Workforce. The Nuffield Trust (1998).
Report of the Royal Commission into the NHS, Merrison report, HMSO (1979).
National Health Service: Hospital Catering in England, House of Commons Public Accounts Committee, 49th Report, HMSO (1994).
Pennington Report on 1996 outbreak of infection with E. coli, Edinburgh: The Stationery Office (1997).
Report of the Committee of Inquiry into an Outbreak of Food Poisoning at Stanley Royd Hospital, HMSO (1986).

Report of the Taskforce on the Strategy for Research in Nursing, Midwifery and Health Visiting, Department of Health (1993).

Safety and Health at Work, Report of the Committee: 1970–72 (The Robens Committee report) (Cmnd 5034) London: HMSO (1972).

Other guidance

Chartered Institute of Building Services, *Lighting Guide – Hospitals and Health Care Buildings,* Publication no. 12, CIBS (1994).

Chartered Institute of Building Services, *Air filtration and natural ventilation,* GS A4 (1988).

Commission for Racial Equality, *Code of Practice – Race Relations,* London: CRE (1983).

Ergonomics Research Unit, *Back pain in Nurses, Summary and Recommendations,* Guildford: University of Surrey, The Robens Institute (1986).

Illuminating Engineering Society, *The IES Code for Interior Lighting,* London: IES (1977).

National Institute of Occupational Safety and Health, USA, *Waste Anaesthetic Gases and Vapours,* NIOSH Report (1977).

UK Central Council for Nursing, Midwifery and Health Visiting: *Code of Professional Conduct,* revised edition (1992). *The Scope of Professional Practice* (1992). *Complaints about Professional Conduct* (1993). *PREP and You: Factsheets* (1995). *Position statement on clinical supervision for nursing and health visiting* (1996). *Issues arising from professional conduct complaints* (1996). *Scope in Practice* (1997). All available free from the Distribution Department, UKCC, 23 Portland Place, London W1N 4JT.

Whitley Councils for the Health Services (Great Britain) General Councils, (The Whitley Handbook) *Conditions of Service* (1984).

Trade union and pressure group publications

GMB

Hazards in the Health Service. An A to Z Guide for GMB Safety Representatives (undated).

Safety Reps Handbook (1995).

Safety Reps Kit (1995).

Safety Reps Guide to Risk Assessment (1996).

Labour Research Department (LRD)

Finding out about your pension (1997).

Stress, Bullying and Violence – a trade union guide (1997).

Health and Safety Law – a guide for union reps (1997).

State Benefits 1997 (1997).

Maternity Rights – an LRD guide to the law and best practice (1997).

Special leave – a bargainer's guide (1997).

European Works Councils – negotiating the way forward (1997).

Hazardous substances at work – a safety reps guide (1996).

Working Time Directive – LRD's Guide to the European Directive (1996).

Hazardous substances at work (1996).

Stress at Work (1995).

Women's health and safety (1996).

Office health and safety – a guide for union reps (1995).
HIV, AIDS and the Workplace (1995).
Human Resource Management (1995).
Tackling Harassment at Work (1994).
Risk assessment and hazards control (1993).
VDUs and Health and Safety (1991).

Royal College of Midwives

Handle with Care. A Midwife's Guide to preventing back injury (1997).
RCM Health and Safety Representatives Briefings and Bulletins.

Royal College of Nursing

AIDS. Nursing Guidelines (1994).
Introduction to Hepatitis B and Nursing Guidelines for Infection Control (1987).
Safety Representatives' Manual (1991).
Model Policy on Bullying, re-order no. 000 763 (1997).
Nursing a Grievance?, Bullying & harassment advice leaflet, re-order no. 000 742 (1997).
Clinical Effectiveness: A Royal College of Nursing Guide, re-order no. 000 682 (1996).
Clinical Guidelines: What you need to know, re-order no. 000 579 (1997).
Counselling and Advisory Service: Your questions answered, re-order no. 000 533 (1995).
In the Balance: Registered Nurse Supply and Demand, I. Seccombe and G. Smith, RCN/ IES Report 315, ISBN 1-85184-241-1 (free summary document also available) (1996).
Taking Part: Registered Nurses and the Labour Market in 1997, I. Seccombe, and G. Smith RCN/IES Report 338, ISBN 1-85184-266-7 (free summary document also available) (1997).
Infection Control: Guidelines on Infection Control, re-order no. 000 375 (1994).
Disability Discrimination Act: Guide to the Disability Discrimination Act 1996, RCN Labour Relations Department (1996).
Hazards of Nursing: Personal Injuries at Work, re-order no. 000 692 (1996). Also summary leaflet, re-order no. 000 693 (1996).
Health and Safety at Work leaflets: 'Safety Representatives' Re-order No 000 215. (no date); 'Reporting Accidents' re-order no. 000 344 (1995); 'Accidents at Work: your financial rights', re-order no. 000 344 (1995); 'Your Rights and Responsibilities', re-order no. 000627 (1997); 'Hazards for Pregnant Nurses. An A-Z Guide', re-order no. 000 (1995); 'Shifting the Balance: Towards best practice in shift working and patient care', re-order no. 000 733 (1997).
Back Care: Code of Practice for the Handling of Patients, re-order no. 000 126 (1993).
Back Care: Introducing a Safer Patient Handling Policy, re-order no. 000 603 (1996).
Back Care: RCN Code of Practice for Patient Handling. re-order no. 000 604 (1996).
Back Care: Manual Handling Assessments in Hospitals and the Community, re-order no. 000 605 (1996).
'Back Injured Nurses: A Profile', discussion paper by I. Seccombe and J. Ball. (1992).
Work Injury: An RCN Guide for Work Injured Nurses, re-order no. 000 405 (1994): a new edition is in preparation.
Injury Claims: Your Personal Injury Claim: An explanatory guide for members, RCN Legal Services.
London Needs all its Nurses, re-order no. 000 212 (1993).
Maternity Rights: A Beginner's Guide to New Maternity Rights, RCN Labour Relations Department (1994).
Health Assessment: Advice for Occupational Health Nurses, re-order no. 000 536 (1995).

Health Assessment: Advice to Managers, re-order no. 000 555 (1995).
Job Evaluation: Guidelines for Occupational Health Nurses (1994).
'Occupational Health Nursing Guidelines' 15 fact sheets, Society of Occupational
    Health Nursing (1996).
Opportunities for Developing Professional Practice, re-order no. 000 336 (1993).
Towards Professional Practice, re-order no. 000 040 (1996).
Occupational Health Nursing, newsletter of the RCN Society of Occupational Health
    Nursing (quarterly).
RCN Nursing Update Learning Units:
Approaching with care: Violence at Work, Unit 038 (1993).
Best practice in counselling skills, Unit 049 (1994).
Heart Health: prevention, Unit 074 (1997).
Holding Together: staff support, Unit 048 (1994).
Immunisation: to protect yourself, Unit 052 (1996).
An Immunisation Need: the nursing response, special unit, no number (1994).
Infection Control: surveying the risks, Unit 051 (1995).
MRSA, Unit 073 (1997).
Setting Standards of Care, Unit 013 (1994).
A Shadow from the Past: Tuberculosis Today, Unit 067 (1996).

Royal Society for the Prevention of Accidents

Health and Safety: guide to sources of information (4th edition). Lists all sources of
    occupational safety and health information including journals and Internet sites.

Trades Union Congress

O'Neill, R. *Asthma at Work: causes, effects and what to do about them* (1997).
Hazards at Work: TUC Guide to Health and Safety (1997).

Transport and General Workers Union

Trade unionists and eco-auditing (1996).

Unison

Bullying at Work – guidance for safety representatives, Stock no. 1201 (1996).
Bullying at Work – guidelines for Unison branches, stewards and safety representatives,
    Stock no. 1281 (1997).
Campaigning on Health and Safety: A handbook for Unison safety representatives, Stock
    no. 1352 (1997).
*Health and Safety: a guide for members working in private and voluntary sector nursing
    homes*, Stock no. 1280 (1997).
The Management of Health and Safety at Work Regulations 1992, Stock no. 918 (1994).
The Workplace Health, Safety and Welfare Regulations 1992, Stock no. 919 (1994).
Display Screen Equipment Regulations 1992, Stock no. 920 (1994).
The Provision and Use of Work Equipment Regulations 1992, Stock no. 921 (1994).
Personal Protective Equipment at Work Regulations 1992, Stock no. 922 (1994).
Stress at Work -- a trade union response, Stock no. 1226 (1996).
Women's health and safety: a trade union guide (with the LRD) Stock no. 818 (1996).
Work -- it's a risky business, guide to risk assessment for Unison health and safety
    representatives, Stock no. 1351 (1997).

Leaflets

Scriptographic Publications (Channing House, Butts Road, Alton, Hants GU34
1ND. Tel.: 01420 544534. Fax 01420 541743) publish many leaflets including:
'About preventing back problems', 'Employee's guide to preventing slips, trips and
falls', 'The joy of fitness', 'Risk assessment', 'Sexual harassment in the workplace',
'Equal opportunities', 'The dangers of smoking', 'Assisting a wheelchair user',
'Using hoists', 'Patient safety in the home', 'Hazardous materials in health-care
premises', 'Universal precautions', 'Injuries from sharps', 'Stress and the health
care worker'. 'Smoking at work', 'Hepatitis B', 'HIV and Aids in health care',
'Working with display screen equipment'.

Journals

Hazards: indispensable quarterly information on workplace and health and safety. PO
Box 199, Sheffield, South Yorkshire S1 1FQ. Tel.: 0114 276 5695. Fax: 0114 276
7257. E-mail: editor@hazards.org

Health and Hygiene: quarterly journal of the Royal Institute of Public Health and
Hygiene. Tel.: 0171 580 2731.

Health and Safety Record: published quarterly by the Transport and General Workers
Union.

Health and Safety at Work: Monthly journal published by Tolley Publishing Co. Tel.:
0181 636 9141.

London Food News: bulletin published by the London Food Commission, 3rd Floor,
5–11 Worship Street, London, EC2A 2BH. Tel.: 0171 837 2250.

Nursing Standard: weekly general magazine published by the Royal College of
Nursing.

Nursing Times: weekly, frequently carries news, features and research on health and
safety and nurses' wellbeing. Sold in newsagents.

Occupational Health: monthly, from Reed Business Information. Tel.: 0181 652
4669.

Occupational Health Bulletin: produced by the Institute of Occupational Health,
University of Birmingham, Edgbaston, Birmingham B15 2TT.

Occupational Health Nursing: official journal of the American Association of
Occupational Health Nurses, monthly. AAOHN, 50 Lennox Point, Atlanta,
Georgia 30305, USA. Tel.: 00 1 404 262 1162.

Occupational Health Review: bimonthly from Industrial Relations Services, Tel.: 0171
354 5858.

The Daily Hazard: newsletter published by the London Hazards Centre, Dalby
Street, NW5. Tel. 0171 267 3387.

Workers' Health International Newsletter: published by Hazards Publications (see above
for details). For subscription details e-mail sub@hazards.org

Appendix 2   Organisations

This appendix lists useful organisations that are relevant in some way to nurses' health, safety and well-being.

Government and statutory bodies

Commission for Racial Equality: produces codes of practice and leaflets relevant to NHS employment. Elliot House, 10–12 Allington Street, London SW1E 5EH. Tel.: 0171 828 7022.

Department of Health (DoH): government health ministry for England and some UK functions, where the secretary of state for health has his/her office, supported by a minister of state and a number of junior ministers. Also houses the chief nursing and medical officers. Richmond House, 79 Whitehall, London SW1A 2NS. Tel.: 0171 210 3000.

Department of Health and Social Services, Northern Ireland: the only part of the UK where health and social services are linked in one government department, under the secretary of state for Northern Ireland. Operates through four health and social services boards. Dundonald House, Upper Newtownards Road, Belfast BT4 3SF. Tel.: 01232 520500.

Environmental Health Departments: see your local phone book.

Equal Opportunities Commission, Overseas House, Quay Street, Manchester M3 3HN. Tel 0161-833 9244.

Government Bookshops: for HMSO and other official publications. The Stationery Office Publications Centre, 51 Nine Elms Lane, London SW8 5DR. Tel.: 0171 873 9090. General inquiries: fax: 0171 873 8416.
Belfast: 16 Arthur Street, Belfast, BT1 4GD. Tel.: 01232 238451.
Birmingham: 68/69 Bull Street, Birmingham, B4 6AD. Tel.: 0121 236 9696.
Bristol: Southey House, 33 Wine Street, Bristol BS1 2BQ. Tel.: 0117 926 4306.
Edinburgh: 71 Lothian Road, Edinburgh, EH3 9AZ. Tel.: 0131 228 4181.
London: 49 High Holborn, London, WC1V 6HB. Tel.: 0171 873 0011.
Manchester: 9–21 Princess Street, Manchester, M60 8AS. Tel.: 0161 834 7201.

Health Education Authority (HEA): has the status of a special health authority; its overall role is to encourage the public to adopt a healthier lifestyle. It is required to advise the government on health education issues, and has run campaigns on workplace health. Hamilton House, Mabledon Place, London WC1H 9TX. Tel.: 0171 222 5300.

Health Education Board for Scotland (HEBS): similar role to the HEA in England. Woodburn House, Canaan Lane, Edinburgh EH10 4SG. Tel.: 0645 125442.

Health Promotion Authority for Wales: has a similar role to the HEA in England. Ffynnon-las, Ty Glas Avenue, Llanishen, Cardiff CF4 5DZ. Tel.: 01222 752222.

Health and Safety Executive: a public body that sets standards and monitors the implementation of health and safety legislation in the workplace, particularly in the NHS. The HSE has public inquiry points in different regions. 2 Southwark Bridge Road, London SE1 9HS. Tel.: 0171 717 6000. For HSE area offices, see your local phone book.

Health and Safety Commission: established by the 1974 Health and Safety at Work Act to secure the health, safety and welfare of people at work. Oversees the Health and Safety Executive. Rose Court, 2 Southwark Bridge, London SE1 9HS. Tel.: 0171 717 6000.

National Health Service Executive (NHSE): closely linked with the DoH, the NHSE is the headquarters of the NHS in England; it is responsible for the effective management of the NHS and advises ministers on policy. Quarry House, Quarry Hill, Leeds LS2 7UE. Tel.: 0113 2545000.

Scottish Office: government department responsible for the administration of government business in Scotland. (It will be superseded by the Scottish parliament in 2000, following elections in 1999.) Dover House, Whitehall, London SW1A 2AU. Tel.: 0171 270 3000.

Scottish Health Department: the Scottish equivalent of the DoH in England, working under the Scottish Office and the direction of the secretary of state for Scotland. Scotland's chief nursing officer is based there. St Andrew's House, Regent Road, Edinburgh EH1 3DE. Tel.: 0131 556 8400.

United Kingdom Central Council (UKCC): regulatory body for nursing, midwifery and health visiting in the UK; maintains a register of all qualified staff. Its prime responsibility is to protect the public through establishing and improving standards of nurse education, maintaining professional standards and investigating misconduct. It has mechanisms to ensure humane treatment for nurses whose alleged misconduct arises through problems such as stress, illness or addiction. 23 Portland Place, London W1N 3AF. Tel.: 0171 637 7181.

Welsh Office: government department responsible for the administration of government business in Wales, at the direction of the Welsh secretary of state. The NHS Directorate, which is part of the Welsh Office, sets the policy agenda for the five Welsh health authorities and 30 trusts. The chief nursing officer for Wales is based there. (It will be replaced by a Welsh parliament in 2000, following elections in 1999.) Crown Buildings, Cathays Park, Cardiff CF1 3NQ. Tel.: 01222 825111.

Professional associations and trade unions

Association of Occupational Health Nurse Practitioners (UK): Publishes *Occupational Health Today*, for members only. Victoria House, Desborough Street, High Wyecombe, Bucks HP11 2NF. Tel.: 01494 601083.

British Association for Counselling (BAC): Charity and professional association to promote counselling and improve standards of training. Send SAE for free information. 1 Regent Place, Rugby, Warwickshire CV21 2PJ. Tel.: 01788 578328.

Community and District Nursing Association (CDNA), 8 University House, Ealing Green, London W5 5ED. Tel.: 0181 231 2776.

Community Practitioners' and Health Visitors' Association (CPHVA): TUC-affiliated union. Lobbies on H&S and well-being issues for nurses working in the community. 50 Southwark Street, London SE1 1UN. Tel 0171 717 4000.

Community Psychiatric Nurses Association (CPNA), c/o Brian Rogers, Cals Meyn, Grove Lane, Hinton, Chippenham SN14 8HF. Tel.: 0117 937 3365.

GMB (was General, Municipal, Boilermakers and Allied Trades Union): large, general, TUC-affiliated union with some NHS members. Its national and regional H&S officers are an important resource. Publishes useful literature, including a valuable A–Z handbook of NHS hazards. 22-24 Warple Road, London SW19 4DD. Tel.: 0181 947 3131.

Infection Control Nurses' Association (ICNA): publishes bimonthly supplement in *Nursing Times*. c/o Fitwise, Drumcross Hall, Bathgate, Edinburgh EH48 4JT. Tel.: 01506 811077.

NHS Confederation: influential grouping of NHS authorities and trusts. Has tackled H&S issues, including good publications on violence and an authoritative *NHS Security Manual*. Birmingham Research Park, Vincent Drive, Edgbaston, Birmingham B15 2SQ. Tel.: 0121 471 4444.

Royal College of Midwives (RCM): independent trade union for midwives; has about 400 health and safety reps; runs training courses for them; produces publications on issues such as bullying and manual handling, and an updated Health and Safety Handbook. 15 Mansfield Street, London W1M 0BE. Tel.: 0171 312 3535.

Royal College of Nursing (RCN): independent trade union whose officials include experts on health and safety and occupational health. It has 1600 safety reps. Its Society of Occupational Health Nursing lobbies for better OH services in the NHS and better training for OH nurses. It also has forums for occupational health nurses in the NHS, and for occupational health managers. See also entry for WING below. 20 Cavendish Square, London W1M 0AB. Tel.: 0171 409 3333.

Scottish Health Visitors Association (SHVA): now merged with Unison. Douglas House, 60 Belford Road, Edinburgh EH4 3UQ. Tel.: 0131 226 2662.

Society of Occupational Medicine, Royal College of Physicians, 6 St Andrews Place, London NW1 4LB. Tel.: 0171 486 2641.

Trades Union Congress (TUC): umbrella body for trade unions. Some activity on H&S matters, including NHS-linked committees looking at relevant issues, and publications. Runs safety reps' training courses, which supplement those run by all the major unions. Also supports the TUC Centenary Institute for Occupational Health (Keppel Street, London WC1. Tel.: 0171 580 2386). Congress House, Great Russell Street, London WC1 3LS. Tel.: 0171 636 4030.

Transport and General Workers Union (T & G): giant, general, TUC-affiliated union. Not many NHS staff in membership, but strong on H&S matters, with a national health and safety coordinator. Currently focusing on linking traditional H&S focus with environmental issues. Piloted roving safety reps scheme relevant to small workplaces such as care homes. Transport House, 16 Palace Street, London SW1. Tel.: 0171 828 7788. Fax: 0171 630 5861.

UK Occupational Health Nurses' Research Forum: encourages the development of research in OH nursing. c/o Institute of Occupational Health, University of Birmingham, Egbaston, Birmingham B15 2TT. Tel.: 0121 414 6015.

Unison: the UK's largest public sector union, with large health service membership. TUC-affiliated. Wide network of safety reps backed up by national and regional experts. Campaigns and produces material on a wide range of health and safety issues. 1 Mabledon Place, London SW1H 9AJ. Tel.: 0171 388 2366.

Self-help, support and advice

Alcoholics Anonymous, 11 Redcliffe Gardens, London, SW10 9BG. General Service Centre, PO Box 1, Stonebow House. Tel.: 01904 644026. London Regional Telephone Service (10 am–10 pm): 0171 352 3001.

Liberty (National Council for Civil Liberties), 21 Tabard Street, London, SE1 4LA. Tel.: 0171 403 3888.

Nurseline: independent advice, information and support service for all nurses and midwives, provided by the RCN (but you do not have to be an RCN member to use the service). First Floor, 8–10 Crown Hill, Croydon, Surrey CR0 1RZ. Tel.: 0181 681 4030.

Nurses Welfare Service: provides support and help to nurses who appear before the professional conduct committee at the UKCC. Does not offer money directly (apart from travelling expenses when needed) but does offer counselling, advice and support. Victoria Chambers, 16–18 Strutton Ground, London SW1P 2HP. Tel.: 0171 222 1563/4.

Royal National Pension Fund for Nurses (RNPFN): offers pensions, life assurance and other financial services exclusively for members of the caring professions and their spouses. Burdett House, 15 Buckingham Street, London WC2N 6ED. Tel.: 0171 839 6785.

Terrence Higgins Trust: provides information on AIDS and help and advice to sufferers and anyone who is worried about the disease. 52–54 Grays Inn Road, London WC1X. Tel 0171 831 0330. Helpline: 0171 833 2971 (7–10 pm weekdays, 3–10 pm weekends).

Work Injured Nurses Group (WING): self-help group run by its members and coordinated by the RCN. Not open to non-RCN members. Administrator, WING, 8–10 Crown Hill, Croydon, Surrey CR0 1RZ. Tel.: 0181 649 9536. WING advisor direct line: 01832 733177. e-mail croydon.office@RCN.ORG.UK

Others

British Nutrition Foundation, 52–54 High Holborn, London WC1V 6IR. Tel.: 0171 404 6504. Fax: 0171 235 4904.

British Standards Institute: will answer enquiries on their published standards. 389 Chiswick High Road, London W4 4AL. Tel.: 0181 996 9000.

City Centre: advice and information for office workers, including health and safety and equal opportunities. 32–5 Featherstone Street, London EC1Y 8QX. Tel. and fax: 0171 608 1338.

Disability Alliance Educational and Research Association, Universal House, 88–94 Wentworth Street, London E1 7SA. Tel.: 0171 247 8776/8763.

Disabled Living Foundation: advice on living with disability, especially equipment. 380–384 Harrow Road, London, W9 2HU. Tel.: 0171 289 6111.

English Sports Council: wide range of activities, including advice on sports facilities and planning. PO Box 480, Crystal Palace National Sports Centre, Ledrington Road, London SE19 2BQ. Tel.: 0181 778 8600.

Institute of Occupational Health, University of Birmingham: academic centre which aims to improve the health and well-being of employed people through research, teaching and consultancy. It welcomes inquiries from nurses. Edgbaston, Birmingham B15 2TT. Tel.: 0121 414 6030, fax.: 0120 414 6217. It is also a WHO Collaborating Centre for occupational health.

King's Fund: independent health charity to support the health care of the people of London (but also works across the UK) by influencing health policy and stimulating good practice. Activities include grant-giving, policy research, service development and audit programmes, and information services for people working in and with the health service. 11–13 Cavendish Square, London W1M 0AN. Tel.: 0171 307 2400

Labour Research Department: publications and research centre for trade unionists. 78 Blackfriars Road, London SE1 8HF. Tel.: 0171 928 3649.

London Food Commission: carries out independent research; supplies information and advice on all aspects of food and catering; publishes a range of impressive material, including *The Food Magazine*. 94 White Lion Street, London N1 9PF. Tel.: 0171 837 2250.

London Hazards Centre: provides information and advice to London-based trade unions and community groups organising against hazards. Publishes regular newsletter, *The Daily Hazard.* Interchange Studios, Dalby Street, London NW5 3NQ. Tel.: 0171 267 3387.

Royal Institute of Public Health and Hygiene: an examining body; food hygiene and safety examinations (for catering staff, businesses and so on). 28 Portland Place, London W1N 4DE. Tel.: 0171 580 2731/636 1208.

Suzy Lamplagh Trust: Campaigns for better security for vulnerable staff at work. 14 East Sheen Avenue, London SW14 8AS. Tel.: 0181 392 1839.

U.S. Centers for Disease Control and Surveillance: U.S. government agency which publishes research and information on health and disease. 1600 Clifton Road N.E., Atlanta, Ga 30333, USA.

U.S. National Institute of Occupational Safety and Health: a branch of the U.S Centers for Disease Control and Surveillance, undertakes and publishes research and U.S. exposure limits. Robert Taft Laboratory, 4647 Columbia Pathway, Cincinatti, Ohio 45226, USA.

Appendix 3 An A to Z of hazards

Adverse incident An event that produces, or has the potential to produce, unwanted effects involving the safety of patients, staff or others.

Anaesthetic gases Waste gases produced during the process of patient anaesthesia, and dispersed by scavenging systems.

Asbestos A fibrous mineral used extensively in building and ventilation, long known to cause lung damage through asbestosis, mesothelioma and lung cancer.

Asthma An allergic respiratory disease characterised by constricted respiratory passages, producing acute coughing and wheezing episodes, and chronic disability and death.

Back injury Mechanical and /or neurological damage to the spinal column, ranging from herniated discs to nerve compression.

Bullying The abuse of power in personal or professional relationships.

Chemicals Hazardous substances used extensively in health care environments, in medications, and in environmental /instrument cleansing/sterilisation – *see also* glutaraldehyde.

Clinical waste Includes used equipment, protective clothing, bed linen and disposable items such as syringes and needles. These are often contaminated and are potential sources of infection to staff and patients.

Computers Electrical equipment with potential direct hazard from low-level radiation or eyestrain, and indirect risk of repetitive strain injury – *see also* RSI and VDUs.

Cytotoxic drugs Potent chemicals used in the treatment of cancers, with potential hazards from accidental handling, spillage or ingestion of aerosol spray.

Dermatitis Allergic skin irritations caused by contact with drugs, chemicals and toxic substances, including latex products – *see also* latex.

Drugs Biochemical substances used in the treatment of infection and physical and mental illness, and in symptom relief such as pain – sometimes with potent side-effects or addictive qualities.

Enteric infections Infections of the intestinal tract by bacteria such as salmonella and *E. coli*, generally caused by poorly prepared or stored food or faulty hand hygiene.

Electrical hazards Any unsafe or potentially unsafe/lethal electrical equipment, including wiring, lighting and infusion pumps.

Equipment A wide range of clinical technology with the potential for misuse, abuse or harm to staff and patients. *Medical devices* is another term describing the instruments, apparatus, appliances, materials or other articles used to diagnose, prevent, monitor, treat or alleviate disease or disability.

Fire The 'fire triangle' of heat, air and fuel is a potential cause of massive damage, injury and loss of life in clinical and residential settings.

Glutaraldehyde A highly toxic chemical used for cold sterilisation of instruments, especially endoscopes; there is no safe exposure level and substitution with a safer alternative is necessary.

Hepatitis Inflammation of the liver. Viral hepatitis is caused by any one of at least five viruses. Hepatitis A, often transmitted by the faecal–oral route, can occasionally be fatal and most commonly occurs in children and young adults. Hepatitis B is transmitted by blood or blood products, contaminated instruments and needles, or sexually, and has a higher mortality rate.

Humidifier fever A disease caused by the breeding of amoebae in the water reservoirs of air-conditioning systems and spread by aerosol spray from contaminated ducts.

Human immunodeficiency virus (HIV) A virus spread through infected blood or blood products, but mainly through sexual contact. Results acutely in the production of antibodies, and may chronically result in AIDS (Acquired Immune Deficiency Syndrome), where lymphocytes are destroyed, the body's immune response is suppressed and further symptoms and infections may occur.

Injuries Any damage, physical or psychological, to people; work/industrial injuries being those caused by or occurring at work. For nurses some of the most common injuries are musculo-skeletal injuries, RSI, stress-related illnesses after traumatic incidents, harassment and violence.

Ionising radiation The production of electrically charged particles (ions) caused by specific types of radiation (electromagnetic waves). These particles cause damage when passed through living tissue, intentionally to tumours but also inevitably to healthy cells, so careful precautions are needed for patients and staff.

Laser A device that concentrates high energies into an intense narrow beam of electromagnetic radiation, used in microsurgery, cauterisation and diagnosis. Commonly used in ophthalmology, gynaecology and dermatology.

Latex Natural and synthetic rubber products used in many clinical procedures and settings. They can produce allergic responses, sensitisation and acute anaphylaxis; hypoallergenic substances should be substituted whenever possible, and risk assessment procedures carried out.

Legionnaires' disease An infection of the lungs caused by the *legionella* bacterium. Symptoms include malaise, muscle pain, fever, dry cough, chest pain and breathlessness. It is generally spread through contaminated air-conditioning, showers, humidifiers and stagnant water supplies.

Lighting Artificial lights, especially fluorescent, may cause tiredness or eye strain and provoke migraine. Poor lighting increases the risk of accidents, and exacerbates security risks to staff and the public.

Medical devices See equipment.

Mental health problems Nurses' mental health may be undermined by factors such as excessive stress, poor working conditions, violence, racism, sexism, bullying, harassment and poor management practices.

Mercury A toxic, vaporous mineral traditionally used in clinical observation of temperature (thermometers) and blood pressure (sphygmomanometers). It is a dangerous substance and there are numerous practical alternatives.

MRSA Methicillin–resistant *Staphylococcus aureus* derives from a genus of bacteria which occur commonly on the skin and moist areas such as skin folds, nasal passages and the perineum. It is resistant to the most powerful antibiotics, leading to numerous episodes of hospital-acquired infection; strict infection control programmes and surveillance policy and practice are needed.

Noise Unwanted sound may cause unnecessary stress and distraction, leading to illness, accidents and injury. Sound above defined levels has been shown to cause hearing loss.

Racial harassment Bullying, victimisation and professional side-lining of staff because of their ethnic origin is widespread in UK health services, and results in demoralisation and loss of staff.

Racism The belief in and practice of discrimination against individuals and ethnic groups because of race. Whether unconscious or conscious, it often leads to harassment and bullying.

Reproductive hazards   Hazards which adversely affect the ability to conceive (men and women), have a healthy pregnancy and produce a healthy baby are surprisingly common in health care environments. They include ionising radiation, chemical hazards (anaesthetic gases, mercury), manual moving and handling, biological agents (chicken pox, rubella, herpes, hepatitis, cytomegalovirus), stress and shift work.

RSI   Repetitive work with legs, hands, or arms may result in repetitive strain injury, also known as work-related upper limb disorders (WRULDs) or occupational over-use syndrome (OOS). It is manifested in muscle, nerve and tendon injury, pain and disability.

Salmonella   A genus of bacteria found in the intestines. Two species of *salmonella* cause food poisoning and gastro-enteritis (salmonellosis), while another species transmitted in contaminated water and food causes typhoid fever.

Sexism   A set of beliefs and attitudes based on the premise that one sex is innately superior – in most societies, the male. Its effects are pervasive in health services and nursing, a profession numerically dominated by women, suffers greatly from it.

Sexual harassment   Bullying behaviour by someone, usually male, using his hierarchical position or gender to exercise power in the work environment, whether over opposite-sex subordinates, superiors, colleagues or patients.

Sharps   Hypodermic needles, broken ampoules, scalpel blades and similar clinical equipment. These, often contaminated with body fluids, are potential sources of accidental injury such as 'needlestick injury' and infections such as hepatitis and HIV.

Shift work   The patterned variations in working hours may cause insomnia, fatigue, stress, loss of appetite, constipation and menstrual disorders.

Sick building syndrome   An environmentally caused occupational illness, in particular related to poor ventilation and lighting of work environments. Symptoms include lethargy, dry mouth, skin disorders, eye irritation and headaches.

Stress   Generally used to describe the adverse psychological effects of poor working conditions, job insecurity, poor management, harassment and bullying. Common manifestations include constant anxiety, depression, insomnia, fatigue and low morale.

Temperature   Extremes of environmental temperature at work affect individual mood, judgement and decision-making, and can aggravate physical health problems.

Tuberculosis   (TB) An infectious disease caused by *Mycobacterium tuberculosis*, most commonly in the lungs. It is becoming more common again in British urban society, especially among homeless people, some immigrant communities and people with compromised immune systems such as those with HIV.

VDUs   Prolonged use of video display units or display screen equipment (DSE) in workplace computers may cause eye strain, RSI and ill health related to low-level radiation.

Violence   Physical and psychological attacks on health staff are an increasing problem, especially in accident and emergency departments.

Workload   Excessive and difficult emotional and physical work, staff shortages, unpaid overtime and high patient throughput are common in nursing and lead to many mental and physical health problems.

Working environment   The health care workplace is filled with potential and actual hazards.

X-rays   Extremely short electromagnetic radiation used for diagnosis in radiography and radiotherapy. They are a reproductive hazard to both sexes if adequate safety procedures are not observed.

Index